RADIATION PROTECTION
IN
MEDICAL RADIOGRAPHY

RADIATION PROTECTION

IN

MEDICAL RADIOGRAPHY

FIFTH EDITION

MARY ALICE STATKIEWICZ SHERER, AS, RT (R), FASRT

PAULA J. VISCONTI, PhD, DABR

E. RUSSELL RITENOUR, PhD, DABR, FAAPM, FACR

with 228 illustrations

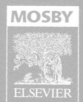

MOSBY

ELSEVIER

MOSBY
ELSEVIER

11830 Westline Industrial Drive
St. Louis, Missouri 63146

Notice

Knowledge and best practice in this field are constantly changing. As new research and experience broaden our knowledge, changes in practice, treatment and drug therapy may become necessary or appropriate. Readers are advised to check the most current information provided (i) on procedures featured or (ii) by the manufacturer of each product to be administered, to verify the recommended dose or formula, the method and duration of administration, and contraindications. It is the responsibility of the practitioner, relying on their own experience and knowledge of the patient, to make diagnoses, to determine dosages and the best treatment for each individual patient, and to take all appropriate safety precautions. To the fullest extent of the law, neither the Publisher nor the Authors assumes any liability for any injury and/or damage to persons or property arising out or related to any use of the material contained in this book.

The Publisher

Previous editions copyrighted 2002, 1998, 1993, 1983

ISBN-13: 978-0-323-03600-9
ISBN-10: 0-323-03600-7

Executive Editor: Jeanne Wilke
Managing Editor: Mindy Hutchinson
Senior Developmental Editor: Linda Woodard
Associate Developmental Editor: Christina Pryor
Publishing Services Manager: Melissa Lastarria
Project Manager: Rich Barber
Designer: Julia Dummitt

Printed in Canada

Last digit is the print number: 9 8 7 6 5 4 3 2 1

Working together to grow
libraries in developing countries

www.elsevier.com | www.bookaid.org | www.sabre.org

ELSEVIER   BOOK AID International   Sabre Foundation

ABOUT THE AUTHORS

Mary Alice Statkiewicz Sherer, AS, RT (R), FASRT, the primary author of this text, is a private radiography education, radiation safety, and medical publishing consultant. She also works as an instructor for the Limited Scope X-Ray Program at High-Tech Institute, a career college located in Nashville, Tennessee. Before assuming this position in January 2004, Ms. Sherer was employed for 13 years at Summit Medical Center in Hermitage, Tennessee, where she performed diagnostic imaging procedures, and also served as that department's Compliance/Education Coordinator. Prior to that time, Ms. Sherer was employed at Memorial Hospital of Burlington County (now Virtua Memorial Hospital of Burlington County) in Mount Holly, New Jersey, where she served for more than 16 years as radiography program director, and then as educational administrative assistant for the Department of Radiology.

After earning an ARRT certification in 1965, Ms. Sherer filled several technical and teaching positions in the New Jersey area, and in 1980, graduated with an associate degree in science from the College of Allied Health Professions, Hahnemann Medical College and Hospital of Philadelphia (now Hahnemann University). She has been an active and leading member of several professional organizations, having served on committees and task forces of the American Society of Radiologic Technologists, as president of the 28th Mid-Eastern Conference of Radiologic Technologists, and as president and chairman of the Board of Directors of the New Jersey Society of Radiologic Technologists. Services to the ASRT include functioning as chairman of the Radiologic Technology editorial review board for the membership year 1989-1991 and participating as a member of the Committee on Memorial Lectures for the membership years 1989-1991 and 1991-1993. For her services and contributions to the profession of Radiologic Technology, in June 1990, Ms. Sherer was elevated to Fellow of the American Society of Radiologic Technologists. She continues to hold this professional honor.

In addition to being the primary author of the first edition of *Radiation Protection for Student Radiographers*, and the second, third, and fourth editions of *Radiation Protection in Medical Radiography*, and also this edition, Ms. Sherer co-authored the textbook *Radiation Protection for Dental Radiography*, which was published by Multi-Media Publishing, Denver, in 1984. Articles written by Ms. Sherer have been published in *Radiologic Technology; The Journal of the American Society of Radiologic Technologists;* and *ADVANCE for Radiologic Science Professionals,* a national biweekly newspaper published by Merion Publications, King of Prussia, Pennsylvania. She has also served as a consultant to *ADVANCE.* In 1999, Mosby produced *Radiobiology and Radiation Protection,* the fourth program in *Mosby's Radiographic Instructional Series,* a CD-ROM (and slide series) presentation consisting of eight modules, approximately 1 hour each in duration. A *Study Guide* and an *Instructor's Manual* accompanied the audiovisual materials. Ms. Sherer served as chief consultant for the development of the program and as a technical reviewer.

Paula J. Visconti, PhD, DABR, is the director of medical physics at Virtua Memorial Hospital of Burlington County in Mount Holly, New Jersey. She has served as the radiation safety officer for the entire Virtua Health System in Southern New Jersey, which comprises four hospitals. Dr. Visconti received her PhD in experimental atomic physics from the City University of New York in 1971. She was a full-time instructor in the Physics Department at the City College of New York for several years thereafter. Dr. Visconti began her career in medical physics at Montefiore Hospital and Medical Center in New York City, where she remained for 5 years as an associate physicist. During that time, she lectured extensively in radiologic physics to both diagnostic radiology residents and student radiographers.

Dr. Visconti is a member of the Society of the Sigma Xi, the American Association of Physicists in Medicine, the American College of Medical Physics, and the American College of Radiology and is certified in therapeutic radiological physics by the American Board of Radiology.

E. Russell Ritenour, PhD, DABR, FAAPM, FACR, is professor and chief of the physics section, Department of Radiology, University of Minnesota Medical School and is director of graduate studies in biophysical sciences and medical physics, University of Minnesota Graduate School. Dr. Ritenour received his PhD in physics from the University of Virginia and completed a post-doctoral fellowship sponsored by the National Institutes of Health in medical physics at the University of Colorado Health Sciences Center. He stayed on the faculty at Colorado for 10 years, serving as director of the graduate medical physics training program, until moving to the University of Minnesota in 1989.

Dr. Ritenour has served as radiation safety officer for several hospitals and research facilities, served as consultant to the U.S. Army for resident training programs, and has written a number of audiovisual training programs and educational websites for radiologic technologists, radiology residents, and medical physicists. He is co-author of four books, two of which are now in their fifth editions. Dr. Ritenour is past president of the Rocky Mountain Chapter of the Health Physics Society and a frequent contributor to that society's website's feature, "Ask the Expert." He has chaired education and training committees of the American College of Radiology and the American Association of Physicists in Medicine and has served as board examiner and written examination committee chair for the American Board of Radiology for more than 10 years. In 2001, Dr. Ritenour was made a Fellow of the American Association of Physicists in Medicine. He is also a fellow of the American College of Radiology. Recently, Dr. Ritenour was elected president of the American Association of Physicists in Medicine effective January 1, 2006.

REVIEWERS

Mary J. Carillo, RT(R)(M)(CDT), MBA/HCM
Faculty, Diagnostic Medical Imaging
Gateway Community College
Phoenix, Arizona

Michael P. Covone, MEd, RT(R), CT
Assistant Professor
Pennsylvania College of Technology
Williamsport, Pennsylvania

Catherine S. DeBaillie, RT(R), BS
Instructor
Trinity College of Nursing and Health Sciences
Rock Island, Illinois

Charles Francis, MEd, RT(R)(QM)
Department Chair
Associate Professor Radiographic Science
Idaho State University
Pocatello, Idaho

Donna Goetz, MS, RT(R)(M), LRT
Associate Professor
Bronx Community College
Bronx, New York

Mari P. King, EdD, RT(R), CDT
Health Sciences Division Chair
Associate Professor of Medical Imaging
College Misericordia
Dallas, Pennsylvania

Barbara A. Koontz, MA, RT(R)(M)
Radiography Program Manager
Polk Community College
Winter Haven, Florida

Jean M. Korth, BS, RT(R)
Program Director
Mary Lanning Memorial Hospital
School of Radiologic Technology
Hastings, Nebraska

Josephine Marie Latini, MS, RT(R)(M), FASRT
Multi-phasic Chief Technologist
Geisinger Health System
Lock Haven, Pennsylvania

Vicki Armstrong Lemaster, RT(R)(CVT)
Co-Director Radiology
Director CVT
Spencerian College
Louisville, Kentucky

Nancy Moffet, BS, RT(R)(CT)(M)
Professor of Radiologic Technology
New Hampshire Technical Institute
Concord, New Hampshire

Gloria J. Mongelluzzo, MEd, RT(R)(M)
Program Director
Conemaugh Memorial Medical Center
Johnstown, Pennsylvania

Debra J. Poelhuis, RT(R)(M), MS
Director Health Careers
Montgomery County Community College
Pottstown, Pennsylvania

John G. Radtke, MA, RT(R), RTNM
Professor Radiology, Nuclear Medicine
Los Angeles City College
Charles Drew University
Los Angeles, California

Jayme S. Rothberg, MS, RT(R)(M)
Associate Professor
Radiography Program Coordinator
Pasco-Hernando Community College
New Port Richey, Florida

Francine J. Todd, BEd, MEd, (R), ARRT
Interim Program Director
Associate of Applied Science in Radiologic
Technology Degree Program
Bowling Green State University
Firelands College
Huron, Ohio

Diana Sue Wederman, BS, RT(R)
Clinical Coordinator
Trinity College of Nursing and Health Sciences
Rock Island, Illinois

Christine E. Wiley, MEd, ARRT (R)(M)
Program Director
Professor
North Shore Community College
Danvers, Massachusetts

In memory of my parents,
Felix J. and Elizabeth M. Krohn,
To my sons,
Joseph F. Statkiewicz, Christopher R. Statkiewicz, and Terry R. Sherer, Jr., with love,
And
To all with whom I may share my knowledge.

FOREWORD

The new fifth edition of this now classic textbook continues to provide comprehensive and timely coverage of radiation protection for radiography students and radiographers. Over the years the book has also become a primary reference book for medical physicists and residents in radiology. The book has earned a distinctive reputation as one that is readable and understandable, with the text supported by excellent illustrations and detailed tables. The addition of an accompanying workbook with this new edition adds considerable value.

The authors, a highly experienced radiographer/physicist team who have been working together for 25 years, have included the latest information on radiation protection on the expanding use of digital imaging and the use of fluoroscopic equipment by non-radiologists. A new and very timely section covers radiation emergencies and the use of radiation as a terrorist weapon—including "dirty bombs." This section also includes current information on the cleanup of a contaminated urban area and the latest EPA limits. This should be of interest to professionals at many different levels, including nurses, emergency room personnel, and even the general public.

The authors' experience in this field is brought forth in this new edition by including separate coverage of molecular and cellular radiation biology and a new detailed chapter on the effects of radiation on organ systems. Radiation quantities and units, a difficult area to comprehend, has been simplified. A new chapter entitled "Radioisotopes and Radiation Protection" covers the medical use of radioisotopes in nuclear medicine, radiation therapy, and the latest use of this radiation source in positron emission tomography (PET) and computed tomography (CT).

The area of radiation protection and biology continues to expand, with more information, especially with the increased doses for many procedures, needed by the profession. The American Registry of Radiologic Technologists (ARRT) has expanded the number of questions in this topic area on their examination for the radiographer. Reducing the harmful effects of ionizing radiation to imaging personnel, to patients, and to the general public is paramount. The authors have done a commendable job of revising their book for the fifth time to enable radiography students and other professionals to obtain comprehensive and timely information on the safe use of radiography equipment and isotopes.

Eugene D. Frank, MA, RT(R) FASRT, FAERS
Director, Radiography Program
Riverland Community College
Austin, Minnesota
Retired, Assistant Professor of Radiology
Mayo Clinic College of Medicine
Rochester, Minnesota

PREFACE

CONTENT

Thoroughly updated and revised, the fifth edition of *Radiation Protection in Medical Radiography* again offers student and practicing radiographers, radiology residents, medical physicists, and physicians the essential information on the biological effects of ionizing radiation and radiation protection to ensure the safe use of x-rays in diagnostic imaging. It also presents radiation physics relevant to radiation protection; cell structure; effects of radiation on humans at the molecular, cellular, and systemic levels; radiation quantities and units; regulatory and advisory limits for human exposure to radiation; the implementation of patient and personnel radiation protection practices for diagnostic x-ray procedures; radiation monitoring; and radioisotopes and radiation protection.

The fifth edition contains practical material that describes the way radiographers deal with the day-to-day implementation of radiation safety, regulations, and theory. The latest information concerning regulations and guidelines from the major standards-setting and advisory agencies, including the National Council on Radiation Protection and Measurements (NCRP) and the International Commission on Radiological Protection (ICRP), is discussed. The authors have endeavored to present this material in a succinct but reasonably complete fashion to meet the needs of the various members of the health care sector. With each new edition, the authors have also expanded the scope of the material covered in the text to provide the reader with a broader base of knowledge.

NEW TO THIS EDITION

The order of arrangement of the chapters has been changed to accommodate general revision of existing material, division of the original radiation biology chapter into two separate chapters, and the inclusion of a new chapter that offers advanced and important information on radioisotopes and radiation protection. Several new illustrations (diagrams and photos) have been added to complement new, updated, or expanded material. New tables have been included in some chapters while other existing tables have been updated to reflect the most current data.

Additional information boxes have been created to call attention to important information. Many existing boxes have also been revised. Throughout the book numerous subheadings have been added to aid the reader in locating specific material in the text. Several new terms have also been added to the glossary, while others have been expanded or updated. Chapter 1 now includes a new section on particulate radiation and updated and expanded information on Chernobyl. To facilitate greater understanding for the reader, complex material on radiation quantities and units, covered in Chapter 3, has been simplified. As stated above, the original radiation biology chapter has been separated into two individual chapters, to make presentation of the material by the instructor and mastery of the material by the learner easier. Additional information has been added to our discussion of repair enzymes and hormones and antibodies in Chapter 4. Information on the Human Genome Project has also been updated in this chapter, and a new section covering the topic of multiple births has been added. Chapter 5 now covers molecular and cellular radiation biology, while Chapter 6 addresses radiation effects on organ systems. Discussion on action limits has been added in Chapter 7, and other related subject matter has been expanded. Chapter 8 now includes discussion on digital imaging with emphasis on digital radiography and computed radiography. Under the section on high-level-control interventional procedures, we have added a discussion about the use of fluoroscopic equipment by non-radiologist physicians. The order of arrangement of materials in Chapter 9 has been changed to emphasize the cardinal principles of time, distance, and shielding earlier in the chapter. There is also expanded discussion addressing the use of the C-arm fluoroscope. Chapter 9 ends with a discussion on diagnostic x-ray suite protection design that includes an updated section on new approaches to shielding with emphasis on new information from NCRP Report #147. Chapter 10 provides expanded discussion on the optically stimulated luminescence (OSL) dosimeter that includes a new subsection on OSL energy discrimination. Chapter 11 contains both new and advanced information about radioisotopes and radiation protection.

Medical usage of radioisotopes in radiation therapy, nuclear medicine, positron emission tomography, and computed axial tomography (PET/CT) are covered in the first half of the chapter. The second half of Chapter 11 presents information on radiation emergencies discussing the use of radiation as a terrorist weapon. Discussion includes informative information about contamination from a radioactive dispersal device or "dirty bomb," and the process of decontamination. Additional material describing cleanup of a contaminated urban area, including limits of radioactive contamination set by the Environmental Protection Agency (EPA), follows. The final subject matter in this chapter covers medical management of persons suffering from radiation bioeffects resulting from surface contamination and internal contamination.

LEARNING ENHANCEMENTS

Each chapter begins with an outline, followed by key terms and learning objectives. An introductory paragraph provides an overview of the material to be covered in each chapter. Chapter content is followed by a bulleted summary, references, general discussion questions, and multiple-choice review questions, all of which can be used by the reader to assess acquired knowledge or by the instructor to stimulate discussion. Bold print has been used to focus the reader's attention on the key terms of each chapter. These key terms are defined in the glossary at the end of the book along with other relevant terms. Throughout the text,

information boxes are present to call the reader's attention to important information. The back matter of the book contains a series of appendices that provide support material for the text and provide additional relevant information.

Information has been presented as clearly and concisely as possible in a style that builds from basic to more complex concepts. Radiographs, photographs, tables, information boxes, and graphs reinforce and enhance learning and retention of material. Examples are included after discussions of difficult concepts to aid comprehension.

ANCILLARIES

Workbook

A workbook to accompany the text is also available. The workbook contains a variety of exercises for each of the 11 chapters in the book. Examples include matching terms with their definitions, crossword puzzles, labeling of diagrams, true or false statements, short answer, fill-in-the-blanks, short answer essay questions, multiple choice review questions and a post-test. Utilization of the workbook will provide a challenging experience for the learner. It will reinforce learning and help students to remember important concepts and material covered in each chapter of the book. The answers for the exercises are located in the back of the workbook.

Instructor's Electronic Resource

The instructor's electronic resource, available with this edition, will assist the educator in preparing lesson plans and presenting material. Included on the CD-ROM are key terms and their definitions, chapter objectives, instructional chapter outlines, suggested activities, general discussion questions, a test bank containing multiple choice questions, and electronic images from the textbook.

Evolve

Evolve is an interactive learning environment designed to work in coordination with *Radiation*

Protection in Medical Radiography, fifth edition. All of the material included in the Instructor's Electronic Resource is also available on Evolve. Instructors may use Evolve to provide an Internet-based course component that reinforces and expands the concepts presented in class. Evolve may be used to publish the class syllabus, outlines, and lecture notes; set up "virtual office hours" and e-mail communication; share important dates and information through the online class calendar; and encourage student participation through chat rooms and discussion boards. Evolve allows instructors to post exams and manage their grade books online. For more information, visit http://evolve.elsevier.com/Sherer/radiationprotection or contact an Elsevier sales representative.

USING THE BOOK

In general, the presentation of the fifth edition presumes that the reader has some background in physics, human anatomy, and medical and imaging terminology. Basic knowledge of simplified mathematics, units of measurement (metric and English), basic atomic structure, the physical concepts of energy, electric charge, subdivision of matter, electromagnetic radiation, x-ray production (both quality and quantity), and the process of ionization is useful but not mandatory. The reader may build on this knowledge by assimilating information presented in this text.

To facilitate a working knowledge of the principles of radiation protection, study materials presented in the fifth edition remain sophisticated enough to be true to the complexity of the subject yet simple and concise enough to permit comprehension by all readers. For student radiographers and radiology residents, this text is best used in conjunction with formal instruction from a qualified instructor. The practicing radiographer, medical physicist, and physician may use this book as a self-teaching instrument to broaden and reinforce existing knowledge of the subject matter and also always as a means to acquaint themselves with changing concepts and new material. The book can serve as a resource for continuing education because it provides an extensive range of information.

By mastering the material covered in this radiation protection text and its ancillaries and by applying this knowledge in the performance of radiologic procedures, the reader will help to ensure the safety of patients and all diagnostic imaging personnel.

Mary Alice Statkiewicz Sherer

ACKNOWLEDGMENTS

The production of this book would not be possible without the ongoing encouragement and support of family, friends, professional colleagues, and the staff members of Elsevier-Mosby, Inc., who have been involved with this project. To my family—sons Joseph, Christopher, and Terry—a very special acknowledgment and thanks is given. The constant love and support you provide gives me the strength and determination to accomplish my goals in life. I also want to acknowledge my youngest son, Terry, for serving as a research assistant to me during the preparation of this edition. I appreciate the countless hours he has spent finding various materials on the internet, in books, and in professional journals to enhance this publication. He has also assisted with typing and editing of the computerized manuscript before submission for publication. In addition to my sons, my family also includes my very special furry little friends, my dogs: Pixie Lee, Precious, and Tips. They are always nearby when I am working on my writing and are such a great comfort and joy. They are remembered for their loyalty and unconditional love.

To my many caring friends and professional colleagues, thank you for the support you have given me. Special acknowledgment is given to Lisa Bacon, former President, High-Tech Institute, Nashville Campus; Susan Houston, RT(R), X-Ray Program Manager; fellow instructors; and the 3rd and 4th Session X-Ray Program Students for ongoing support and encouragement. Gratitude and deep appreciation is expressed to my co-worker and friend, Judy Altheide, and also to my friend, Bonnie Barnes, for continuing support and encouragement. I truly appreciate and cherish your friendships.

The technical integrity of this edition and the earlier editions can be attributed to the collaborative efforts of two brilliant medical physicists, Paula J. Visconti, PhD, and E. Russell Ritenour, PhD. Their significant contributions to the new edition and previous editions ensure an accurate, timely, and well-rounded publication. I am deeply indebted to both Dr. Visconti and Dr. Ritenour for many technical recommendations, contribution of materials, and many hours of discussion. Both are also acknowledged for critical review of all chapter drafts and other materials in the text. Although it is not possible to list each piece of information contributed, acknowledgment is given for specific materials in this edition. For example, in Chapter 11, Dr. Visconti is acknowledged for new material on the medical usage of radioisotopes and radiation protection in radiation therapy, nuclear medicine, positron emission tomography, and computed axial tomography (PET/CT) and an accompanying diagram. The section in this chapter on radiation emergencies—use of radiation as a terrorist weapon that includes discussion on contamination from a radioactive dispersal device or "dirty bomb," and the process of decontamination, was written by Dr. Ritenour. He has also presented information covering cleanup of a contaminated urban area and medical management of persons suffering from radiation bioeffects. Both physicists have also contributed information to the new section on particulate radiation in Chapter 1. They have also provided several new definitions for terms added to our glossary.

Dr. Visconti has expanded discussion on repair enzymes and hormones and antibodies covered in Chapter 4 and has also updated and enhanced the section on the Human Genome Project. In Chapter 9, she revised the section on new approaches to shielding by placing emphasis on new NCRP report #147. Dr. Visconti has also contributed material on the subject of energy discrimination relating to the optically stimulated luminescence (OSL) dosimeter that is discussed in Chapter 10. "The Pregnant Patient" (fetal dose) section that now appears in Chapter 8 was also written by Dr. Visconti.

The fourth edition of *Radiation Protection for Medical Radiography* contained complex material on radiation quantities and units in Chapter 3. Dr. Ritenour has simplified this material, making that technical information much easier to comprehend. Emphasis is now placed on the use of equivalent dose and effective dose for radiation protection purposes. In Chapter 4, Dr. Ritenour has written a new section explaining multiple births. In Chapter 7, he has also contributed a new section on action limits and has expanded existing information on other related subject matter. In Chapter 8, Dr. Ritenour enhanced the section on digital imaging by writing new material on digital radiography. He has also contributed new illustrations for some of the chapters in this edition. Dr. Ritenour previously contributed certain material in Chapter 1 on radiation and the electromagnetic spectrum with an accompanying figure and table. He was also responsible for supplying information on the radiation safety officer (RSO) (e.g., requirements and responsibilities) that now appears in Chapter 7.

The participation of both Dr. Visconti and Dr. Ritenour by the updating of old materials and development of new materials helps to maintain the ongoing credibility of this text. Paula and Russ, thank you sincerely for all that you have done to make this book a successful and valued publication.

My gratitude also extends to the staff of Elsevier-Mosby who have been involved with the production of this text. Special acknowledgment is given to executive editor, Jeanne Wilke; managing editor, Mindy Hutchinson; senior developmental editor, Linda Woodard; associate developmental editor, Christina Pryor; and production editor, Rich Barber, for assistance in the preparation of this manuscript and for continuing support. Their publishing expertise has guided this manuscript from its initial stages to the development to the final product.

The time and effort expended by the reviewers is very much appreciated. The recommendations and suggestions made it possible for the authors to see the manuscript from another point of view. Through their constructive feedback, we have been able to strengthen various areas of the text. We also sincerely appreciate their many positive comments and encouraging words. They have all contributed to the overall success of this writing project. Since this edition contains some of the photographs from the third and fourth editions, thanks is again given to the individuals who participated in the photo shoot held in the radiology department of Anna Jacques Hospital in Newburyport, Massachusetts.

Special thanks is given to Judith Tunstall, RT(R) (CT), the radiographer/model. Her participation in this capacity helps to make our visual material current and fashionable. Ms. Tunstall's efforts in obtaining permission for the original photo shoot are still very much appreciated. We also continue to thank Tom Lochhaas, the photo shoot coordinator, for his efforts.

Shadow shield photos used in the third and fourth editions were originally shot at the Mayo Clinic in Rochester, Minnesota. Eugene D. Frank, MA, RT(R), FASRT, was responsible for arranging for that photo shoot. Since these photos are also included in this edition, I am indebted to Gene for the continued use of the photos. Furthermore, I want to acknowledge Gene and also thank him for writing the foreword to this edition. The authors sincerely appreciate his continuing support for the text. Mr. Frank has also been exceptionally helpful to us by reviewing the fourth edition of the book and by making numerous recommendations for the addition of new materials and update of existing technical and general information. Gene, thank you. We appreciate your efforts to help us enhance this text.

Appreciation is extended to those who have given permission to reproduce illustrations, diagrams, quotations, and pictures from their work. Their material enhances this manuscript. In particular, special thanks for the use of materials is given to Stewart C. Bushong, ScD; Philip W. Ballinger, MS, RT(R), FAERS, and Eugene D. Frank, MA, RT(R), FASRT; and Professor Elizabeth LaTorre Travis. We also want to thank Evelyn O. Talbott, DRPH, of the Department of Epidemiology, University of Pittsburgh in Pittsburgh, Pennsylvania, who provided information on mortality among the residents affected by the TMI accident. Dr. Talbott was the principal investigator of the 13-year study of people who lived within 5 miles of TMI at the time of the accident. The information she supplied enabled us to update our discussion of this topic in Chapter 1 of the fourth edition, and also utilize this information in this edition. Photographs of Chernobyl in Chapter 1 obtained from the U.S. Department of

Energy with the help of Mr. Gary Petersen and Mr. Tim Ledbetter continue to be appreciated. We also express gratitude to Judith Mangan, Marketing Technical Coordinator at Landauer, Inc., for providing written material on radiation dosimetry reports and photographic materials on the Luxel optically stimulated luminescence (OSL) dosimeter and the extremity dosimeter, now described in Chapter 10. We also want to thank Mr. Robert Hayward, Marketing Manager, Brachytherapy, Implant Sciences Corporation, Wakefield, Massachusetts, for providing us with an illustration of an I-125 implant seed and a photo of I-125 implant seeds as seen before encapsulation. These materials appear in Chapter 11 of the textbook. Gratitude is also expressed to Mark Rzeszotarski, PhD, Associate Professor of Radiology, Department of Radiology, MetroHealth Medical Center, Cleveland, Ohio, for the use of C-arm fluoroscope illustrations used in Chapters 8 and 9. For the use of a figure that depicts the concept of linear energy transfer, thanks is given to William R Hendee, E. Russell Ritenour, and John Wiley & Sons. We have placed this illustration in Chapters 3 and 5 of this text.

Acknowledgments and thanks for permission to reproduce photographic materials are also given to the National Council on Radiation Protection and Measurements in Bethesda, Maryland; the U.S. Department of Energy, Office of LWR Safety and Technology and the Office of Nuclear Energy in Washington, D.C.; the U.S. Department of Energy, Nevada Operations Office in Las Vegas, Nevada; and the U.S. Environmental Protection Agency, Washington, D.C. Special thanks for the use of photographic materials with permission is also given to Mr. Tom Conkling, Head of the Engineering Library, Pennsylvania State University. The permission to use photographic materials produced by Elsevier-Mosby, Inc., is also acknowledged and appreciated. Many manufacturers of products and commercial suppliers provided technical information about their products and gave permission for the reproduction of photographs and other illustrations. Thanks for the use of these materials is given to the following companies: Baird Corporation in Bedford, Massachusetts; Dosimetry Corporation of America in Cincinnati, Ohio; Emberline Instruments in Santa Fe, New Mexico; Landauer, Inc., in Glenwood, Illinois; Machlett Labs, Inc., in Stamford, Connecticut; Nuclear Associates in Hicksville, New York; Solon Technologies, Inc., in Solon, Ohio; Victoreen, Inc., in Solon, Ohio; and X-Rite, Inc., in Grandville, Michigan.

Those who seek to learn within the field of medical imaging are the future of the profession. To the radiography students and radiology residents who will use this text, it is my hope that the materials contained in this edition will greatly contribute to enhancing your knowledge of radiation protection and radiation biology.

Finally, as I have stated in preceding editions, a very special remembrance is noted to my parents, the late Felix and Elizabeth (Markovitch) Krohn, for all they did for me. Their many words of wisdom and lifelong personal encouragement remain with me. The education they made possible helped me gain the knowledge necessary to prepare this and previous editions. My accomplishments serve as a tribute to them.

Mary Alice Statkiewicz Sherer

CONTENTS

RADIATION PROTECTION

IN

MEDICAL RADIOGRAPHY

1

Introduction to Radiation Protection

KEY TERMS

as low as reasonably achievable (ALARA)
background equivalent radiation time (BERT)
biologic damage
biologic effects
cellular damage
diagnostic efficacy
effective dose (EfD)
electromagnetic spectrum

electromagnetic wave
equivalent dose (EqD)
genetic damage
ionization
ionizing radiation
manmade, or artificial, radiation
natural background radiation
occupational and nonoccupational dose limits

optimization for radiation protection (ORP)
organic damage
radiation
radiation dose
radiation protection
radionuclide
radon
rem
sievert (Sv)

OBJECTIVES

After completing this chapter, the reader will be able to perform the following:

- Identify consequences of ionization in human cells.
- Give examples of how radiologic technologists and radiologists can exercise control of radiant energy while performing imaging procedures.
- Discuss the concept of effective radiation protection.
- Discuss the need to safeguard against significant and continuing radiation exposure.
- Explain the justification and responsibility for radiologic procedures.
- Explain how diagnostic efficacy of a radiographic procedure can be maximized.

Continued

Although radiation in all of its manifestations has been ever-present on our planet since the beginning of time, its use in the healing arts did not begin until the discovery of x-rays in 1895. Scientists experimenting with the newly discovered mysterious rays gradually became aware of their value to the medical community both as a diagnostic and as a therapeutic tool. The ability of x-rays to cause injury in normal biologic tissue soon became apparent as well. Hence, since the early 1900s both the beneficial and destructive potential of x-rays have been known. X-rays are a form of **ionizing radiation.** Ionizing radiation produces positively and negatively charged particles (ions) when passing through matter. The production of these ions is the event that may cause injury in normal biologic tissue. Consequences of ionization in human cells are listed in Box 1-1 and are discussed in Chapter 5 of this text.

By using the knowledge of radiation-induced hazards that has been gained over many years and by employing effective methods to limit or eliminate those hazards, humans can safely control the use of "radiant energy." An example of controllable radiant energy is the radiation produced from an x-ray tube (Fig. 1-1). Radiologic technologists and radiologists are educated in the safe operation of radiation-producing imaging equipment. They use protective devices whenever possible, follow established procedures, and select technical exposure factors that significantly reduce radiation exposure to patients and to themselves. Through these good practices, they minimize the possibility of causing damage in healthy biologic tissue.

EFFECTIVE RADIATION PROTECTION

Diagnostic imaging professionals have an ongoing responsibility to ensure radiation safety during all medical radiation procedures. They fulfill this obligation by adhering to an established radiation protection program. **Radiation protection** may be defined simply

*Each of these consequences is fully discussed in subsequent chapters.

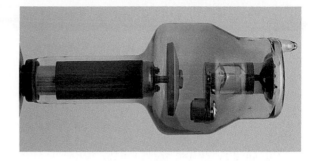

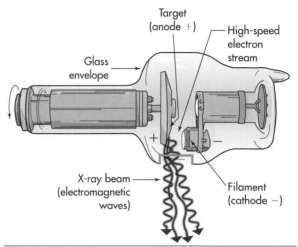

FIG. 1-1. Radiant energy is emitted from the x-ray tube in the form of waves (or particles). This energy can be controlled by the selection of equipment components and devices made for this purpose and by the selection of appropriate technical exposure factors.

as effective measures employed by radiation workers to safeguard patients, personnel, and the general public from *unnecessary* exposure to ionizing radiation. This is any radiation exposure that does not benefit a person in terms of diagnostic information obtained or any radiation exposure that does not enhance the quality of the study. Effective protective measures take into consideration both human and environmental physical determinants, technical elements, and procedural factors. They consist of tools and techniques used to minimize radiation exposure while producing optimal diagnostic images.

Need to Safeguard Against Significant and Continuing Radiation Exposure

Biologic Effects

The need for safeguarding against significant and continuing radiation exposure is based on evidence of harmful **biologic effects** (i.e., damage to living tissue of animals and humans exposed to radiation). Various methods of radiation protection may be applied to ensure safety for persons employed in radiation industries, including medicine, and for the population at large. In medicine, when radiation safety principles are correctly applied during imaging procedures, the energy deposited in living tissue by the radiation can be limited, thereby reducing the potential for biologic effects. This book focuses on radiation protection

for patients, diagnostic imaging personnel, and the general public. Biologic effects are also discussed extensively in Chapters 5, 6, and 7.

JUSTIFICATION AND RESPONSIBILITY FOR RADIOLOGIC PROCEDURES

Benefit vs. Risk

Radiation exposure should *always* be kept at the lowest possible level for the general public. However, when illness or injury occurs or when a specific imaging procedure for health screening purposes is prudent, a patient may elect to assume the risk of exposure to ionizing radiation to obtain essential diagnostic medical information. A prime example of such a voluntary assumption of risk occurs when women elect to undergo screening mammography to detect breast cancer in its early stages (Fig. 1-2). Because mammography continues to be the most effective tool for diagnosing breast cancer early, when the disease can best be treated,[1] its use contributes significantly to improving the quality of life for women. When ionizing radiation is used in this fashion for the welfare of the patient, the directly realized benefits of the exposure to this radiant energy far outweigh any slight risk of inducing a radiogenic malignancy or any genetic defects (Fig. 1-3).

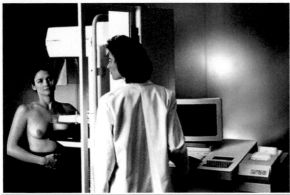

FIG. 1-2. Mammography continues to be the most effective tool for diagnosing breast cancer. A patient may elect to assume the risk of exposure to ionizing radiation to obtain essential diagnostic medical information. Mammography may be used as a screening tool or it can be used as a diagnostic procedure. In either instance, the directly realized benefit, in terms of medical information obtained, far outweighs any slight risk of possible biologic damage. (From *Mosby's radiographic instructional series,* St. Louis, 1999, Mosby.)

Diagnostic Efficacy

Diagnostic efficacy is the degree to which the diagnostic study accurately reveals the presence or absence of disease in the patient. It is maximized when essential radiographs are produced under recommended radiation protection guidelines. Efficacy is a vital part of radiation protection in the healing arts. It provides the basis for determining whether an imaging procedure or practice is justified (Box 1-2). The referring physician carries the responsibility for determining this medical necessity for the patient. After ordering an x-ray examination or procedure, the referring physician must accept basic responsibility for protecting the patient from non-useful radiation exposure. The physician exercises this responsibility by relying on qualified imaging personnel. As health care professionals, radiographers accept a portion of the respon-

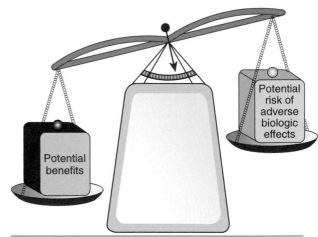

FIG. 1-3. The potential benefits of exposing the patient to ionizing radiation must far outweigh the potential risk of adverse biologic effects.

BOX 1-2					
Achievement of Diagnostic Efficacy					
Imaging procedure or practice justified by referring physician	→	Minimal radiation exposure	→	Optimum radiograph(s) produced	→ Presence or absence of disease revealed = Diagnostic efficacy

sibility for patient welfare by providing quality imaging services. The radiographer and participating radiologist share in keeping patient medical radiation exposure at the lowest level possible. In this way imaging professionals help ensure that both **occupational and nonoccupational dose limits,** the upper boundary doses of ionizing radiation that result in a negligible risk of bodily injury or genetic damage, remain well below maximum allowable levels. This can best be accomplished by using the *smallest* radiation exposure that will produce useful radiographs, and by producing optimal radiographs with the *first* exposure. Repeated examinations made necessary by technical error or carelessness (Fig. 1-4) must be avoided because they significantly increase radiation exposure for both the patient and the radiation worker.

AS LOW AS REASONABLY ACHIEVABLE (ALARA) PRINCIPLE

Concepts of Radiologic Practice

ALARA is an acronym for **as low as reasonably achievable.** This term is synonymous with the term **optimization for radiation protection (ORP).** The intention behind these concepts of radiologic practice is to keep radiation exposure and consequent dose to the lowest possible level (Fig. 1-5). The rationale for this comes from evidence compiled by scientists over the past century.[2] At the time of this publication, radiation protection guidelines are rooted in the philosophy of ALARA. Therefore, this philosophy, *as low as reasonably achievable,* should be a main part of every health care facility's personnel radiation control program, and should also be established and maintained for patients. Radiation-induced cancer does not have a threshold—that is, a dose level below which individuals would have no chance of sustaining this disease. Therefore, because no threshold exists for radiation-induced malignant disease, radiation exposure should always be kept ALARA for all medical imaging procedures. For radiographers and radiologists participating in diagnostic x-ray procedures, the ALARA concept should serve as a guide for the selection of technical radiographic and fluoroscopic exposure factors for all patient imaging procedures.

Responsibility for Maintaining ALARA in the Medical Industry

Both employers of radiation workers and the workers themselves have a responsibility for radiation safety in the medical industry. For the welfare of patients and the workers, facilities providing imaging services must have an effective radiation safety program. This requires a firm commitment to radiation safety by all participants. It is the responsibility of the employer to provide the necessary resources and appropriate environment in which to execute an ALARA program. A written policy statement describing this program and identifying the commitment of management to keeping all radiation exposure ALARA must be available to all employees in the workplace. To determine how radiation exposure in the workplace might be lowered, management should perform periodic exposure audits.[3] Radiation workers with appropriate education and work experience must function with awareness of rules governing the work situation. They are required to perform their occupational practices in a manner consistent with the ALARA principle (Box 1-3). When radiation is safely and prudently used in the imaging of patients, the benefit of the exposure can be maximized while the potential risk of biologic damage can be minimized. Additional information on the ALARA concept can be found in Chapter 7.

PATIENT PROTECTION AND PATIENT EDUCATION

Educating Patients about Radiologic Procedures

Facilities that provide radiologic services have a responsibility to ensure the highest quality of service. An important part of this occurs when imaging personnel educate patients about radiologic procedures. Patients not only should be aware of what a specific procedure involves and what type of cooperation is required, but also they must be informed of what needs to be done, if anything, as a follow-up to their examination. Through appropriate and effective communication, patients can be made to feel that they are active participants in their own health care (Fig. 1-6).

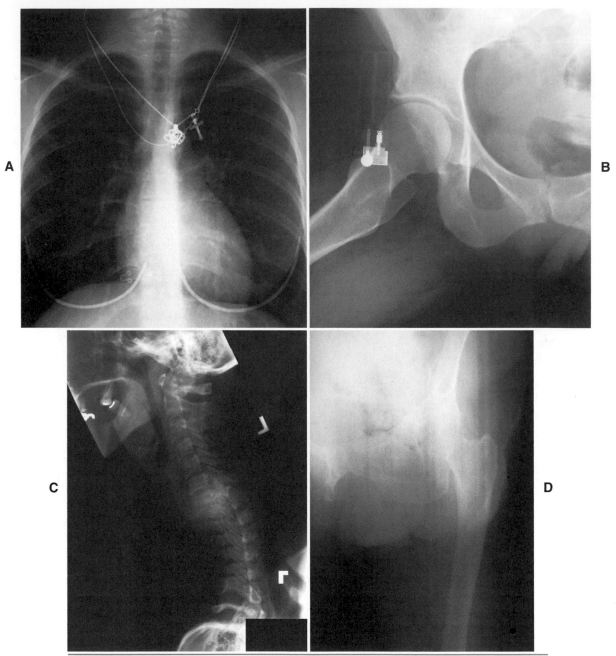

FIG. 1-4. A, Posteroanterior chest radiograph requiring a repeat examination because of multiple external foreign bodies (several necklaces and an under-wire bra) that should have been removed before the radiographic examination. **B,** Anteroposterior radiograph of a right hip requiring a repeat examination because of poor collimation and the presence of an external foreign body (a cigarette lighter) overlying the anatomy of concern. The patient's slacks with the pocket containing the lighter should have been removed before the radiographic examination. **C,** Double exposure (two lateral projections of the cervical spine) requiring a repeat examination. **D,** Radiograph of left hip demonstrating an "off-level" grid error. This occurs when the patient's weight is not evenly distributed on the grid, causing the grid to tilt so that it is not properly aligned to the x-ray tube.

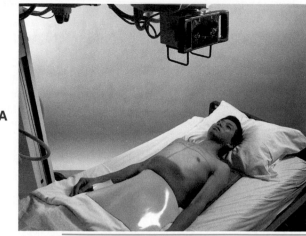

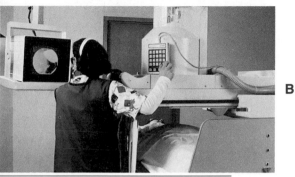

FIG. 1-5. **A,** Patient protection. **B,** Radiographer protection. Medical radiation exposure should always be kept as low as reasonably achievable (ALARA) for the patient and for imaging personnel. (**A** from Ballinger PW, Frank ED: *Merrill's atlas of radiographic positions and radiologic procedures,* ed 10, St. Louis, 2003, Mosby. **B** from *Mosby's radiographic instructional series,* St. Louis, 1999, Mosby.)

BOX 1-3

Responsibilities for an Effective Radiation Safety Program

Employers' Responsibilities
- Implement and maintain an effective radiation safety program in which to execute ALARA by providing:
  - necessary resources
  - appropriate environment for ALARA program
- Make a written policy statement describing the ALARA program and identifying the commitment of management to keep all radiation exposure ALARA available to all employees in the workplace.
- Perform periodic exposure audits to determine how to lower radiation exposure in the workplace.

Radiation Workers' Responsibilities
- Be aware of rules governing the workplace.
- Perform duties consistent with ALARA.

ALARA, As low as reasonably achievable.

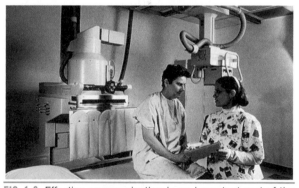

FIG. 1-6. Effective communication is an important part of the patient-radiographer relationship. Patients need to be educated about radiologic procedures so that they can understand what the procedure involves and what type of cooperation is required. The radiographer must answer patient questions about the potential risk of radiation exposure honestly. To create understanding and reduce fear and anxiety for the patient, the radiographer can provide an example that compares the amount of radiation received for a specific procedure with natural background radiation received over a given period of time. (From *Mosby's radiographic instructional series,* St. Louis, 1999, Mosby.)

Risk of Radiologic Examination vs. Potential Benefit

In general terms, risk can be defined as the probability of injury, ailment, or death resulting from an activity. In the medical industry with reference to the radiation sciences, risk is the possibility of inducing a radiogenic cancer or genetic defect after irradiation. Typically, people are more willing to accept a risk if they perceive that the potential benefit to be obtained is greater than the risk involved. Regarding exposure to ionizing radiation, patients who have an understanding of the medical benefit from an imaging procedure are more likely to overcome any radiation phobia and be willing to assume a small risk of possible biologic damage. Greater understanding of biologic effects associated with diagnostic radiology was gained throughout the 20th century. The medical imaging industry presently continues to build upon this knowledge. This information coupled with better design and sophistication of medical imaging equipment and improved radiation safety standards has greatly reduced risk from imaging procedures for both patients and radiographers. When radiographers use their knowledge and answer patient questions about the risk of radiation exposure honestly, they can do much to alleviate any patient apprehension and fears during a routine radiologic examination.

Background Equivalent Radiation Time (BERT)

Another way radiographers can improve understanding and reduce fear and anxiety for the patient is to use the **background equivalent radiation time (BERT)**. This method compares the amount of radiation received, for example, from a patient's chest radiograph or from a radiograph of any other part of the anatomy, with natural background radiation received over a given period of time such as days, weeks, months, or years (Table 1-1). BERT is based on an annual U.S. population exposure of approximately 3 millisieverts per year (approximately 300 millirems per year).* Using the BERT method in this context has the following advantages:

1. BERT does not imply radiation risk; it is simply a means for comparison.

TABLE 1-1

Typical Adult Patient Effective Dose (EfD) and BERT Values

Radiologic Procedure	EfD		BERT (Amount of Time to Receive the Same EfD from Nature)
	mSv	mrem	
Dental, intraoral	0.06	6	1 wk
Chest radiograph	0.08	8	10 days
Thoracic spine	1.5	150	6 mo
Lumbar spine	3.0	300	1 yr
Upper GI series	4.5	450	1.5 yr
Lower GI series	6.0	600	2 yr

Adapted from IPSM Report No. 53: *Patient dosimetry techniques in diagnostic radiology*, York, UK, 1988, Institute of Physics and Engineering in Medicine, p 53, and Table A7, p 117.
BERT, background equivalent radiation time; GI, gastrointestinal; mrem, millirem; mSv, millisievert.

2. BERT emphasizes that radiation is an innate part of our environment.
3. The answer given in terms of BERT is easy for the patient to comprehend.

RADIATION

Types of Radiation

Radiation may be defined as energy in transit from one location to another. By this definition, there are many types of radiation. One example is mechanical vibration of materials. Such mechanical vibrations can travel through the air or other materials to interact with structures in the human ear and produce the sensation we call *sound*. Ultrasound is the mechanical

---

*The millisievert (mSv), a subunit of the sievert, is equal to 1/1000 of a sievert. The sievert is the International System of Units unit of measure for the radiation quantity, equivalent dose. The millirem (mrem), a subunit of the rem, is equal to 1/1000 of a rem. The rem is the traditional unit of measure for the radiation quantity, equivalent dose.

TABLE 1-2

The Electromagnetic Spectrum*

Use	Frequency	Wavelength	Energy
AM radio	0.54-1.6 MHz	0.6-0.2 km	2-7 neV
FM radio	88-108 MHz	3.4-3 m	370-440 neV
Television	54 MHz-0.8 GHz	5.6-0.4 m	220 neV-3.3 μeV
Microwaves	0.1-100 GHz	3 m-3 mm	0.4 eV-0.4 meV
Infrared	100 GHz-400 THz	3 mm-0.7 m	0.4 meV-1.6 eV
Visible	400-700 THz	0.7-0.4 m	1.6-2.8 eV
Ultraviolet	1-100 PHz	300-3 nm	4-400 eV
X-rays	100 PHz-100 EHz	3 nm-3 am	0.4-400 keV
Gamma rays	100 EHz-infinity	3-0 am	400 keV-infinity

*Frequency (in units of hertz [Hz] or cycles per second), wavelength (in meters), and energy (in electron volts [eV]). Each frequency within the spectrum has a characteristic wavelength and frequency. Some of the uses of different frequency ranges are listed. Note that higher frequencies are associated with shorter wavelengths and higher energies. The values shown here are typical representations. See Appendix E for an explanation of the abbreviations (M, G, T, P, μ, etc.).

vibration of a material in which the rate of vibration does not stimulate the human ear sensors and therefore is beyond the range of human hearing. Another example of radiation is the **electromagnetic wave.** Radio waves, microwaves, visible light, and x-rays are all representative of this form of radiation. In electromagnetic waves, electric and magnetic fields fluctuate rapidly as they travel through space. A limited range of frequencies of this fluctuation is interpreted by its interaction with the human system as visible light. Within this range, small variations in frequency—the number of cycles or wavelengths of a simple harmonic motion per unit of time—are interpreted as different colors. However, frequencies both above and below the visible range exist and have many uses. Electromagnetic waves are also characterized by their wavelength, which is simply the physical distance between successive maximum values of electric and magnetic fields.

The Electromagnetic Spectrum

The full range of frequencies and wavelengths of electromagnetic waves is known as the **electromagnetic spectrum.** Table 1-2 shows the electromagnetic spectrum in frequency (in units of hertz [Hz] or cycles per second), wavelength (in meters), and energy (in electron volts [eV]). Each frequency within the spectrum has a characteristic wavelength and energy. Some of the uses of different frequency ranges are listed. Note that higher frequencies are associated with shorter wavelengths and higher energies; therefore the wavelength ranges from largest to smallest, whereas frequencies and energy cover the corresponding smallest to largest ranges. Precise frequency ranges attributed to different parts of the electromagnetic spectrum may vary in different references, and there is substantial overlap of ranges (note that FM radio falls completely within the television range). Calculation of the wavelength and energy of electromagnetic radiation is as follows.

The speed of light (c), wavelength (λ), and frequency (ν), are related by the equation:

$$c = \lambda\nu, \text{ where } c = 3 \times 10^8 \text{ m/sec}$$

Therefore, if the frequency of an electromagnetic wave is known, the wavelength may be calculated as follows:

$$\lambda = \frac{c}{\nu}$$

EXAMPLE: Find the wavelength of a 0.5 MHz radio wave.

$$\lambda = \frac{3 \times 10^8 \text{ m/sec}}{0.5 \times 10^6 \text{ sec}^{-1}} = 6.0 \times 10^2 \text{ m} = 0.6 \times 10^3 \text{ m} = 0.6 \text{ km}$$

The energy (in electron volts, eV) of an electromagnetic wave may be calculated using the frequency (ν) and Planck's constant (h) as follows:

$$E = h\nu, \text{ where } h = 4.14 \times 10^{-15} \text{ eV-sec}$$

EXAMPLE: Find the energy of an x-ray having a wavelength of 100 PHz.

$$E = (4.14 \times 10^{-15} \text{ eV-sec})(100 \times 10^{15} \text{ sec}^{-1}) =$$
$$414 \times 10^0 \text{ eV} = 414 \text{ eV} \sim 0.4 \text{ keV}$$

Ionizing and Nonionizing Radiation

For our purposes in the study of radiation protection, the electromagnetic spectrum can be divided into two parts: ionizing and nonionizing (Fig. 1-7). Of the entire range of electromagnetic radiations included in the electromagnetic spectrum, only x- and gamma radiation are classified as ionizing radiations. Ultraviolet radiation, visible light, infrared rays, microwaves, and radio waves are considered to be nonionizing because they do not have sufficient kinetic energy to eject electrons from the atom.

If electromagnetic radiation has a high enough frequency, it can transfer sufficient energy to the electrons to remove them from the atoms to which they were attached. This process, called **ionization,** is the

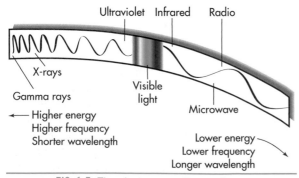

Ultraviolet   Infrared   Radio

X-rays

Visible
light

Gamma rays

← Higher energy
Higher frequency
Shorter wavelength

Microwave

Lower energy
Lower frequency
Longer wavelength →

FIG. 1-7. The electromagnetic spectrum.

foundation of the interactions of x-rays with human tissue. It makes them valuable for creating images but has the undesirable result of potentially producing some damage in the biologic material. The amount of energy transferred to electrons by ionizing radiation is the basis of the concept of **radiation dose.** Thus, a radiation quantity such as equivalent dose, described in the following section, applies *only* to ionizing radiation such as x-rays. Equivalent dose cannot be used to specify the amount of energy imparted to a potato in a microwave oven or to a sunbather on the beach because no ionization is produced by microwaves or sunlight.*

Particulate Radiation

In addition to electromagnetic radiation, there is another category of ionizing radiation called *particulate radiation*. This radiation includes alpha particles, beta particles, neutrons, and protons. These subatomic particles are ejected from atoms at very high speeds. They possess sufficient kinetic energy to be capable of causing ionization. However, no ionization occurs when the subatomic particles are at rest.

Alpha particles are emitted from nuclei of very heavy elements such as uranium and plutonium during the process of radioactive decay. Radioactive decay is a naturally occurring process in which unstable nuclei relieve that instability by various types of nuclear spontaneous emissions, one of which is the emission of charged particles. Alpha particles each contain two protons and two neutrons. They are simply helium nuclei (i.e., helium ions). Alpha particles have a large mass (approximately four times the mass of a hydrogen atom) and a positive charge twice that of an electron. This permits them to have the potential of transferring very substantial kinetic energy to orbital electrons of other atoms.[4]

Particulate radiations vary in their ability to penetrate matter. Compared with beta particles, alpha

---

*Actually, a small amount of ionizing radiation is produced by the sun in the form of solar flares. However, this amount is negligible, and the small amount of ionizing radiation is not what produces the sensation of heat or the chemical changes that produce suntan and sunburn. These are the result of nonionizing infrared and ultraviolet radiation.

particles are less penetrating. Because alpha particles lose energy quickly as they travel a short distance in biologic matter (i.e., into the superficial layers of the skin), they are considered virtually harmless as an external source of radiation. A piece of ordinary paper can absorb them or function as a shield. However, as an internal source of radiation, the reverse is true. If emitted from a radioisotope deposited in the body, for example, in the lungs, alpha particles can be absorbed in the relatively radiosensitive epithelial tissue and can be very damaging to that tissue. It is in a way analogous to what a bowling ball does to a set of pins.

Beta particles, also known as beta rays, are identical to high-speed electrons except for their origin. Electrons originate in atomic shells, whereas beta particles, like alpha particles, are emitted from the nuclei of radioactive atoms, but radioactive atoms that relieve their instability in a different fashion. This process of *beta decay* along with some therapeutic uses of beta radiation is discussed in Chapter 11. Beta particles are approximately 8000 times lighter than alpha particles. They have a small mass and a negative charge. Because they have a much smaller footprint, they are capable of penetrating biologic matter to a greater depth than alpha particles and with far less ionization along their paths. (It should be noted that some high-speed electrons are not beta radiation. These are produced in a radiation oncology treatment machine called a linear accelerator. These electrons are most often used to treat superficial skin lesions in small areas and to deliver radiation boost treatments to breast tumors at tissue depth typically not exceeding 5 to 6 centimeters.) As previously stated, alpha rays can be absorbed by a piece of ordinary paper because they interact so readily with matter, losing their kinetic energy quite rapidly as a consequence. Beta rays with a lesser probability of interaction, however, can penetrate matter more deeply and therefore cannot be stopped by an ordinary piece of paper. Either a thick block of wood or a 1-mm-thick lead shield would be required to absorb them.

Protons are positively charged components of an atom. They have a very small mass, which, however, exceeds that of an electron by a factor of 1800. The number of protons in the nucleus of an atom constitutes its atomic number, or "Z" number. The atomic number identifies an element and determines its placement in the periodic table of elements (see Appendix

D). *Neutrons* are the electrically neutral components of an atom and have approximately the same mass as a proton. If two atoms have the same number of protons but a different number of neutrons in their nuclei, they are referred to as *isotopes*.

Radiation Dose Specification: Equivalent Dose (EqD)

Equivalent dose (EqD) is a *quantity* that attempts to take into account the variation in biologic harm that is produced by different types of radiation. It enables the calculation of the **effective dose (EfD),** a dose that takes into account the dose for all types of ionizing radiation (alpha, beta, gamma, x-ray, etc.) to organs or tissues in the human body (skin, gonadal tissue, thyroid, etc.) being irradiated and the overall harm or the weighting factor of those biologic components for developing a radiation-induced cancer (or for the reproductive organs, the risk of **genetic damage** [radiation damage to generations yet unborn]). Since effective dose takes into account all of the organ weighting factors, it represents the whole body dose that would give an equivalent biologic response. In the International System of Units (SI), the unit of equivalent dose (EqD) is the **sievert (Sv).** In the traditional system, the unit of measure is the **rem.** One sievert equals 100 rem. Both occupational and nonoccupational dose limits are expressed as effective dose and may be stated in Sv (rem). Effective dose, equivalent dose, and other units of dosimetry are discussed in substantial detail in Chapter 3.

Biologic Damage Potential

Ionizing radiation produces **biologic damage** while penetrating body tissues primarily by ejecting electrons from the atoms composing the tissues. Destructive radiation interaction at the atomic level results in molecular change, and this in turn can cause **cellular damage,** leading to abnormal cell function or loss of cell function. If excessive cellular damage occurs, the living organism exhibits genetic or somatic changes such as mutations, cataracts, and leukemia. Changes in blood count are a classic example of **organic damage,** resulting from significant exposure to ionizing radiation. An equivalent dose as low as 0.25 Sv

(25 rem) delivered to the whole body may cause a decrease within a few days in the number of lymphocytes (white blood cells that defend the body against foreign invaders by producing antibodies to combat disease) in the blood. Table 1-3 provides some basic information on the known biologic effects of different radiation equivalent doses that result when radiation exposures are delivered to the whole body over a time period of less than a few hours (acute exposures). Because the potential to cause biologic damage from different radiation equivalent doses to the whole body exists, the use of ionizing radiation should be limited whenever possible.

Sources of Radiation

Human beings are continuously exposed to sources of ionizing radiation. Some people are exposed to a wide variety, whereas others are exposed to a limited number. Sources of ionizing radiation may be natural or manmade (artificial). Table 1-4 provides a quick reference for average annual radiation equivalent doses for the U.S. resulting from both natural background and manmade sources of radiation.

TABLE 1-3

Radiation Equivalent Dose (EqD) and Subsequent Biologic Effects Resulting from Acute Whole Body Exposures*

Radiation EqD

Sv	rem	Subsequent Biologic Effects
0.25	25	Blood changes (e.g., measurable hematologic depression, decreases in the number of lymphocytes present in the circulating blood)
1.5	150	Nausea, diarrhea
2.0	200	Erythema (diffuse redness over an area of skin after irradiation)
2.5	250	If dose is to gonads, temporary sterility
3.0	300	50% chance of death; lethal dose for 50% of population over 30 days (LD 50/30)
6.0	600	Death

*Radiation exposures are delivered to the entire body over a time period of less than a few hours.
Modified from *Radiologic Health*, unit 4, slide 17, Denver, Multi-Media Publishing (slide program).

TABLE 1-4

Average Annual Radiation Equivalent Dose (EqD) for the United States*

Category	Type of Radiation	Dose		Percentage of EqD (%)
		mSv	mrem	
Natural	Radon	1.98	198	55
	Cosmic, terrestrial, internal	0.97	97	27
		2.95	295	82
Manmade	Medical x-rays	0.4	40	11
	Nuclear medicine	0.14	14	4
	Consumer products	0.11	11	3
		0.65	65	18
Other	Occupational	0.009	0.9	0.002
	Fallout	<0.011	<1.1	<0.3
	Nuclear fuel cycle	0.0005	0.05	0.0001
	Miscellaneous	0.0006	0.06	0.0002
	environmental sources	0.02	2.11	0.30

Adapted from National Council on Radiation Protection and Measurements (NCRP): *Report No. 93, ionizing radiation exposure of the population of the United States*, Bethesda, Md, 1987, NCRP.
*Overall 360 mrem (100%). All percentages listed are percentages of 360 mrem (~1 mrem/day). (360 mrem = 0.36 rem = 3.6 mSv.)

Natural Radiation

Natural sources of ionizing radiation have always been a part of the human environment since the formation of the universe. Ionizing radiation from environmental sources is called **natural background radiation** and has three components:

1. Terrestrial radiation from radioactive materials in the crust of the earth
2. Cosmic radiation from the sun (solar) and beyond the solar system (galactic)
3. Internal, from radionuclides, radioactive atoms that make up a small percentage of the body's tissue

If any of these natural sources become increased because of accidental or deliberate human actions, they are termed *enhanced natural sources.*

Terrestrial Radiation Long-lived radioactive elements such as uranium-238, radium-226, and thorium-232 that emit densely ionizing radiations are present in variable quantities in the crust of the earth. These sources of ionizing radiation are classified as *terrestrial*

radiation. The quantity of terrestrial radiation present in any area depends on the composition of the soil or rocks in that geographic area. Approximately 55% of the gross common exposure of human beings to natural background radiation comes from **radon** (Fig. 1-8). Geologic formations or soil containing granite, shale, phosphate, and pitchblende produce higher concentrations of radon than other commonly encountered materials. It is by far the largest contributor to background radiation. The average U.S. resident receives approximately 1.98 mSv (198 mrem) per year from indoor and outdoor levels of radon. Radon, the first decay product of radium, is a colorless, odorless, heavy radioactive gas that along with its decay products, polonium-218 and polonium-214 (solid form), is always present to some degree in the air. Because it is a gas, radon can percolate up through the soil. It enters buildings through cracks or holes in their frameworks. In homes, it may gain access through crawlspaces under the living areas, through floor drains and sump

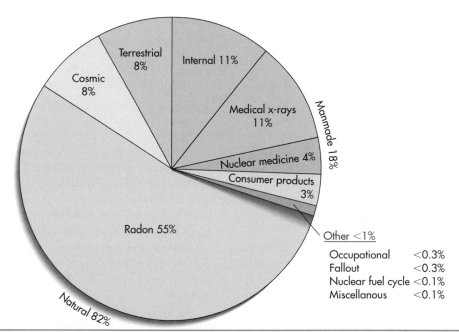

FIG. 1-8. Various radiation sources contribute to the total average effective dose for inhabitants of the United States. This diagram demonstrates the percentage contribution of each natural and manmade radiation source. (From National Council on Radiation Protection and Measurements [NCRP]: *Report No. 93, ionizing radiation exposure of the population of the United States,* Bethesda, Md, 1987, NCRP.)

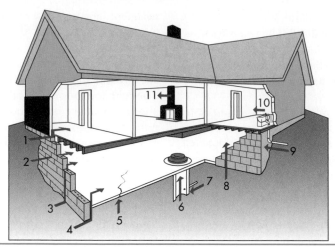

FIG. 1-9. Radon gas can penetrate up through soil and enter a home through holes or cracks in its framework, crawlspaces under the living areas, floor drains, sump pumps, and porous cement block foundations. *1,* Spaces behind brick veneer on top of block foundation; *2,* pores and cracks in concrete block foundation; *3,* open top of block foundation walls; *4,* floor to wall joints; *5,* cracks in concrete floor; *6,* exposed soil as in basement sump; *7,* weeping drain tile draining into open sump; *8,* mortar joints; *9,* loose-fitting pipe wall penetration; *10,* well water from some wells; *11,* building materials such as stone. (Courtesy U.S. Environmental Protection Agency, Washington, DC.)

pumps, and through porous cement block foundations (Fig. 1-9). In many cases, a pressure gradient exists between a house and the soil on which it rests so that the house draws on the ground like a vacuum cleaner. Commonly used building materials such as bricks, concrete, and gypsum wallboard contain radon. These construction materials are classified as earth-based materials.[4]

Radon concentrations in a particular structure vary across days and seasons. In the cooler months, when homes and buildings are tightly closed, radon levels are usually higher. This is the best time to perform tests for radon.*

High indoor concentrations of radon have the potential to cause serious health hazards for humans. After being inhaled, this airborne radioactive gas produces daughter radioactive isotopes that remain for lengthy periods in the epithelial tissue of the lungs. As these secondary isotopes decay, they give off radiation

that may injure lung tissues, thereby increasing the risk for lung cancer. The severity of this risk depends on how concentrated the radon is and the length of time that the person is exposed to the gas.[5] Smokers exposed to high radon levels face a higher risk of lung cancer than do nonsmokers. One reason for this may be that smokers have already been exposed to higher concentrations of radioactivity from the lead-210 (^{210}Pb) and polonium-210 (^{210}Po) isotopes contained in tobacco and tobacco smoke. An isotope is an atom that contains a different number of neutrons but the same number of protons in its nucleus as does the reference atom (e.g., helium-3 and helium-4, whose nuclei contain one and two neutrons, respectively). Radioactive isotopes of atoms that make up biologic materials may be used in medical imaging nuclear medicine studies.

The Environmental Protection Agency (EPA) considers radon to be the second leading cause of lung cancer in the U.S. It is responsible for approximately 20,000 cancer deaths per year. (For more information on the EPA, see Chapter 7.) The EPA recommends that action be taken to reduce elevated levels of radon

---

*Detection kits are relatively easy to use and may be purchased at retail stores or obtained at minimal cost from the National Safety Council in Washington, D.C., by calling 1-800-SOS-RADON.

to below 4 picocuries* per liter (pCi/L) of air (a concentration that specifies the number of radioactive processes per second that occur on average in 1 L of air). A radon concentration of 4 pCi/L results in a yearly equivalent dose to the lung of approximately 0.05 mSv (5 mrem).[6] This level of radon presence is considered statistically safe by the EPA. The EPA estimates that 10% of the homes in the U.S. exceed the recommended limit of 4 pCi/L. Hence, accurate radon testing and appropriate structural repair, if required, are essential to reduce the risk of lung cancer from radon.

Cosmic Radiation Cosmic rays are of extraterrestrial origin and result from nuclear interactions that have taken place in the sun and other stars. The intensity of cosmic rays varies with altitude relative to the earth's surface. The greatest intensity occurs at high altitudes, and the lowest intensity occurs at sea level. The earth's atmosphere and magnetic field help shield it from cosmic rays. The shielding is diminished at higher elevation where less atmosphere separates the earth from cosmic rays. The average U.S. inhabitant receives an equivalent dose of approximately 0.3 mSv (30 mrem) per year from extraterrestrial radiation. Cosmic radiations consist predominantly of high-energy protons; as a result of interactions with molecules in the earth's atmosphere, these protons may be accompanied by alpha particles, atomic nuclei, mesons, gamma rays, and high-energy electrons. These other forms of radiation are collectively referred to as *secondary cosmic radiation*. The gamma rays among them are energetic enough to penetrate several meters of lead.

Terrestrial and Internal Radiation The tissues of the human body contain many naturally existing radionuclides that have been ingested in minute quantities from various foods or inhaled as particles in the air. A **radionuclide** is an unstable nucleus that emits one or more forms of ionizing radiation to achieve greater stability. These forms of ionizing radiation may include alpha particles (helium nuclei), beta particles (electrons), and gamma rays (similar to x-rays, but usually higher energy in the range of a million electron volts [MeV]). Certain types of radioactive decay also affect the distribution of

electrons around the atom, resulting in the emission of x-rays. Potassium-40 (^{40}K), carbon-14 (^{14}C), hydrogen-3 (^{3}H; tritium), and strontium-90 (^{90}Sr) are examples of radioactive nuclides that exist in small quantities within the body. Radionuclides in the soil and air also add to the human radiation dose burden. The average member of the general population receives more than 0.67 mSv (67 mrem) per year from combined exposure to radiations from the earth's surface (terrestrial) and radiation within the human body. In total, the radon (1.98 mSv [198 mrem]), cosmic ray radiations (0.3 mSv [30 mrem]), terrestrial, and internally deposited radionuclides (0.67 mSv [67 mrem]) that comprise the natural background radiation in the U.S. result in an estimated average annual individual equivalent dose of approximately 2.95 mSv (295 mrem) (see Table 1-4).

Manmade (Artificial) Radiation

Ionizing radiation created by humans for various uses is classified as **manmade, or artificial, radiation.** Sources of artificial ionizing radiation include the following:
1. Consumer products containing radioactive material
2. Air travel
3. Nuclear fuel for generation of power
4. Atmospheric fallout from nuclear weapons
5. Nuclear power plant accidents
6. Medical radiation

Manmade radiation contributes about 0.65 mSv (65 mrem) to the average annual radiation exposure of the U.S. population. Of this equivalent dose, 0.4 mSv (40 mrem) results from medical diagnostic x-ray procedures, 0.14 mSv (14 mrem) results from nuclear medicine imaging, and 0.11 mSv (11 mrem) results from consumer products (see Table 1-4). Of course, an individual may or may not have these procedures in a given year, but these figures represent an "average share" of dose that would be true if the total medical radiation dose were shared equally among all individuals. A qualified medical physicist can calculate an individual's actual medical radiation exposure from x-ray examinations if she or he is provided with the technical details (x-ray tube voltage used, exposure time, etc.) pertaining to the studies.

Consumer Products Containing Radioactive Material Consumer products containing radioactive

---

*1 picocurie = 10^{-12} curie.

material include airport surveillance systems; early televisions; electron microscopes; shoe fitting fluoroscopes used in the early 1950s; ionization type smoke detector alarms; phonograph record static eliminators; some timepieces with luminous dials and numbers containing promethium-147, radium-226, strontium-90, and tritium; and video display terminals that use cathode-ray tubes. These products contribute a small fraction of the total average equivalent dose to each member of the general population.

When color television monitors were first made available to consumers, radiation exposure levels from these devices was substantial. As a result of technologic advances during the last 40 years and strict regulations imposed within the U.S. by the Food and Drug Administration (FDA) regarding such devices, the radiation exposure to the general public may now be considered negligible.

Porcelain used for making dentures provides a common present-day example of a consumer product that contains radioactive material. Porcelain contains potassium-40 and is usually "doped" with uranium to give a more natural color to the denture.[3] Artificial teeth made in the U.S. are estimated to give the tissues of the oral cavity an average dose of 600 mSv/yr (60,000 mrem/yr) whereas dental porcelain made in Great Britain has been reported to have dose rates 10 times higher.[3]

Air Travel The normal use of the airplane at high elevations brings many humans in closer contact with high-energy extraterrestrial radiation and consequently increases exposure. A flight on a typical commercial airliner results in an equivalent dose rate of 0.005 to 0.01 mSv/hr (0.5 to 1 mrem/hr).

Sunspots are dark spots that occasionally appear on the surface of the sun. They indicate regions of increased electromagnetic field activity and are sometimes responsible for ejecting particulate radiation into space. This radiation normally constitutes a small fraction of our dose from cosmic radiation here on earth. However, the solar contribution to the cosmic ray background increases during periods of high sunspot activity.

If a person spends 10 hours flying aboard a commercial aircraft during a period of normal sunspot activity, that individual will receive a radiation equivalent dose that is about equal to the dose received from one chest radiograph. During a solar flare, this dose can be 10 to as much as 100 times higher. Awareness of these increases in radiation exposure is important information for the general public. However, this increase in radiation exposure carries an immeasurably small health risk. With this knowledge, a person choosing air travel during such periods of high sunspot activity and solar flares can make an intelligent decision whether or not the potential benefit of the air travel outweighs the small increased health risk.

Nuclear Fuel for Generation of Power Nuclear power plants that produce nuclear fuel for the generation of power do not contribute significantly to the annual equivalent dose of the U.S. population. The nuclear fuel cycle contributes approximately 0.0001% to the total average annual equivalent dose for persons living in the U.S.

Atmospheric Fallout from Nuclear Weapons An accurate estimate of the total annual equivalent dose from fallout cannot be made because actual radiation measurements do not exist. The *dose commitment* (the dose that may ultimately be delivered from a given intake of radionuclide)[7] may be estimated by using a series of approximations and simplistic models that are subject to considerable speculation. The actual radiation dose to the global population from atmospheric fallout from nuclear weapons testing is not received all at once. It is instead delivered over a period of years at changing dose rates. The changes in the dose rates depend on factors such as characteristics of the fallout field and the elapsed time since the test occurred. No atmospheric nuclear testing has occurred since 1980.

When spread over the inhabitants of the United States, fallout from nuclear weapons tests (Fig. 1-10) and other environmental sources contributes less than 0.0116 mSv (1.16 mrem) annually to the equivalent dose of each person. This annual equivalent dose is considered to have a negligible impact on the U.S. population.

Nuclear Power Plant Accidents Although nuclear power benefits humans by creating a needed power supply of electricity, unfortunate accidents involving nuclear reactors can occur. This can lead to additional, unplanned radiation exposure for humans and the environment. Examples of two nuclear power

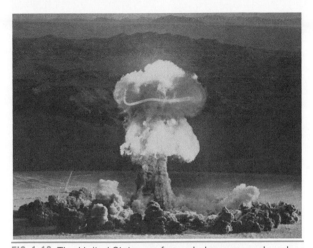

FIG. 1-10. The United States performed above-ground nuclear weapons tests before 1963. During the Priscilla Test, this atomic cloud resulted when a 37-kiloton testing device exploded from a balloon at the Nevada test site on June 24, 1957. The atomic cloud top, which contained manmade ionizing radiation, ascended approximately 43,000 feet. (Courtesy U.S. Department of Energy, Nevada Operations Office, Las Vegas, Nev.)

plant accidents are addressed in the discussion that follows.

Three Mile Island-2 (TMI-2) On March 28, 1979, the TMI-2 pressurized water reactor, situated on an island in the Susquehanna River located about 15 miles southeast of Harrisburg, Pennsylvania (Fig. 1-11, A), suffered a loss of coolant that resulted in severe overheating (at a temperature greater than 5000° F) of the radioactive reactor core. Consequently, a significant melting of the core occurred. The U.S. Department of Energy estimated that about 40% of the material in the TMI-2 nuclear reactor core reached a molten state. Approximately 15% of the melted uranium dioxide fuel of the core actually flowed through the undamaged portions of the core and settled on the bottom of the reactor vessel. This melted material in the nuclear reactor core and bottom of the reactor vessel formed crusts on its outside surfaces and in time cooled to re-solidified debris (Fig. 1-11, B). Although significant melting of the core and flowing of the molten radioactive material into intact

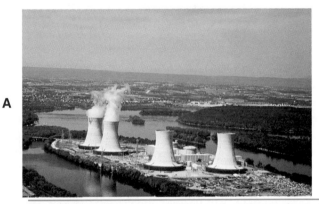

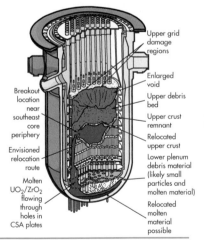

FIG. 1-11. **A,** Nuclear power stations such as the one located on Three Mile Island (TMI) near Harrisburg, Pennsylvania, house nuclear reactors. The large round containment buildings holding the reactors retain radioactive liquids and gases even in a high-pressure environment. **B,** TMI-2 end-state core conditions, illustrating the damage to the radioactive nuclear reactor core after the loss of coolant accident on March 28, 1979. Some of the original core mass formed an upper layer of debris. A hard crust supports this material. Zones of previously molten material and standing fuel rod segments account for some of the core mass lying beneath the upper debris bed. The lower reactor vessel head contains some of the melted core material. Closed-circuit television, mechanical probing, and core-boring operations contributed to assessing the TMI-2 end-state core conditions. (**A,** courtesy Pennsylvania State University Engineering Library; **B,** courtesy U.S. Department of Energy, Washington, DC.)

portions of the reactor vessel occurred, fortunately no "melt-through" of the reactor vessel resulted.

Although the potential existed for release of significant amounts of radioactive material, according to the General Public Utilities Nuclear Corporation (GPU), the quantity of radiation that actually escaped during the accident (approximately 15 curies of iodine-131 [^{131}I]) was not sufficient to cause health problems for persons occupationally exposed or for the 2 million people living within 50 miles of the plant.* The average dose that the exposed population living within a 50-mile radius of the TMI nuclear power station received was 0.08 mSv (8 mrem). According to conventional methods of risk assessment, if 0.08 mSv (8 mrem) is used as an upper limit dose of ionizing radiation, it can be predicted that no more than one additional case of fatal cancer may occur in this population as a result of radiation exposure from this accident.[8] Therefore excess cancer deaths are not expected to be detected in this population as a consequence of the radiation dose it received.

Beginning at the time of the accident and continuing through 1992, the University of Pittsburgh followed more than 32,000 people who lived within 5 miles of TMI and were exposed to the low-level radioactivity released by the accident. Researchers found no link between radiation released (primarily xenon and iodine radioisotopes) during the TMI accident and cancer deaths among persons residing in the area. During the 13-year study of the people who lived within 5 miles of TMI at the time of the accident, only one death occurred as a consequence of thyroid cancer, and this death was not attributed to radiation exposure.[9]

Because most radiation-induced cancers have a latent period of 15 years or more, continued monitoring of the health of the exposed residents is needed. Studies are expected to continue to obtain the necessary data to further evaluate the mortality experience.

Chernobyl An explosion at a nuclear power plant in Chernobyl (near Kiev in Ukraine in the former Soviet Union) (Fig. 1-12) on April 26, 1986

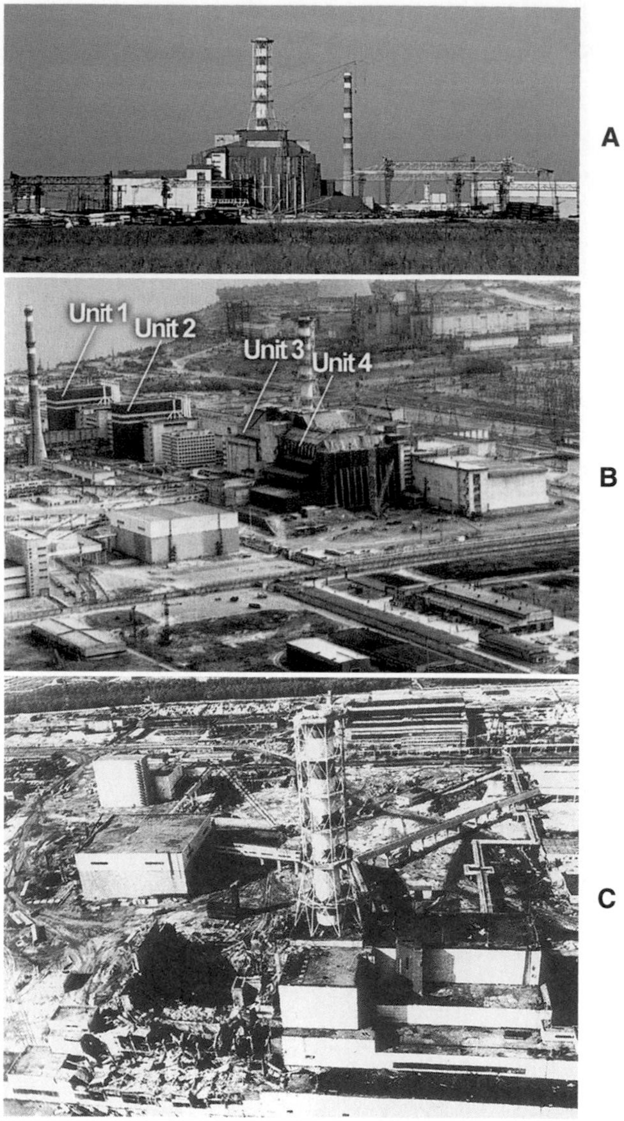

FIG. 1-12. A, Nuclear power plant in Chernobyl, former Soviet Union, site of the 1986 radiation accident. **B,** Aerial view of the four identical units of the Chernobyl nuclear power plant before the accident. Graphics point out each of the reactors. **C,** Chernobyl nuclear power plant following the explosion of Unit 4 on April 26, 1986. (**A,** courtesy Ken Graham Photography; **B** and **C,** courtesy U.S. Department of Energy.)

---

*^{131}I is a radioactive isotope that emits both beta particles (fast electrons) and energetic gamma rays with the most common beta emission (89.3%) having 192 keV mean energy and the most common gamma emission (81.2%) having 365 keV energy.

resulted in the release of a number of radioactive nuclides, including 46 megacuries of ^{131}I, 136 megacuries of xenon radioisotopes, and 2.3 megacuries of cesium-137 (^{137}Cs). This is far more than one million times the amount of radioactive material released at TMI. More than 200 people working at the Chernobyl plant received a whole-body equivalent dose exceeding 1 Sv (100 rem). More than two dozen workers died as a result of explosion-related injuries and the effects of receiving doses greater than 4 Sv (400 rem). The average equivalent dose to the approximately quarter of a million individuals living within 200 miles of the reactor was 0.2 Sv (20 rem), with thyroid doses (from drinking milk containing radioactive iodine) in some individuals exceeding several sieverts. Adverse health effects from radiation exposure are expected to occur for many years as a consequence of the total collective equivalent dose received by the affected population.

The ETHOS project Beginning in 1996, a 3-year pilot research project called the ETHOS Project[10] was launched in the Republic of Belarus. This project was supported by the radiation project research program of the European Commission (DG XII). In the aftermath of the Chernobyl accident, the local citizens of the contaminated territories were empowered to make their own decisions to facilitate reconstruction of their overall quality of life. They have also been given the authority to manage their radiologic risk in the same way that the rural communities manage natural risk.[10,11] The aim of the ETHOS Project is to rebuild acceptable living conditions by actively involving the local population in the reconstruction process. This process encompasses dealing with the aspects of daily living that have been changed or threatened as a consequence of radioactive contamination. One example is the establishment of guidelines for the amount of ash that is allowed to build up in wood stoves and fireplaces before cleaning is recommended. The ash is residue that remains after burning wood from trees that have taken up radioactive materials from the soil. The ash contains radioactive materials and is more compact than the piles of wood from which it came. The elimination of use of wood from the surrounding forests would pose an unreasonable economic hardship on the population and is unnecessary as long as appropriate guidelines are set. Through this program local citizens are engaging in cooperative problem-solving as they reconstruct their environment.

Thyroid cancer, leukemia, and breast cancer Thyroid cancer continues to be the main adverse health effect of the 1986 Chernobyl nuclear power accident. Children and adolescents living in the Ukraine region of Russia, where dose was heaviest following the disaster, continue to be the focus of the disease. Over 1700 cases of thyroid cancer were diagnosed in the period between 1990 and 1998.[12] Most of these cases are attributed to the radiation dose delivered when ^{131}I was taken up by the thyroid gland, although previous studies of atomic bomb survivors and Pacific Island inhabitants exposed to fallout predicted only 10 or so extra cases of thyroid cancer.[13] Since the time of the Chernobyl accident, there has also been an increase in the incidence of breast cancer directly attributed to the radiation exposure.[14,15] Some early research indicated no other increases in the effects that are generally associated with radiation exposure (leukemia, congenital abnormalities, or adverse pregnancy outcomes).[16] For example, the World Health Organization found no increase of leukemia by 1993 in the population hit hardest by fallout from Chernobyl.[17] Later studies have begun to show some of the expected effects. It was reported that there has been about a 50% increase in leukemia cases in children and adults in the Gomel region since the Chernobyl disaster.[18,19] Also, reported in June of 2001 at the 3rd International Conference held in Kiev, in the Russian liquidators who worked during 1986 and 1987 at the Chernobyl power station complex, there was a statistically significant rise in the number of leukemia cases.[20,21] Some time will be required before all the implications of these findings, if they continue to be substantiated, will be understood. Additional information about the Chernobyl catastrophe and its resulting health effects may be found in Chapter 6.

Human beings are unable to control natural background radiation; however, exposure from artificial sources must be limited to protect the general population from further biologic damage.

Medical Radiation Medical radiation exposure results from the use of diagnostic x-ray machines and radiopharmaceuticals in medicine. Diagnostic medical x-ray and nuclear medicine procedures are the *two largest sources* of artificial radiation, collectively accounting for 15% of the total average effective dose of the U.S. population (see Fig. 1-8). These two types of medical radiation account for about 0.54 mSv (54 mrem) of the average annual individual effective dose of ionizing radiation (see Table 1-4). The total average annual effective dose from manmade and natural radiation, including radon, is 3.6 mSv (360 mrem). Although the amount of natural background radiation remains fairly constant from year to year, the frequency of exposure to manmade radiation in medical applications is rapidly increasing among all age groups in the U.S. for a number of reasons. Because of medicolegal considerations, physicians in general are relying more on radiologic diagnoses to assist them in patient care. Greater accuracy in radiologic diagnosis resulting from educational and technologic improvements makes this increased use understandable. However, to reduce the possibility of the occurrence of genetic damage in future generations, this increase in frequency of radiation exposure in medicine must be counterbalanced by limiting the amount of patient exposure in individual imaging procedures. This can best be accomplished through efficient application of radiation protection measures on the part of the radiographer.

Because of the large variety of radiologic equipment, differences in imaging procedures and in individual radiologist and radiographer technical skills, the patient dose for each examination varies according to the facility providing imaging services. The amount of radiation received by a patient may be indicated in terms of entrance skin exposure (ESE) and glandular dose, bone marrow dose, and gonadal dose. In pregnant females, fetal dose also may be estimated. A more complete discussion of the amount of radiation received by a patient may be found in Chapter 8. Tables 1-5 through 1-9 indicate permissible patient ESEs and skin and glandular, bone marrow, gonadal, and fetal doses for several different radiologic examinations.

TABLE 1-5

Permissible Skin Entrance Exposures for Various Radiographic Examinations

Examination	Entrance Skin Exposure (mR per Projection)*
Chest (posteroanterior)	10-25
Skull (lateral)	105-240
Abdomen (AP)	375-700
Retrograde pyelogram	475-830
Cervical spine (AP)	35-165
Thoracic spine (AP)	295-485
Extremity	10-330
Dental (bite wing and periapical)	230-425

Modified from Ballinger PW, Frank ED: *Merrill's atlas of radiographic positions and radiologic procedures*, ed 10, vol 1, St. Louis, 2003, Mosby.
*These ranges are liberal and reflect the imaging equipment and techniques used in state-of-the-art technology.
AP, anteroposterior; mR, milliroentgens.

TABLE 1-6

Typical Entrance Skin Exposure and Mean Glandular Dose for Screen-Film Mammography Examinations

Examination	Entrance Skin Exposure*	Mean Glandular Dose†
Screen-film (nongrid)	800	150
Screen-film (4:1 grid)	1200	200
Magnification (1.5×)	1600	300

Modified from Ballinger PW, Frank ED: *Merrill's atlas of radiographic positions and radiographic procedures*, ed 10, vol 1, St. Louis, 2003, Mosby.
*Per projection in milliroentgens (mR).
†Approximate mean glandular dose per projection (in millirads). The millirad (mrad) is equal to 1/1000 of a rad. The rad is the traditional unit of absorbed dose. See Chapter 3 for further information.

TABLE 1-7

Typical Bone Marrow Doses for Various Radiographic Examinations*

X-Ray Examination	Mean Marrow Dose (mrad)
Skull	10
Cervical spine	20
Chest	2
Stomach and upper GI tract	100
Lumbar spine	60
Intravenous urography	25
Abdomen	30
Pelvis	20
Extremity	2

Modified from Ballinger PW, Frank ED: *Merrill's atlas of radiographic positions and radiologic procedures*, ed 10, vol 1, St. Louis, 2003, Mosby.
*These values are based on typical protocols that are average patient and filming protocols.
GI, gastrointestinal; mrad, millirad.

TABLE 1-9

Typical Fetal Dose Factors as a Function of Skin Entrance Exposure

X-Ray Examination	Fetal Dose Factor (mrad/R)
Skull	<0.01
Cervical spine	<0.01
Full-mouth dental	<0.01
Chest	2
Stomach and upper GI tract	25
Lumbar spine	250
Intravenous urography	265
Abdomen	265
Pelvis	265
Extremity	<0.01

Modified from Ballinger PW, Frank ED: *Merrill's atlas of radiographic positions and radiologic procedures*, ed 10, vol 1, St. Louis, 2003, Mosby.
GI, gastrointestinal; mrad/R, millirads/roentgen.

TABLE 1-8

Typical Gonadal Doses from Various Radiographic Examinations*

X-Ray Examination	Gonadal Dose (mrad)†	
	Male	Female
Skull	<1	<1
Cervical spine	<1	<1
Full-mouth dental	>1	<1
Chest	<1	<1
Stomach and upper GI tract	<2	40
Lumbar spine	175	400
Intravenous urography	150	300
Abdomen	100	200
Pelvis	300	150
Extremity	<1	<1

Modified from Ballinger PW, Frank ED: *Merrill's atlas of radiographic positions and radiologic procedures*, ed 10, vol 1, St. Louis, 2003, Mosby.
*These values are based on typical protocols that are average patient and filming protocols.
†In some radiologic examinations, the female gonadal dose is greater than the dose received by the male because the female reproductive organs are located within the pelvic cavity, unlike the male reproductive organs, which are located outside and below the pelvic cavity. The distribution of biologic tissue overlying the ovaries also affects the dose received for a given radiologic examination.
GI, gastrointestinal; mrad, millirads.

SUMMARY

➤ Ionizing radiation has both a beneficial and a destructive potential.

➤ Healthy normal biologic tissue can be injured by ionizing radiation, therefore it is necessary to protect humans against significant and continuous exposure.

➤ X-rays are a form of ionizing radiation; therefore, their use in medicine for the detection of disease and injury requires protective measures.

➤ To safeguard patients, personnel, and the general public, effective radiation protection measures should always be employed when performing diagnostic imaging procedures.

➤ Radiation exposure should always be kept ALARA to minimize the probability of any potential damage to people.

➤ Referring physicians should justify the need for every radiation procedure and accept basic responsibility for the protection of the patient from ionizing radiation.

➤ The benefits of exposing patients to ionizing radiation should far outweigh any slight risk of inducing radiogenic cancer or genetic effects after irradiation.

➤ Radiographers should select the smallest radiation exposure that produces the best radiographic results and should avoid errors that result in repeated radiographic exposures.

➤ Imaging facilities must have an effective radiation safety program that provides patient protection and patient education.

➤ BERT is used to compare the amount of radiation a patient receives from a radiologic procedure with natural background radiation received over a specific period of time.

➤ Ionizing radiation produces electrically charged particles that can cause biologic damage on molecular, cellular, and organic levels in humans.

➤ Equivalent dose (EqD) is a quantity that attempts to take into account the variation in biologic harm produced by different types of radiation. It enables the calculation of the effective dose.

➤ Effective dose (EfD) takes into account the dose of all types of ionizing radiation to human organs and tissues and the weighting factor of those body parts for developing a radiation-induced malignancy (or for the reproductive organs, the risk of genetic damage).

➤ Both occupational and nonoccupational dose limits are expressed as effective dose.

➤ Sievert (Sv) and rem are the units of equivalent dose and effective dose.

➤ Sources of ionizing radiation may be natural or manmade.

■ Natural sources include radioactive materials in the crust of the earth, cosmic rays from the sun and beyond the solar system, internal radiation from radionuclides deposited in humans through natural processes, and terrestrial radiation in the environment.

■ Manmade sources include consumer products containing radioactive material, air travel, nuclear fuel, atmospheric fallout from nuclear weapons, nuclear power plant accidents, and medical radiation from diagnostic x-ray machines and radiopharmaceuticals in nuclear medicine procedures.

References

1. Women's breast health: annual reminder needed for mammography, *RT Image* 17:35, 2004.
2. National Research Council, Commission of Life Sciences, Committee on Biological Effects on Ionizing Radiation (BEIR V), Board on Radiation Effects Research: *Health effects of exposure to low levels of ionizing radiations*, Washington, DC, 1989, National Academy Press.
3. Gollnick DA: *Basic radiation protection technology*, ed 4, Altadena, CA, 2000, Pacific Radiation Corporation.
4. Bushong SC: *Radiologic science for technologists: physics, biology, and protection*, ed 8, St. Louis, 2004, Mosby.
5. Read AB: Radon gas the invisible threat, *RT Image* 5:12, 1992.
6. National Council on Radiation Protection and Measurements (NCRP): *Report No. 94, exposure of the population in the United States and Canada from natural background radiation*, Washington, DC, 1987, NCRP.
7. National Council on Radiation Protection and Measurements (NCRP): *Report No. 93, ionizing radiation exposure of the population of the United States*, Bethesda, Md, 1987, NCRP.
8. Bushong SC: *Radiologic science for technologists: physics, biology and protection*, ed 8, St. Louis, 2004, Elsevier Mosby.
9. Talbott EO, Youk AO, McHugh KP et al: Mortality among the residents of the Three Mile Island accident area: 1979-1992, Research Triangle Park, NC, *Environ Health Perspect* 108:545, 2000.
10. Dubreuil GH, Lochard J, Giraard P et al: Chernobyl post-accident management: the Ethos project, *Health Phys* 77:361, 1999.
11. Ollagnon H: *Approche patrimoniale de gestion du risqué naturel*, Paris, 1992, Etude de CEMAGREFF.
12. United Nations Scientific Committee on the Effects of Atomic Radiation (UNSCEAR): 2000 report to the General Assembly, with Scientific Annexes, UNSCEAR 2000: sources and effects of ionizing radiation, New York, 2000, United Nations.
13. Lazole E: Thoughts and lessons from the Chernobyl accident, *Health Physics Society Newsletter* 28:10, 2000.
14. European Commission, OCHA et al, International Conference: Fifteen years after accident: Lessons Learned. Executive Summary, Kiev, April 2001.
15. Chernobyl Info. Available at: http://www.chernobyl.info/. Accessed June 30, 2004 and January 2, 2005.
16. Stone R: Living in the shadow of Chernobyl, *Science* 292:420, 2001.

17. Walker SJ: Permissible dose: a history of radiation protection in the twentieth century, Berkeley and Los Angeles, California, 2000, University of California Press.

18. Otto Hug Strahleninstit: Information, Ausgabe 9/2001 K, 2001.

19. Chernobyl Info. Available at: http://www.chernobyl. info/. Accessed June 30, 2004 and January 2, 2005.

20. Conclusions of 3rd International Conference, Health Effects of the Chernobyl Accident. *Int Jf Radiation Med* 3:3-4, 2001.

21. Chernobyl Info. Available at: http://www.chernobyl. info/. Accessed June 30, 2004 and January 2, 2005.

GENERAL DISCUSSION QUESTIONS

1. What are the consequences of ionization in the human cell?
2. When is medical radiation exposure considered unnecessary?
3. How can the background equivalent radiation time (BERT) method be used to eliminate a patient's fears about medical radiation exposure?
4. Describe how radiographers can use the ALARA concept in the performance of their daily responsibilities.
5. Explain the use of the radiation quantity, equivalent dose (EqD).
6. What are enhanced natural sources of radiation?
7. How does radon affect the epithelial tissue of the lungs in humans?
8. How can a flight on a typical commercial airliner result in radiation exposure for a passenger?
9. What consumer products contain radioactive materials?
10. What is the main adverse health effect of the 1986 Chernobyl nuclear power plant accident?

REVIEW QUESTIONS

1. A patient may elect to assume the risk of exposure to ionizing radiation to obtain essential diagnostic medical information when:
   1. Illness occurs
   2. Injury occurs
   3. A specific imaging procedure for health screening purposes is prudent
   A. 1 and 2 only
   B. 1 and 3 only
   C. 2 and 3 only
   D. 1, 2, and 3

2. Effective measures employed by radiation workers to safeguard patients, personnel, and the general public from unnecessary exposure to ionizing radiation defines:
   A. Diagnostic efficacy
   B. Optimization
   C. Radiation protection
   D. The concept of equivalent dose (EqD)

3. Which of the following is a method that can be used to answer patient questions about the amount of radiation received from a radiographic procedure?
   A. ALARA concept
   B. BERT
   C. BRET
   D. EPA

4. The term *optimization for radiation protection (ORP)* is synonymous with the term:
   A. As low as reasonably achievable (ALARA)
   B. Background equivalent radiation time (BERT)
   C. Equivalent dose (EqD)
   D. Diagnostic efficacy (DE)

5. Which of the following are natural sources of ionizing radiation?
   A. Medical x-radiation and cosmic radiation
   B. Radioactive elements in the crust of the earth and in the human body
   C. Radioactive elements in the human body and a diagnostic x-ray machine
   D. Radioactive fallout and environs of atomic energy plants

6. **An equivalent dose as low as 0.25 Sv (25 rem) delivered to the whole body may cause which of the following within a few days?**
   A. An increase in the number of lymphocytes in the circulating blood
   B. A decrease in the number of lymphocytes in the circulating blood
   C. A drop immediately to zero in the lymphocyte count
   D. A large increase in the number of platelets

7. **The degree to which the diagnostic study accurately reveals the presence or absence of disease in the patient defines which of the following terms?**
   A. Radiation protection
   B. Radiographic pathology
   C. Effective diagnosis
   D. Diagnostic efficacy

8. **Which of the following is the total average annual effective dose from manmade and natural radiation?**
   A. 0.3 mSv (30 mrem) per year
   B. 0.6 mSv (60 mrem) per year
   C. 1.8 mSv (180 mrem) per year
   D. 3.6 mSv (360 mrem) per year

9. **An effective radiation safety program requires a firm commitment to radiation safety by:**
   1. **Facilities providing imaging services**
   2. **Radiation workers**
   3. **Patients**
   A. 1 and 2 only
   B. 1 and 3 only
   C. 2 and 3 only
   D. 1, 2, and 3

10. **Which of the following is recognized as the *main* adverse health effect from the 1986 Chernobyl nuclear power accident?**
    A. Increase in the incidence of leukemia in adults
    B. Increase in the incidence of leukemia in children
    C. Increase in the incidence of thyroid cancer in adults
    D. Increase in the incidence of thyroid cancer in children and adolescents

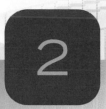

Interaction of X-Radiation with Matter

2

KEY TERMS

absorbed dose (D)
absorption
attenuation
Auger electrons
characteristic photon
coherent scattering
Compton scattered electron
Compton scattering
contrast media (positive, negative)

effective atomic number
exit, or image-formation, photons
fluorescent yield
mass density
milliampere-seconds (mAs)
pair production
peak kilovoltage (kVp)
photodisintegration
photoelectric absorption

photoelectron
primary radiation
radiographic contrast
radiographic density
radiographic fog
radiographic image receptor
small-angle scatter

OBJECTIVES

After completing this chapter, the reader will be able to perform the following:

- Differentiate between peak kilovoltage (kVp) and milliampere-seconds (mAs) as technical exposure factors.
- Describe the process of absorption and explain the reason why absorbed dose in atoms of biologic matter should be kept as small as possible.
- Differentiate between primary radiation; exit, or image-formation, radiation; and scattered radiation.
- List two types of x-ray photon transmission and explain the difference between them.
- Discuss the way x-rays are produced and explain the range of energies present in the x-ray beam.
- List the events that occur when x-radiation passes through matter.
- Discuss the probability of photon interaction with matter.

Continued

- Describe and illustrate by diagram the x-ray photon interactions with matter that are important in diagnostic radiology.
- List the x-ray photon interactions with matter that occur above the energy range used in diagnostic radiology.
- Describe the impact of positive contrast media on photoelectric absorption and identify its effects regarding absorbed dose in the body structure that contains it.
- Describe the effect of kVp on radiographic image quality and patient absorbed dose.

In this chapter, basic physics concepts that relate to radiation absorption and scatter are reviewed. The processes of interaction between radiation and matter are emphasized because a basic understanding of the latter is necessary for radiographers to optimally select technical exposure factors such as **peak kilovoltage (kVp),** the highest energy level of photons in the x-ray beam, and **milliampere-seconds (mAs),** the product of electron tube current and the amount of time in seconds that the x-ray tube is activated. kVp controls the quality, or penetrating power, of the photons in the x-ray beam and, to some degree, also affects the quantity, or number of photons, in the beam. The product of milliamperes (mA), which is the x-ray tube current, and time (seconds [s], during which the x-ray tube is activated) is the main determinant of how much radiation is directed toward a patient during a selected x-ray exposure. Because the level of energy (beam quality) and number of x-ray photons are controlled by technique factors selected by the radiographer, the radiographer is actually responsible for the dose the patient receives during an imaging procedure. With a suitable understanding of these factors, radiographers can select appropriate techniques that can minimize the dose to the patient and produce a radiograph of acceptable quality.

SIGNIFICANCE OF X-RAY ABSORPTION IN BIOLOGIC TISSUE

X-rays are carriers of man-made, electromagnetic energy. If x-rays enter a material such as human tissue,

they may interact with the atoms of the biologic material or pass through without interaction. If they interact, electromagnetic energy is transferred from the x-rays to the atoms of the biologic material. This transference of electromagnetic energy to the atoms of the material is called **absorption** (Fig. 2-1), and the amount of energy absorbed per unit mass is referred to as the **absorbed dose (D).** The more electromagnetic energy received by the atoms of the patient's body, the greater the possibility of biologic damage in the patient; thus, the amount of electromagnetic energy transferred should be kept as small as possible. Without the phenomenon of absorption and the differences in the absorption properties of various body structures, it would not be possible to produce diagnostically useful radiographs in which different anatomic structures could be perceived and distinguished. The radiographer also benefits when patient dose is minimal because less radiation is scattered from the patient.

X-RAY BEAM PRODUCTION AND ENERGY

Production of Primary Radiation

A diagnostic x-ray beam is produced when a stream of high-speed electrons bombards a positively charged target in a highly evacuated glass tube. In general radiography, this target, also known as the *anode,* is usually made of tungsten (a metal), or rhenium tungsten (a metal alloy). These materials have high melting points and high atomic numbers. As the electrons interact with the atoms of the target, x-ray photons (particles

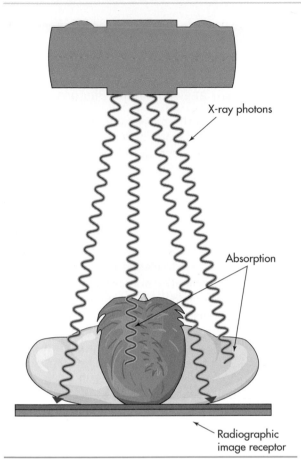

FIG. 2-1. X-ray photons can interact with atoms of the patient's body and transfer energy to the tissue. This transference of electromagnetic energy to the atoms of the material is called *absorption*.

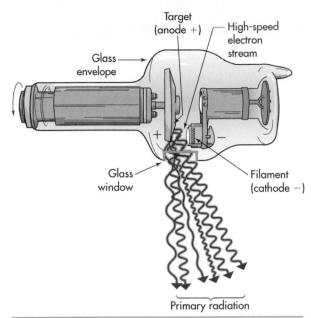

FIG. 2-2. Primary radiation emerges from the x-ray tube target and consists of x-ray photons of various energies. It is produced when the positively charged target is bombarded with a stream of high-speed electrons and these electrons interact with the atoms of the target.

associated with electromagnetic radiation that have neither mass nor electric charge and travel at the speed of light) emerge from the target with a broad range of energies and leave the x-ray tube through a glass window. The glass window permits passage of all but the lowest energy components of the x-ray spectrum. It therefore acts as a filter by removing diagnostically useless, very-low-energy x-rays. In addition to this, a certain thickness of added aluminum is placed within the collimator assembly to intercept the emerging x-rays before they reach the patient. This aluminum "hardens" the x-ray beam (i.e., raises its effective energy) by removing low-energy components that

would serve only to increase patient dose. The combination of the x-ray tube glass wall and the added aluminum placed within the collimator may be called the *permanent inherent filtration* of the x-ray unit. The emerging x-ray photon beam is collectively referred to as **primary radiation** (Fig. 2-2).

Energy of Photons in a Diagnostic X-Ray Beam

Although all photons in a diagnostic x-ray beam do not have the same energy, the most energetic photons in the beam can have no more energy than the electrons that bombard the target. The energy of the electrons inside the x-ray tube is expressed in terms of the electrical voltage applied across the tube. In diagnostic radiology, this is expressed in thousands of volts, or kilovolts (kV). Moreover, because the voltage across the tube fluctuates, it is usually expressed in kVp. If an electron is drawn across an electrical potential difference of 1 volt, it has acquired an energy of 1 electron volt (eV). Thus a technique factor of 100 kVp means that the electrons bombarding the target have a maximum energy of 100,000 eV, or 100 keV. X-rays of various energies are produced, but the most energetic x-ray photon can have no more energy than 100 keV. For a typical diagnostic x-ray unit, the energy of the average photon in the x-ray beam is about one third the energy of the most energetic photon. Therefore a 100-kVp beam contains photons having energies of 100 keV or less, with an average energy of about 33 keV.

ATTENUATION

Direct and Indirect Transmission X-Ray Photons

When an x-ray beam passes through an object, it goes through a process called **attenuation.** Attenuation is simply the reduction in the number of primary photons in the x-ray beam through absorption (a total loss of radiation energy) and scatter (a change in direction of travel that may also involve a partial loss of radiation energy) as the beam passes through the object in its path. Some primary x-ray photons will also traverse the object without interacting. This may be called *"direct" transmission.* These noninteracting x-ray photons reach the **radiographic image receptor** (e.g., radiographic film). Other primary photons can undergo Compton and/or coherent interactions (these processes are discussed later in this chapter) and as a result may be scattered or deflected. Such photons may still traverse the object and strike the image receptor. This process is called *"indirect" transmission.* The optimal x-ray image is formed when only direct transmission x-ray photons reach the image receptor. In clinical situations, scattered photons do reach the image receptor and degrade image quality (sharpness of the recorded image). Therefore, several methods— air gaps and radiographic grids are the most common— have been devised to limit the effects of indirectly transmitted x-ray photons. These methods are described in Chapter 8. In radiography, the image receptor covers a broad enough area that x-ray photons scattered from one part of the beam might still strike the image receptor in another area. Consequently the

resulting radiographic image is formed from both directly transmitted x-ray photons and indirectly transmitted (i.e., scattered) x-ray photons.

Primary, Exit, and Attenuated Photons

Fig. 2-3 illustrates the passage of four x-ray photons through an object. Before the four photons produced by the x-ray source enter the object, they are referred to as primary photons. Only two photons emerge from the object and strike the radiographic image receptor below it. They are referred to as **exit, or image-formation, photons.** The two that do not strike the image receptor are attenuated. The term *attenuation* is rather broad; with respect to x-rays, it may be used to refer to any process decreasing the intensity of the primary photon beam that was directed toward a destination. The ultimate destination of the photons in Fig. 2-3 is the image receptor. Therefore photon #3, which has deviated from its path (i.e., it has been "scattered") to the extent that it will not strike the image receptor, is said to have been attenuated. Photon #4 seems to disappear. It has transferred all its energy to the atoms of the object and has therefore been eliminated. Because a photon has no mass, it ceases to exist when it gives up its energy. *Attenuation,* then, refers to both absorption and scatter processes that prevent photons from reaching a predefined destination. Fig. 2-3 shows that the path of photon #2 was bent, but not so much that the photon missed its target. Insofar as photon #2 reaching the image receptor, it is part of the exit, or image-formation, radiation, but the bending of its path represents what is called **small-angle scatter.** Scattered photons in this category have essentially the same energy as the incident photons. Small-angle scatter degrades the appearance of a finished radiograph by blurring the sharp outlines of dense objects. Moreover, because many billions of such scatter events occur, a radiosensitive film darkens overall, interfering with the radiologist's ability to distinguish different structures in the image. This undesirable, additional density is called **radiographic fog.** Reducing the amount of tissue irradiated reduces the amount of fog produced by small-angle scatter. Therefore, adequately collimating the x-ray beam is one way to reduce fog (Fig. 2-4). Other methods used to reduce the image-degrading effects of scatter are discussed later.

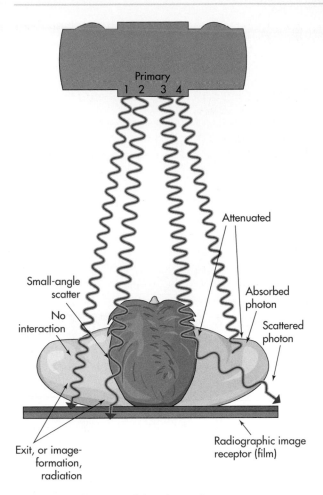

FIG. 2-3. Primary, exit, and attenuated photons. Primary photons (photons #1, #2, #3, and #4) are photons that emerge from the x-ray source. Exit, or image-formation, photons (photons #1 and #2) are photons that pass through the object being radiographed (the patient) and reach the radiographic image receptor (e.g., film). Attenuated photons (photons #3 and #4) are photons that have interacted with atoms of the object (the patient) and been scattered or absorbed such that they do not reach the radiographic image receptor.

PROBABILITY OF PHOTON INTERACTION WITH MATTER

Because the interaction of photons with biologic matter is random, it is impossible to predict with certainty what will happen to a single photon when it enters biologic matter. When dealing with a large number of photons, however, it is possible to predict what will happen on the average, and this is more than adequate to determine the characteristics of the radiograph that results from such numerous interactions (Table 2-1). For example, in an ordinary beam of x-ray photons (which consists of a vast number of such particles) a 50-keV photon on average has a 66% probability of interaction when it travels through 5 cm of soft tissue (see Appendix A); 34% of the time such photons will be likely to just pass through the tissue. Another way to say this is that in a randomly chosen group of 100 50-keV photons traveling through 5 cm of soft tissue, 66 interactions may be expected to occur. Of the 66 interactions, 11% (7 out of the 66 interactions) should be of a type called *photoelectric*. In photoelectric interaction, a photon is completely absorbed by the atoms of the tissue (i.e., removed from the beam). If this were the only interaction possible, irradiating 5 cm of soft tissue with 50-keV photons would create a lighter area on a processed radiographic film, which would be the result of fewer photons reaching that portion of the film. In reality, the process is much more complicated because several additional effects occur, and a typical x-ray beam is composed of photons with a continuous range of energies. Table 2-2 shows the factors that influence the probability of interactions in matter. In the remainder of this chapter, the different interactions of photons with individual atoms and the effect of a particular type of interaction on the radiograph are examined.

PROCESSES OF INTERACTION

Five types of interaction between x-radiation and matter are possible: coherent scattering, Compton scattering, photoelectric absorption, pair production, and photodisintegration. Of these, only two are important in diagnostic radiology: Compton scattering and photoelectric absorption (Box 2-1).

Coherent Scattering (Classical, Elastic, or Unmodified Scattering)

Coherent scattering is sometimes called classical, elastic, or unmodified scattering. It is basically a

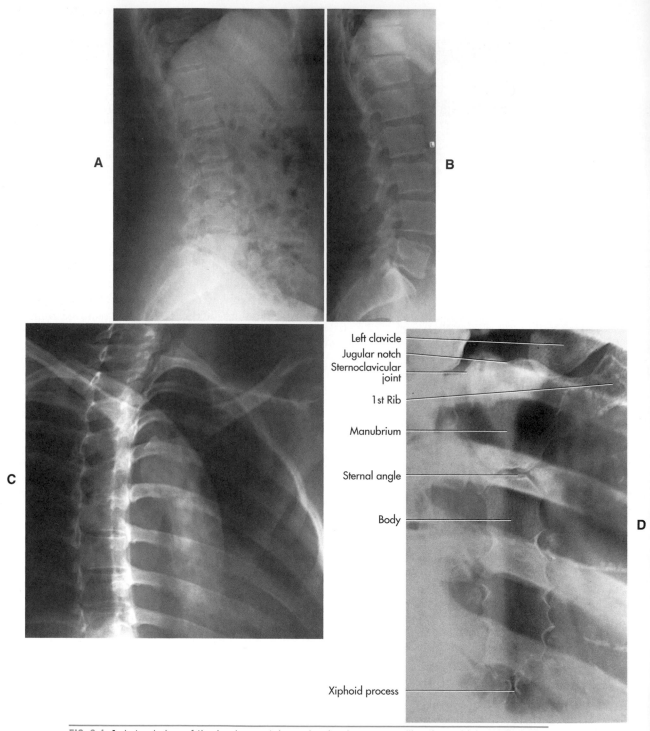

FIG. 2-4. **A,** Lateral view of the lumbar vertebrae showing improper collimation, which results in the production of radiographic fog and a consequent lack of radiographic clarity. **B,** Lateral view of the lumbar vertebrae showing proper collimation, which eliminates radiographic fog and consequently increases radiographic clarity. **C,** Right anterior oblique view of the sternum demonstrating poor collimation. **D,** Right anterior oblique view of the sternum demonstrating good collimation. (**D** from Ballinger PW, Frank ED: *Merrill's atlas of radiographic positions and radiologic procedures,* ed 10, vol 1, St. Louis, 2003, Mosby.)

TABLE 2-1

Interaction of X-Radiation with Soft Tissue: Overview

X-Ray Photon Energy Range	Site of Interaction	X-Ray Photon	Typical Interaction	By-products of Interaction
1-50 kVp	An atom	Energy: unchanged; direction after interaction: slight change (<20 degrees)	Coherent scattering*	None
1-50 kVp	Inner-shell electron (usually K shell)	Energy: absorbed; direction after interaction: not applicable	Photoelectric absorption[†]	Photoelectron (characteristic photon)
60-90 kVp	Outer-shell electron	Energy: reduced; direction after interaction: changed (x-ray photon energy partially absorbed)	Compton scattering[‡]	Compton scattered electron; Compton scattered photon
200 kVp-2 MeV	Outer-shell electron	Energy: reduced; direction after interaction: changed	Compton scattering[§,‖]	Compton scattered electron; Compton scattered photon
Begins at about 1.022 MeV; becomes important at 10 MeV; becomes predominant at 50 MeV and greater	Nucleus of atom	Energy: disappears after interaction with nucleus; transformed into two new particles that annihilate each other; direction after interaction: energy reappears in form of two 0.511-MeV photons, each moving in opposite directions	Pair production	Positive electron (positron); ordinary electron (negatron); two 0.511-MeV photons
Greater than 10 MeV	Nucleus of atom	Energy: absorbed by nucleus after collision with high-energy photon; excess energy in nucleus creates instability that is usually alleviated by emission of a neutron; other emissions possible	Photodisintegration	Neutron; other types of emissions possible if sufficient energy is absorbed by the nucleus: proton or proton-neutron combination (deuteron) or even an alpha particle

*Occurs mostly in this energy range, but still much less probable than photoelectric absorption.
[†]The interaction most responsible for radiation dose in this energy range.
[‡]Both Compton and photoelectric interactions occur in this energy range.
[§]Compton interaction is predominantly responsible for radiation dose in this energy range.
[‖]In this energy range, the scattered particles go on to produce many more Compton and photoelectric interactions on their own.

TABLE 2-2

Factors That Influence the Probability of Interaction of Photons with Energy E in Materials with Density ρ

Interaction	Photon Energy	Atomic Number	Electron Density ρ_e (e/g)	Physical Density ρ (g/cm³)
Photoelectric	$1/E^3$	Z^3	Independent	ρ
Compton	$1/E$	Independent	ρ_e	ρ
Pair production	E	Z	Independent	ρ

BOX 2-1

Importance of Various Interactions of X-Radiation with Matter

Interaction	Where Important
Coherent scattering	Not important in any energy range
Compton scattering	Diagnostic radiology
Photoelectric absorption	Diagnostic radiology
Pair production	Therapeutic radiology
Photodisintegration	Therapeutic radiology

relatively simple process that actually results in no loss of energy as x-rays scatter.

Process of Coherent Scattering

When a low-energy photon (typically less than 30 keV), which may be thought of as a moving electromagnetic wave, interacts with an atom, it may transfer its energy by causing some or all of the electrons of the atom to vibrate momentarily. This is analogous to the behavior of electrons in the antenna of a receiver intercepting a radio signal. Because they are charged particles, each of the atom's vibrating electrons radiates energy in the form of electromagnetic waves. These waves coherently (i.e., cooperatively) combine with each other to form a scattered wave, which represents a scattered photon. Because the wavelengths of both incident and scattered waves are the same, no net energy has been absorbed by the atom (see Appendix B). However, a change in the direction of the emitted photon is very likely. In general, this change in direc-tion is less than 20 degrees with respect to the initial direction of the original photon. This is the net effect of coherent, or unmodified, scattering, also known as *Rayleigh scattering* in honor of the scientist who first explained it, before the concept of the photon was known, by using wave analysis alone. Although coherent scattering is most probable to occur below a 30-kVp generator setting, some unmodified scattering occurs throughout the diagnostic range and may result in small amounts of radiographic fog (Fig. 2-5). This source of fog, however, is not significant in diagnostic imaging. In mammography, coherent scattering does not contribute to radiographic fog because during this imaging procedure, breast tissue is gently but firmly compressed. As a result of this compression, the breast actually becomes relatively thin. This eliminates the production of a large amount of scatter radiation.

In addition to Rayleigh scattering, there is also another kind of coherent scattering known as *Thompson scattering,* in which the low-energy photon interacts with one or more free (i.e., unbound) electrons. As with Rayleigh scattering, the photon energy is absorbed and then re-radiated in a different direction with no change in wavelength of the associated electromagnetic wave. Rayleigh and Thompson scattering play essentially no role in radiography, but they affect optical phenomena such as the sky being blue, clouds white, and the sunset red.[1]

Compton Scattering (Incoherent, Inelastic, or Modified Scattering)

Compton scattering, also known as *incoherent, inelastic,* or *modified scattering,* is responsible for most of the scattered radiation produced during radiologic proce-

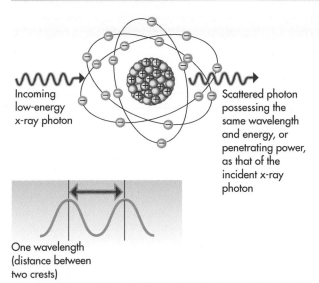

Incoming low-energy x-ray photon

Scattered photon possessing the same wavelength and energy, or penetrating power, as that of the incident x-ray photon

One wavelength (distance between two crests)

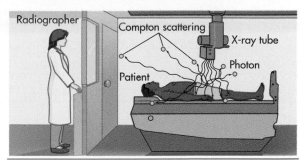

FIG. 2-6. Compton scattering is responsible for most of the scattered radiation produced during a radiologic procedure. (From *Mosby's radiographic instructional series,* St. Louis, 1999, Mosby.)

FIG. 2-5. Coherent scattering. The incoming low-energy x-ray photon interacts with an atom and transfers its energy by causing some or all of the electrons of the atom to vibrate momentarily. The electrons then radiate energy in the form of electromagnetic waves. These waves nondestructively combine with each other to form a scattered wave, which represents the scattered photon. Its wavelength and energy, or penetrating power, is the same as that of the incident photon. Generally the emitted photon may change in direction less than 20 degrees with respect to the direction of the original photon. (Wavelength is the distance from one crest to the next.)

dures (Fig. 2-6). This scatter may be directed forward as small-angle scatter, backward as backscatter, and to the side as sidescatter. The intensity of radiation scatter in various directions is a major factor in planning protection for medical imaging personnel during a radiologic examination (Fig. 2-7).

Process of Compton Scattering

In the Compton process, an incoming x-ray photon interacts with a loosely bound outer-shell electron of an atom of the irradiated object (Fig. 2-8 and Table 2-3). On encountering the electron, the incoming x-ray photon surrenders a portion of its kinetic energy to dislodge the electron from its outer-shell orbit (see Appendix C for an extended discussion of this type of interaction). The freed electron, called a **Compton scattered electron,** possesses excess kinetic energy and

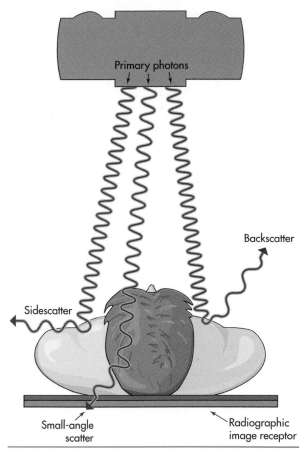

FIG. 2-7. Compton scattering results in all-directional scatter. The scatter created may be directed onward as small-angle scatter, backward as backscatter, and to the side as sidescatter. The intensity of radiation scatter in various directions is a major factor in planning protection for medical imaging personnel during a radiologic examination.

TABLE 2-3
Electron Shell Occupancies for Some Common Atoms

Atom	Symbol	Atomic Number	Shell					
			K	L	M	N	O	P
Hydrogen	H	1	1					
Helium	He	2	2					
Lithium	Li	3	2	1				
Carbon	C	6	2	4				
Oxygen	O	8	2	6				
Sodium	Na	11	2	8	1			
Aluminum	Al	13	2	8	3			
Calcium	Ca	20	2	8	8	2		
Copper	Cu	29	2	8	18	1		
Molybdenum	Mo	42	2	8	18	13	1	
Tungsten	W	74	2	8	18	32	12	2
Lead	Pb	82	2	8	18	32	18	4
Radon	Rn	86	2	8	18	32	18	8

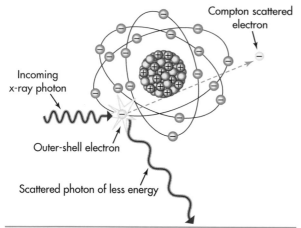

FIG. 2-8. Compton scattering. On encountering a loosely bound outer-shell electron, the incoming x-ray photon surrenders a portion of its kinetic energy to dislodge the electron from its orbit. The energy-degraded x-ray photon then continues on its way but in a new direction. The high-speed electron ejected from its orbit is called a *Compton scattered electron,* or *"recoil" electron.*

is capable of ionizing atoms. It loses its kinetic energy by a series of collisions with nearby atoms and finally recombines with an atom that needs another electron. This usually occurs within a few micrometers of the site of the original Compton interaction.

The x-ray photon that surrendered some of its energy (see Appendix C) to free the electron from its orbit continues on its way but in a new direction. It has the potential to interact with other atoms either by the process of photoelectric absorption (described later) or by Compton scattering. It also may emerge from the patient, in which case it may contribute to degradation of the radiographic image by creating an additional, unwanted density (radiographic fog) or present a health hazard to the radiographer and the radiologist.

In diagnostic radiology the probability of occurrence of Compton scattering relative to that of the photoelectric interaction increases as the energy of the x-ray photon increases. Compton scattering and photoelectric absorption in tissue are equally probable at about 35 keV. Therefore, in a 100-kVp x-ray beam when the photons have an average energy in the range of 30 to 40 keV, a significant number of Compton events occur.

Photoelectric Absorption

Within the energy range of diagnostic radiology that includes mammography (23 to 150 kVp), photoelectric absorption is the most important mode of interaction between x-ray photons and the atoms of the patient's body for producing useful patient images.

Process of Photoelectric Absorption

Photoelectric absorption is an interaction between an x-ray photon and an inner-shell electron (usually in the K shell) tightly bound to an atom of the absorbing medium (Fig. 2-9). To dislodge an inner-shell electron from its atomic orbit, the incoming x-ray photon must be able to transfer a quantity of energy as large as or larger than the amount of energy that binds the electron in its orbit. On interacting with an inner-shell electron, the x-ray photon surrenders all its energy to the orbital electron and ceases to exist. The electron is ejected from its inner shell, creating a vacancy. The ejected orbital electron, called a **photoelectron,** possesses kinetic energy equal to the energy of the incident photon less the binding energy of the electron shell. This photoelectron may interact with other atoms, causing excitation or ionization, until all its kinetic energy has been spent. The photoelectron is usually absorbed within a few micrometers of the medium through which it travels. In the human body, this energy transfer results in increased patient dose and contributes to biologic damage of tissues.

As a result of the photoelectric effect, in general a vacancy exists in the inner shell of the parent atom. To fill this opening, an electron from an outer shell drops down to the vacated inner shell opening by releasing energy (equivalent to the energy level difference between the two shells) in the form of a photon. This photon is termed a **characteristic photon.** It possesses relatively low energy in human tissue and is locally absorbed in the irradiated object. Ensuing vacancies in successive shells are filled and photons emitted in a like fashion until the atom regains electrical equilibrium. The by-products of photoelectric absorption include photoelectrons (those induced by interaction with external radiation and the internally generated Auger electrons) and characteristic x-ray photons (fluorescent radiation). When their energy is locally absorbed in human tissue, both patient dose and the potential for biologic damage increase.

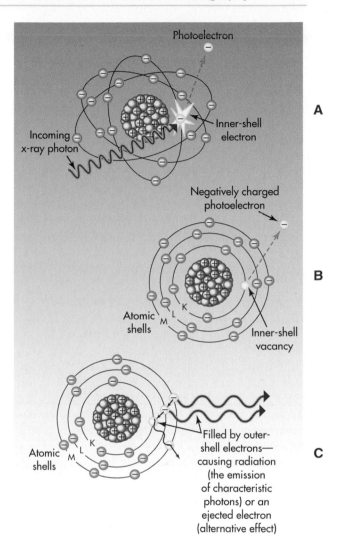

FIG. 2-9. Photoelectric absorption. **A,** On encountering an inner-shell or K-shell electron, the incoming x-ray photon surrenders all its energy to the electron and the photon ceases to exist. **B,** The atom responds by ejecting the electron, called a *photoelectron,* from its inner shell, creating a vacancy in that shell. **C,** To fill the opening, an electron from an outer shell drops down to the vacated inner shell by releasing energy in the form of a characteristic photon. Then, to fill the new vacancy in the outer shell, another electron from the shell next farthest out drops down and another characteristic photon is emitted, and so on until the atom regains electrical equilibrium. There is also some probability that, instead of emission of a characteristic photon, an Auger electron will be ejected.

Auger Electrons

An alternative to the emission of a characteristic photon is a process in which the energy that would have appeared as a photon is instead used to eject an outer-shell electron. Unbound electrons generated in this manner are known as **Auger electrons.** This alternative effect reduces the intensity of characteristic radiation (also known as *fluorescent radiation*) emitted from atoms as a result of photoelectric interactions. The term **fluorescent yield** refers to the number of characteristic x-rays emitted per inner-shell vacancy. The fluorescent yield per photoelectric interaction in general is lower in materials composed of atoms with higher atomic numbers (see Fig. 2-9, C).

Probability of Occurrence of Photoelectric Absorption

The probability of occurrence of photoelectric absorption depends on the energy of the incident x-ray photons and the atomic number (Z) of the atoms composing the irradiated object; it increases markedly as the energy of the incident photon decreases and the atomic number of the irradiated atoms increases, experimentally observed to vary approximately as Z^4/E^3 per atom and Z^3/E^3 per electron where E is the photon energy. Thus in the radiographic kilovoltage range, compact bone (effective atomic number 13.8 [**effective atomic number** is a composite Z number for many different chemical elements composing a material]) with a high content by weight (14.7%) of calcium (Z = 20) undergoes much more photoelectric absorption (approximately 12 times per atom) than an equal mass of soft tissue (effective atomic number approximately 7.4) and air (effective atomic number 7.6). For this reason bone can be exceptionally well demonstrated in diagnostic images because of the "x-ray shadow" that it casts.

Mass Density of Different Body Structures

The density (**mass density** measured in grams per cubic centimeter) of different body structures also influences attenuation. A density increase leads to a corresponding increase in photon absorption. In any given sample of material, both density and atomic number play a role in determining attenuation. For example, if radiography is performed on an equal thickness of bone and soft tissue, the bone, which is approximately twice as dense as soft tissue, will absorb about nine times as many photons in the diagnostic energy range as will the soft tissue. A factor of 4.5 is caused by the higher atomic number of the bone, and a factor of 2 is caused by the higher density of bone. The total effect is 2 × 4.5, for an overall factor of 9 (Fig. 2-10, A).

Body Part Thickness

Thickness of body parts also plays a role. The thickness factor is approximately linear. If two structures have the same density and atomic number, but one is twice as thick as the other, the thicker structure absorbs twice as many photons. Consequently, if a 2-cm-thick bone sample is radiographed next to a 4-cm-thick tissue sample, the density and thickness factors would cancel each other out (Fig. 2-10, B). The bone is half as thick in this example, but it is approximately twice as dense. However, the remaining factor, the higher atomic number of bone, causes the bone to absorb approximately 4.5 times as many photons as the soft tissue.

Difference in Absorption Properties Between Different Body Structures

Such differences in absorption properties between different body structures make diagnostically useful radiographs possible. In other words, the ability to perceive and distinguish between different body structures in a radiograph depends on the presence of differences in the amount of x-radiation these structures permit to pass through them to reach the radiographic image receptor.

The less a given structure attenuates radiation, the darker (i.e., the greater the **radiographic density**, or degree of overall blackening on the finished radiograph) its image on the finished radiograph will be, and vice versa. Thus bone, with a higher effective atomic number and greater mass density than either soft tissue or air cavities, absorbs more radiation and

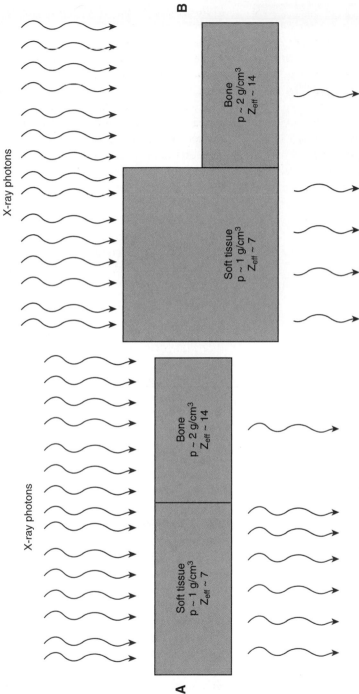

FIG. 2-10. **A,** Equal thicknesses of bone and soft tissue are shown here. The bone absorbs nine times as many photons as the soft tissue. A factor of two is the result of bone being approximately twice as dense as soft tissue. A factor of four and a half is due to the higher atomic number of bone compared to that of soft tissue. Both factors together result in $2 \times 4.5 = 9$ times more absorption in this sample of bone. **B,** In the example shown here, the soft tissue is twice as thick as the bone. This thickness difference approximately cancels out the density difference between the bone and soft tissue. However, because the difference in atomic number still exists, in this example the bone would absorb 4.5 times as many photons as the soft tissue.

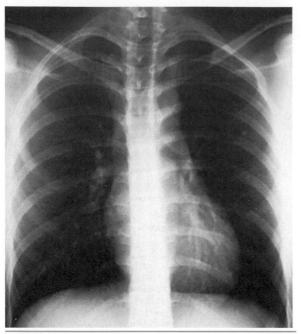

FIG. 2-11. The less a given structure attenuates radiation, the darker (i.e., the greater its radiographic density) its image will be on the finished radiograph, and vice versa. Thus, compact bone, with a higher effective atomic number and greater mass density than either soft tissue or air cavities, absorbs more radiation and appears white on a diagnostic radiograph, whereas soft tissue presents a gray image, and air-containing structures such as the lungs appear black.

appears white on a diagnostic radiograph, whereas soft tissue presents a gray image, and air-containing structures (e.g., lungs, stomach) appear black (Fig. 2-11).

In Fig. 2-12, two posteroanterior (PA) hand radiographs illustrate age-related changes in bone density resulting from changes in calcium content. Radiograph A exhibits substantial quantities of calcium in the bones of a young person. Radiograph B exhibits the demineralized bones of an elderly person. The lack of x-ray absorption results from the decrease in bone calcium. Hence the elderly person's bones are almost transparent in radiographic appearance. Pathologic conditions such as degenerative arthritis also contribute to differences in absorption. Technical radiographic exposure factors must be adjusted to compensate for such changes.

Impact of Photoelectric Absorption on Radiographic Contrast

Within the energy range of diagnostic radiology, the greater the difference in the amount of photoelectric absorption, the greater the contrast in the radiographic image between adjacent structures of differing atomic numbers. However, as absorption increases, so does the potential for biologic damage. For those regions in which the photoelectric absorption occurs most frequently (e.g., in dense-atomic-number areas such as cortical bone), the absorbed dose to the patient may be greater by a factor of 6 to 9 than in adjacent low-atomic-number and less dense regions. Thus, to ensure both radiographic image quality and patient safety, both the radiologist and the radiographer should choose the highest-energy x-ray beam that permits adequate **radiographic contrast.**

Use of Contrast Media to Ensure Visualization of Anatomic Structures

If tissues or structures that are similar in atomic number and mass density must be distinguished, the photoelectric interaction by itself will not be sufficient to produce the contrast needed in that tissue or structure to ensure its visualization in the radiographic image. To resolve the problem, the use of **contrast media** has been adopted. Very simply, positive contrast media consist of solutions containing elements having a higher atomic number than surrounding soft tissue (e.g., barium or iodine based) that are either ingested or injected into the tissues or structures to be visualized. The high atomic number of the contrast media (barium, Z = 56; iodine, Z = 53) significantly enhances the occurrence of photoelectric interaction relative to similar adjacent structures that do not have the contrast media. Also, the inner-shell electrons of iodine and barium have a binding energy that is in the energy range of the x-ray photons that is most commonly used in general-purpose radiography (30 to 40 keV). This means that photoelectric absorption of the photons in the x-ray beam is greatly increased. In the radiographic image, positive contrast–enhanced structures, therefore, will appear lighter than adjacent structures that did not receive the contrast. Fig. 2-13, A presents an

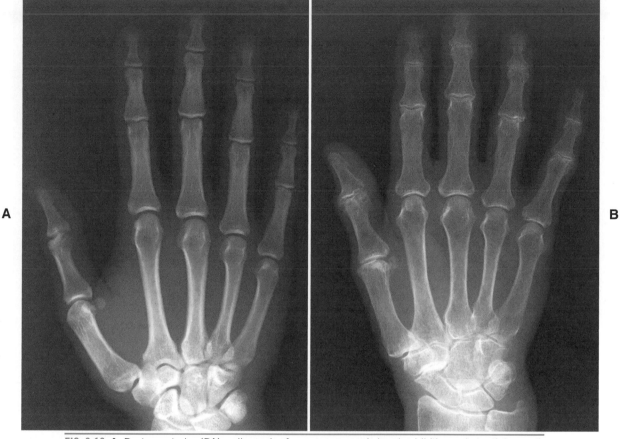

FIG. 2-12. A, Posteroanterior (PA) radiograph of a young person's hand exhibiting substantial quantities of calcium in the bones. **B,** PA radiograph of an elderly person's hand exhibiting demineralized bone as a consequence of a decrease in bone calcium. This and other degenerative changes account for the almost transparent appearance of the bones.

anteroposterior (AP) radiograph of the abdomen without the aid of a positive contrast medium to visualize the urinary system, whereas Fig. 2-13, *B* presents an AP radiograph of the abdomen with a positive contrast medium visualizing the urinary system, thus permitting each contrast-filled structure to be distinguished.

Caution must be exercised in the use of contrast media because some patients may not be able to tolerate their presence. The use of positive contrast medium also leads to an increase in absorbed dose in the body structures that contain it. Negative contrast media such as air or gas are also used for some radio-

logic examinations. These negative agents result in darker areas on the processed radiograph.

Pair Production

Pair production does not occur unless the energy of the incident photon is at least 1.022 megaelectron volts (MeV; a unit of energy equal to one million electron volts). Although this energy range is far above that used in diagnostic radiology, a brief description of pair production is included in this chapter to provide the reader with a broader understanding of the basic interactions of x-radiation with matter.

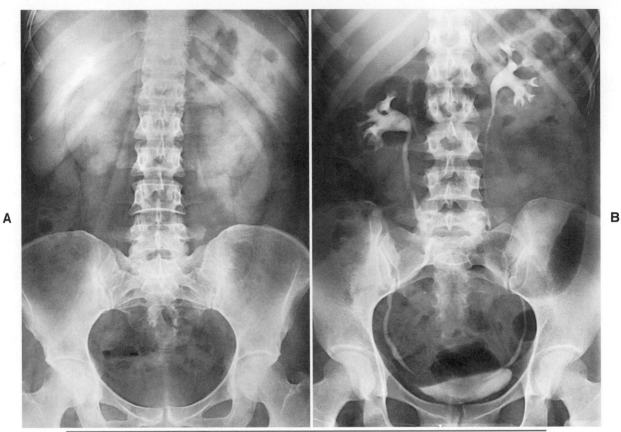

FIG. 2-13. A, Anteroposterior (AP) radiograph of an abdomen without the aid of a positive contrast medium. Parts of the urinary system other than the kidneys, which have their own unique density, are not radiographically demonstrated. **B,** AP radiograph of the abdomen following the intravenous injection of an appropriate positive contrast medium that permits visualization of the entire urinary system, thus allowing each contrast-filled structure to be distinguished. (From Ballinger PW, Frank ED: *Merrill's atlas of radiographic positions and radiologic procedures*, ed 10, vol 2, St. Louis, 2003, Mosby.)

Process of Pair Production

In pair production (Fig. 2-14) the incoming photon strongly interacts with the nucleus of an atom of the irradiated object and disappears. In the process, the energy of the photon is transformed into two new particles: a negatron (an ordinary electron) and a positron (a positively charged electron). The negatron and the positron have the same mass and magnitude of charge; the only difference is in the "sign" of their electrical charges. The incoming photon must have enough energy to produce the combined mass of these two particles. The minimum energy required to produce an electron-positron pair is 1.022 MeV (Box 2-2). For this reason, pair production does not occur at lower energies. The electron loses its kinetic energy by exciting and ionizing atoms in its path. The electron eventually loses enough energy that it may be captured by an atom in need of another electron.

As far as is known, no large quantities of positrons freely exist in the universe. The positron is classified as a form of antimatter. It interacts destructively

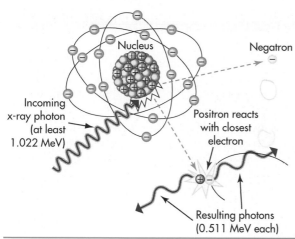

FIG. 2-14. Pair production. The incoming photon (equivalent in energy to at least 1.022 MeV) strongly interacts with the nucleus of the atom of the irradiated object and disappears. In the process, the energy of the photon is transformed into two new particles: a negatron (electron) and a positron. The negatron eventually recombines with any atom that needs another electron. The positron interacts destructively with a nearby electron. During the interaction, the positron and the electron annihilate each other, with their rest masses being converted into energy, which appears in the form of two 0.511-MeV photons, each moving in the opposite direction.

BOX 2-2

Mass-Energy Equivalent

Mass (electron or positron) = 9.1×10^{-31} kg
$c = 3 \times 10^{8}$ m/s

E (total) = E (electron) + E (positron) =
mc^2 (positron) = 16.38×10^{-14} J

1 MeV = 1.602×10^{-13} J
Therefore, E = $16.38 \times 10^{-14} \div$
1.602×10^{-13} = 1.022 MeV

---

with a nearby electron. During this interaction the positron and the electron annihilate each other, a conversion of matter into energy in accordance with Albert Einstein's famous theory of relativity, mathematically expressed as $E = mc^2$ (c is the speed of light in a vacuum). This energy that appears is carried off by two 0.511-MeV photons moving in opposite directions.

Use of Annihilation Radiation in Positron Emission Tomography (PET)

Annihilation radiation is used in positron emission tomography (PET) (see Chapter 11). In PET scanning, the source of the positrons are atomic nuclei that are unstable because they contain too many protons relative to their number of neutrons. To relieve this instability, the surplus proton is replaced in the nucleus by a neutron while a positron and another particle called a *neutrino* are ejected from the nucleus. This process is called *positron decay*. Within a very short distance (several micrometers or less) the emitted positron interacts with a local electron, and the two mutually annihilate, yielding a pair of photons emerging in opposite directions from the electron-positron interaction site. These annihilation photons are intercepted by a ring of detectors surrounding the patient and are used to build a cross-sectional image of the radioactivity within the patient. Some examples of unstable nuclei used in PET scanning are fluorine-18 (^{18}F), carbon-11 (^{11}C), and nitrogen-13 (^{13}N).

Photodisintegration

Photodisintegration is an interaction that occurs above 10 MeV in high-energy radiation therapy treatment machines. Although this energy range is far above that employed in diagnostic radiology, a short explanation of this interaction is included in this chapter to provide the reader with a more complete understanding of the possible interactions of x-radiation with matter.

Process of Photodisintegration

In photodisintegration a high-energy photon collides with the nucleus of an atom, which absorbs all of the photon's energy. This energy excess in the nucleus creates an instability that in most cases is alleviated by the emission of a neutron by the nucleus. Other types of emissions—a proton or proton-neutron

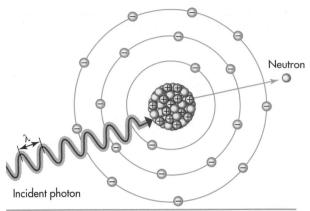

FIG. 2-15. Photodisintegration. An incoming high-energy photon collides with the nucleus of the atom of the irradiated object and absorbs all of the photon's energy. This energy excess in the nucleus creates an instability that is usually alleviated by the emission of a neutron. Also, if sufficient energy is absorbed by the nucleus, other types of emissions are possible, such as a proton or proton-neutron combination (deuteron), or even an alpha particle.

combination (deuteron) or even an alpha particle—are possible if sufficient energy is absorbed by the nucleus. Because emission of charged and/or uncharged particles has occurred from a previously indolent nucleus, we can say that the photodisintegration interaction has made a nucleus radioactive (Fig. 2-15).

SUMMARY

> Biologic damage in the patient may result from the absorption of x-ray energy.
> Variations in x-ray absorption properties of various body structures make radiographic imaging of human anatomy possible.
> Attenuation results when, through the processes of absorption and scatter, the intensity of the primary photons of an x-ray beam decreases as it passes through matter.
> Scattered radiation can result in radiographic fog and can be a biologic hazard to the radiographer.
> The energy absorbed by the patient per unit mass is called the *absorbed dose*.
> Two interactions of x-radiation are important in diagnostic radiology: photoelectric absorption and Compton scattering. The photoelectric effect is

the basis of radiographic imaging, whereas the Compton effect is its bane.
> For each radiographic procedure an optimal kVp and mAs combination exists that minimizes the dose to the patient and produces an acceptable radiograph.
> ▪ Within the energy range of diagnostic radiology that includes mammography (23 to 150 kVp), when kVp is decreased, the number of photoelectric interactions increases and the number of Compton interactions decreases; however, more energy is absorbed by the patient, and patient dose is increased.
> ▪ When kVp is increased, the patient receives a lower dose, but image quality is compromised.
> ▪ kVp selection is usually based on type of procedure and body part being radiographed.
> Radiographers must balance other variables such as film-screen combination, patient thickness, and degree of muscle tissue to arrive at technical exposure factors that will provide an acceptable image yet stay within the standards of radiation protection.
> Coherent scattering is most probable to occur below a 30-kVp generator setting; pair production and photodisintegration occur far above the range of diagnostic radiology.

Reference

1. Hendee WR, Ritenour ER: *Medical imaging physics*, ed 4, Chicago, 2002, John Wiley & Sons.

GENERAL DISCUSSION QUESTIONS

1. Why is it necessary for radiographers to have a basic understanding of the processes of interaction between radiation and matter?
2. How is an x-ray beam produced?
3. Why is tungsten or rhenium tungsten used in the target of the x-ray tube?
4. Describe the function of filtration in a diagnostic x-ray beam.
5. What is attenuation?

6. Why do human bones appear white on a diagnostic radiograph?

7. Describe the interactions between x-radiation and matter that occur within the diagnostic radiology range.

8. In the mathematical expression $E = mc^2$, what dose "c" represent?

9. What type of radiation is used in positron emission tomography?

10. When a high-energy photon collides with the nucleus of an atom during the process of photodisintegration, how much of the photon's energy is absorbed by the nucleus?

REVIEW QUESTIONS

1. **Exit, or image-formation, radiation comprises which of the following?**
   A. Primary photons and Compton-scattered photons
   B. Noninteracting and small-angle scattered photons
   C. Attenuated photons
   D. Absorbed photons

2. **Which of the following contributes *significantly* to the exposure of the radiographer?**
   A. Positrons
   B. Electrons
   C. Compton-scattered photons
   D. Compton-scattered electrons

3. **Which of the following defines attenuation?**
   A. Absorption and scatter
   B. Absorption only
   C. Scatter only
   D. Compton electrons

4. **In the radiographic kilovoltage range, which of the following structures will undergo the *most* photoelectric absorption?**
   A. Air cavities
   B. Compact bone
   C. Fat
   D. Soft tissue

5. **In which of the following x-ray interactions with matter is the energy of the incident photon *partially* absorbed?**
   A. Compton
   B. Photoelectric
   C. Coherent
   D. Pair production

6. **When a high atomic number solution is either ingested or injected into human tissue or a structure to visualize it during an imaging procedure, which of the following occurs?**
   A. Photoelectric interaction becomes greatly decreased, resulting in an increase in the absorbed dose in the body tissues or structures that contain the contrast medium
   B. Photoelectric interaction becomes significantly enhanced, leading to an increase in the absorbed dose in the body tissues or structures that contain the contrast medium
   C. Photoelectric interaction becomes greatly decreased, resulting in a decrease in the absorbed dose in the body tissues or structures that contain the contrast medium
   D. Photoelectric interaction becomes significantly enhanced, leading to a decrease in the absorbed dose in the body tissues or structures that contain the contrast medium

7. **Which of the following characteristics primarily differentiates the probability of occurrence of the various interactions of x-radiation with human tissue?**
   A. Energy of the incoming photon
   B. Direction of the incident photon
   C. X-ray beam intensity
   D. Exposure time

8. **Which of the following influences attenuation?**
   1. **Effective atomic number of the absorber**
   2. **Mass density**
   3. **Thickness of the absorber**
   A. 1 and 2 only
   B. 1 and 3 only
   C. 2 and 3 only
   D. 1, 2, and 3

9. **Radiographic fog results from which of the following interactions between x-radiation and matter?**
   1. **Compton scattering**
   2. **Pair production**
   3. **Photoelectric absorption**
   A. 1 only
   B. 2 only
   C. 3 only
   D. 1, 2, and 3

10. **The interactions of x-ray photons with any atoms of biologic matter are:**
    A. Able to be preplanned to selective atoms in order to limit radiation exposure to those atoms
    B. Only important in therapeutic radiology
    C. Random in nature and therefore the effects of such interactions cannot be predicted with certainty
    D. Unimportant in diagnostic radiology, making radiation protection unnecessary

3 Radiation Quantities and Units

KEY TERMS

absorbed dose (D)
collective effective dose (ColEfD)
coulomb (C)
coulomb per kilogram (C/kg)
effective dose (EfD)
equivalent dose (EqD)
exposure (X)
genetic, or heritable, effects
gray (Gy)

International System of Units
  (SI)
linear energy transfer (LET)
long-term, or late, somatic
  effects
occupational exposure
rad
radiation weighting factor (W_R)

rem
roentgen (R)
short-term somatic effects (acute
  or early effects)
sievert (Sv)
somatic damage
tissue weighting factor (W_T)
traditional units

OBJECTIVES

After completing this chapter, the reader will be able to perform the following:

- Explain the concept of skin erythema dose, tolerance dose, and threshold dose.
- List five examples of short-term somatic effects (early or acute effects) and three examples of long-term, or late, somatic effects.
- Differentiate between somatic and genetic effects.
- Differentiate between the following radiation quantities: *exposure, absorbed dose, equivalent dose,* and *effective dose,* and identify the appropriate symbol for each quantity.
- List and explain the International System (SI) and traditional units for radiation exposure, absorbed dose, equivalent dose, and effective dose.
- Describe the function of a tissue weighting factor.
- Given the numeric value for an absorbed dose of radiation stated in gray (rad), the radiation weighting factor for the type and energy of radiation in question, and the tissue weighting factor, determine the effective dose.

Continued

OBJECTIVES—*cont'd*

- State the purpose of the radiation quantity, collective effective dose, and list its International System and traditional unit.
- Explain the importance of linear energy transfer as it applies to biologic damage resulting from irradiation of human tissue.
- State the formula for determining equivalent dose.
- Determine the equivalent dose in terms of SI and traditional units when given the radiation weighting factor and the absorbed dose for different ionizing radiations.
- Explain the concept of effective dose when used for radiation protection purposes.
- State the formula for determining effective dose.

As the potentially harmful effects of ionizing radiation became known, the medical community sought to reduce radiation exposure throughout the world by developing standards for measuring and limiting this exposure. To be able to measure patient and personnel exposure in a consistent and uniform manner, diagnostic imaging personnel should be familiar with the standardized radiation quantities and units discussed in this chapter. Chapter 7 describes the standardized effective dose limits on radiation exposure expressed in these units, which are designed to minimize the associated risk and the potentially harmful effects of such exposure. Equivalent dose limits for tissues and organs are also described.

HISTORICAL EVOLUTION OF RADIATION QUANTITIES AND UNITS

Discovery of X-Rays

On November 8, 1895, while working in a modest laboratory at the University of Wurzburg, in Bavaria, German physics professor Wilhelm Conrad Roentgen (Fig. 3-1) discovered a mysterious ray. While performing an experiment investigating the nature of cathode rays and fluorescent materials, Roentgen passed electricity through a Crookes tube (Fig. 3-2) that he had covered with a shield of black cardboard. As he passed a charge through the pear-shaped, partial vacuum

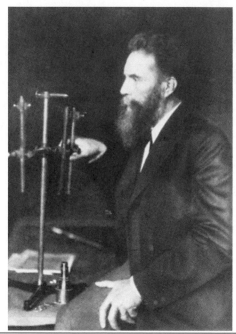

FIG. 3-1. Wilhelm Conrad Roentgen, the discoverer of x-rays. (Courtesy Burndy Library.)

discharge tube, he observed light emanating from a piece of paper coated with barium platinocyanide that was lying on a bench several feet away. Roentgen hypothesized that some type of radiation had been emitted from the Crookes tube that caused the barium platinocyanide to glow. To determine if any object had the ability to obstruct the mysterious rays, he held

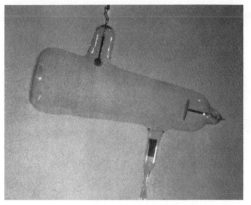

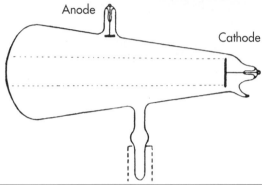

FIG. 3-2. *Top,* Photograph and *bottom,* diagram of the original type of x-ray tube. The cathode stream produced x-rays by impinging on the large area of the glass wall of the tube. (Courtesy Eastman Kodak.)

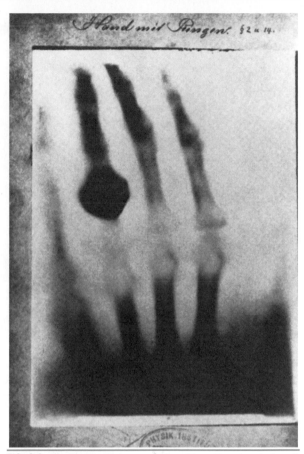

FIG. 3-3. First x-ray picture on film, Mrs. Roentgen's hand. (From Glasser O: *William Conrad Roentgen and the early history of the roentgen rays*, London, 1933, John Bale, Sons, and Danielsson, Ltd.)

various items between the Crookes tube and the fluorescent-coated paper. He found that most materials would allow some of these new rays to pass through. Roentgen called this momentous discovery "x-ray." Roentgen also found that x-rays could expose photographic film. In late November 1895, he took the world's first x-ray picture on film that clearly showed the bones of his wife's hand (Fig. 3-3). In December of 1895, he announced his scientific findings in an abbreviated manuscript titled, "On a New Kind of Ray, a Preliminary Communication," which was presented to the Physical Medical Society of Wurzburg.

First Reports of Injury

In the months that followed the announcement of Roentgen's discovery, experimentation with the new "wonder rays" resulted in acute biologic damage to some patients and pioneer radiation workers. Cases of **somatic** (from the Greek term, *soma*, meaning body) **damage,** biologic damage to the body of the exposed individual caused by exposure to ionizing radiation, were reported in Europe as early as 1896. In the United States, Clarence Madison Dally (Fig. 3-4, A), glassblower, tube maker, assistant, and long-time friend of fluoroscope inventor Thomas A. Edison (Fig. 3-4, B), became the first American radiation fatality. Dally died of radiation-induced cancer in October of 1904 at the age of 39. Because of Clarence Dally's severe injuries and death, Thomas Edison discontinued his x-ray research.

Among physicians, cancer deaths attributed to x-ray exposure were reported as early as 1910. As a result of **occupational exposure,** radiation exposure received by

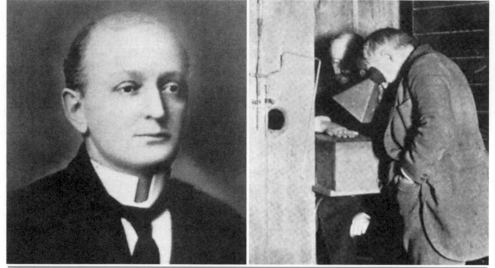

FIG. 3-4. A, Clarence Madison Dally (1865-1904), the first American radiation fatality. **B,** Clarence Madison Dally, assistant to Thomas A. Edison, is seen holding his hand over a box containing an x-ray tube while Edison examines the hand through a fluoroscope that he invented. (From Brown P: *American martyrs to science through the roentgen rays*, Springfield, Ill., 1936, Charles C Thomas.)

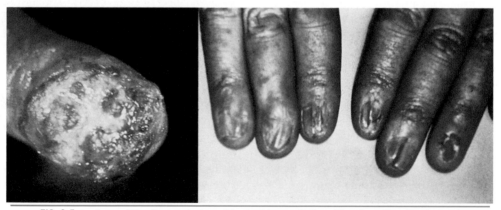

FIG. 3-5. Lesions of the fingers induced by ionizing radiation. (Courtesy Ken Bontrager.)

radiation workers in the course of exercising their professional responsibilities, many radiologists and dentists developed a reddening of the skin, called *radiodermatitis*, caused by exposure to ionizing radiation. Many of these skin lesions on the hands and fingers eventually became cancerous as a consequence of continued exposure to ionizing radiation (Fig. 3-5). Blood disorders such as aplastic anemia, which results from bone marrow failure, and leukemia, an abnormal over-production of white blood cells, were more common among early radiologists than among nonradiologists.

Investigation of Methods for Reducing Radiation Exposure

Alarmed by the increasing number of radiation injuries reported, the medical community decided to investigate methods for reducing radiation exposure. In

1921 the British X-Ray and Radium Protection Committee was formed to perform this task. The committee planned to formulate guidelines for the manufacture and use of radium and x-ray equipment and devices to eliminate the chance of occupational injury. Even though the committee members recognized the danger of excessive radiation exposure, they were handicapped because they did not have measurement techniques or background knowledge of radiobiology. Unfortunately, because they could not agree on a workable unit of radiation exposure, the members of the committee were unable to fulfill their responsibility.

Skin Erythema Dose

From 1900 to 1930 the unit in use for measuring radiation exposure was called the *skin erythema dose*, defined as the received quantity of radiation that causes diffuse redness over an area of skin after irradiation. This amount of absorbed radiation corresponds roughly to a modern dose of several gray (several hundred rads). The radiation units, gray (rad), are discussed later in this chapter. Because the amount of radiation required to produce the erythema reaction varied from one person to another, it was a crude and inaccurate way to measure radiation exposure. Scientists felt compelled to continue searching for a more reliable unit. The new unit selected was to be based on some exactly measurable effect produced by radiation such as ionization of atoms or energy absorbed in the irradiated object.

Early Definition of Quantities and Units

The First International Congress of Radiology was held in London, England, in 1925. This international meeting made possible a collaboration between radiologists from all over the world. Unfortunately, no definite decisions for measuring the effects of ionizing radiation were made based on the recommendations presented. The International Commission on Radiation Units and Measurements (ICRU) was also formed in 1925. In 1928 a Second International Congress of Radiology was held in Stockholm, Sweden. Although the "roentgen" was accepted as a unit of exposure, it was not adequately defined. The congress charged

the ICRU to define this unit of exposure. The congress also established the International X-Ray and Radium Protection Commission, predecessor of the International Commission on Radiological Protection (ICRP), which is discussed in Chapter 7.

Since the early days of radiology, biologic effects in humans caused by exposure to ionizing radiation were only too apparent. These **short-term somatic effects** (also known as **acute** or **early effects**) (Box 3-1), which appeared within minutes, hours, days, or weeks of the time of radiation exposure, were believed to be preventable if doses to radiation workers were limited and kept below a *tolerance level* at which no adverse biologic effects were demonstrated. (A *tolerance dose* is a radiation dose to which occupationally exposed persons could be continuously subjected without any apparent harmful acute effects, such as erythema of the skin.) Hence, the concept of a tolerance dose was developed to protect occupationally exposed persons from acute effects such as erythema of the skin. The general belief was that no adverse effects from radiation exposure would be demonstrated below this *threshold dose*. (A *threshold dose* is a dose of radiation below which an individual has a negligible chance of sustaining specific biologic damage.) The tolerance dose was stated in what at that time was an imprecise

---

BOX 3-1

Effects of Radiation

Short-Term Somatic Effects (Early or Acute)

Nausea	Intestinal disorders
Fatigue	Fever
Diffused redness of the skin	Blood disorders
Loss of hair	Shedding of the outer layer of skin

Long-Term or Late Somatic Effects

Cancer	Formation of cataracts
Embryologic effects (birth defects)	

Genetic Effects (Heritable Effects)
Biologic effects of ionizing radiation on generations yet unborn

measure of exposure. This unit, the roentgen, was the principal guideline for occupational radiation exposure during the 1930s and is discussed later in this chapter.

In 1934 the International X-Ray and Radium Protection Commission recommended a tolerance dose daily limit of 0.2 roentgen. In the United States, the Advisory Committee on X-Ray and Radium Protection, which was formed in 1931 to formulate recommendations for radiation control, also recommended a tolerance dose equal to 0.2 roentgen per day.

In 1936 the Committee reduced this dose to 0.1 roentgen per day. As scientists began to recognize the **long-term, or late, somatic effects** of ionizing radiation that appeared months or years following exposure and the possibility of **genetic, or heritable, effects,** they began to focus on finding ways to minimize the risk of sustaining such damage (see Box 3-1). The search was on for a more reliable unit to replace the tolerance dose.

In 1937 the ICRU finished its assignment from the Second International Congress of Radiology, and although still not accurately defined, the roentgen became internationally accepted as the unit of measurement for exposure to x-radiation and gamma radiation (short wavelength, higher energy electromagnetic waves emitted by the nuclei of radioactive substances). This unit was redefined in 1962 to increase accuracy and acceptability.

In 1946 the U.S. Advisory Committee on X-Ray and Radium Protection became known as the National Committee on Radiation Protection (NCRP). The name of this radiation standards organization underwent another change in 1956 and again in 1964 when it became the National Council on Radiation Protection and Measurements (NCRP). Functions of the NCRP are discussed in Chapter 7.

The General Conference of Weights and Measures, which was responsible for the development and international unification of the metric system, assigned its International Committee for Weights and Measures the responsibility of developing guidelines for the units of measurement in 1948. To fulfill this responsibility, the committee developed the **International System of Units,** from the French "Système international d' unités" **(SI).** This system makes possible the interchange of units among all branches of science throughout the world.

The Modern Era of Radiation Protection

By the early 1950s, maximum permissible dose (MPD) replaced the tolerance dose for radiation protection purposes. MPD basically indicated the largest dose of ionizing radiation that an occupationally exposed person was permitted that was not anticipated to result in major adverse biologic effects as a consequence of radiation exposure. This meant that absorbed doses of ionizing radiation below the established MPD would not result in any appreciable bodily injury or in injury to the reproductive cells. However, some small risk of damage could exist with radiation doses at the MPD level. MPD was expressed in rem (an acronym for "radiation-equivalent man," historically known as "Roentgen-equivalent man"), the traditional unit used for radiation protection purposes at that time. This unit is discussed later in this chapter.

Eventually the concept of "tolerance dose" was no longer accepted as a means for protecting radiation workers from the acute effects of ionizing radiation. This meant that no amount of radiation was considered completely safe. The probability of long-term harm, such as the development of cancer, was expected to decrease as dose decreased, but it was not expected to become zero at any dose. This raised a dilemma: If no amount of radiation was safe, and if it was impossible to design a work environment where the dose was zero (and still be able to perform procedures such as interventional angiography), then what would determine the maximum allowed occupational exposure? The solution was to compare rates of death and accident among various occupations. Insurance companies had been using this method of comparison for many years to determine insurance rates. Some occupations, such as deep sea diving and professional mountaineering, are very hazardous. Other occupations, such as trade or government deskwork, are nonhazardous. However, even in nonhazardous occupations, there is still a small risk of fatality or serious injury (about 1 chance in 10,000 each year[1]). With this in mind, the decision was made to base recommendations for dose limits on the concept that the probability of harm associated with typical film badge readings or that of other dosimeters should be no more than the amount of harm in industries that are generally considered reasonably safe.

By the 1970s, dosimetry and risk analysis had become quite sophisticated. Radiation units were developed that contained factors that accounted for the varied bioeffects of different types of radiation (alpha, beta, gamma, x-radiation, neutrons, etc.). There was also growing recognition that the consequences for the health of the human as a whole organism depended on which organs and organ systems had been irradiated. For example, irradiation of the bone marrow was seen as more significant to the health of an organism than irradiation of the skin. Equal doses of radiation to bone marrow and skin had different consequences. In the late 1970s, dose limits were calculated and established to ensure that the risk from radiation exposure acquired while on the job did not exceed risks encountered in "safe" occupations, such as clerical work, which is approximately 10^{-4} per year.[1]

In 1991 the ICRP revised tissue weighting factors. The revision was based on data from more recent epidemiologic studies of the atomic bomb survivors. The ICRP adopted the term **effective dose (EfD).** Effective dose is based on the energy deposited in biologic tissue by ionizing radiation. It takes into account the type of radiation (x-radiation, gamma, neutron, etc.) and the sensitivity of the tissues exposed to radiation. This quantity is actually a measure of the overall risk arising from the irradiation of biologic tissue. It takes into consideration the exposure to the entire body. Effective dose is expressed in the SI unit, **sievert (Sv),** or in millisievert (mSv), a subunit of the sievert. It can also be expressed in the traditional radiation unit, the **rem.** Further discussion of this radiation quantity and its associated units of measure follows.

Quantities and Units in Use Today

The ICRU adopted SI units for use with ionizing radiation in 1980 and urged full implementation of the units as soon as possible. Many developed countries, particularly in Europe, have already made the transition to SI units. In the United States SI units, the gray, and centigray are used routinely in therapeutic radiology to specify absorbed dose. Even though the NCRP (see Chapter 7) adopted the internationally accepted SI units for use in 1985, **traditional units,** special units associated with radiation protection and dosimetry,

namely the roentgen and the rem, are still widely employed. As previously noted, the **roentgen (R)** is the internationally accepted unit for measurement of exposure to x-radiation and gamma radiation. One roentgen is the photon exposure that under standard conditions of pressure and temperature produces a total positive or negative ion charge of $2.58 \times (10)^{-4}$ coulombs per kilogram of dry air. **Rem** stands for "radiation-equivalent man," the unit for the radiation quantity currently in use, equivalent dose. Rem was previously defined as the dose that is equivalent to any type of ionizing radiation that produces the same biologic effect as 1 rad of x-radiation. One rad corresponds to an energy transfer of 100 ergs per gram of irradiated object.

Fluoroscopic entrance exposure rates are measured in roentgens per minute (R/min), and essentially all radiation survey instruments provide readings in traditional units. In addition, many regulatory criteria are described in terms of traditional units. Because both SI and traditional units are still being used, the current generation of radiation workers must understand both unit systems for the safety of patients and personnel. To help promote the understanding of SI and traditional radiation units, both are presented where applicable throughout this text. The traditional units are usually identified in parentheses after the SI units. Box 3-2 presents an overview of the important dates in the historical evolution of radiation quantities and units and an overview of terminology used in a given period of time to describe radiation dose limitation.

The SI unit of absorbed dose, **gray (Gy)** (discussed later in this chapter), was named after the English radiobiologist Louis Harold Gray (1901-1965), who was instrumental in developing what is arguably the most important theory in all of radiation dosimetry. The *Bragg-Gray theory* (1936) relates the ionization produced in a small cavity within an irradiated medium or object to the energy absorbed in that medium as a result of its radiation exposure. Thus, with the use of appropriate correction factors, the theory essentially links the determination of the absorbed radiation dose in a medium to a relatively simple measurement of ionization charge. Rolf Maximilian Sievert (1896-1966), the Swedish physicist for whom the SI unit of equivalent dose was named, is best known for his method (the Sievert integral) for determining the

BOX 3-2

The Historical Evolution of Radiation Quantities and Units

Year	Event
1895	X-rays are discovered, and the discovery is announced.
1896	Initial cases of somatic damage caused by exposure to ionizing radiation are reported in Europe.
1900	Skin erythema dose becomes the unit for measuring radiation exposure.
1904	Clarence Madison Dally becomes the first American radiation fatality.
1910	First cancer deaths among physicians that are attributed to x-ray exposure are reported.
1921	British X-Ray and Radium Protection Committee is formed to investigate methods for reducing radiation exposure.
1925	First International Congress of Radiology is held in London, England; radiologists from all over the world collaborate, but no definite system for measuring ionizing radiation exposure is identified. International Commission on Radiation Units and Measurements (ICRU) is formed.
1928	ICRU is charged by the Second International Congress of Radiology (Stockholm, Sweden) to define a unit of exposure. The International X-Ray and Radium Protection Commission (predecessor of the ICRP) is established by the Second International Congress of Radiology.
1930s	Tolerance dose is used for radiation protection purposes.
1931	U.S. Advisory Committee on X-Ray and Radium Protection is formed to formulate recommendations for radiation control.
1934	A tolerance dose of 0.2 R per day is recommended.
1936	The tolerance dose is reduced to 0.1 R per day. Bragg-Gray theory is introduced.
1937	Roentgen (R) becomes internationally accepted as the unit of measurement for exposure to x-radiation and gamma radiation.
1946	U.S. Advisory Committee on X-Ray and Radium Protection becomes known as the National Committee on Radiation Protection and Measurements (NCRP).
1948	International System (SI) of units is developed.
1950s	(Early 1950s) Maximum permissible dose (MPD) replaces the tolerance dose for radiation protection purposes.
1962	Roentgen (R) is redefined to increase accuracy and acceptability.
1963	National Committee on Radiation Protection and Measurements becomes the National Council on Radiation Protection (NCRP).
1977	International Commission on Radiological Protection (ICRP) recommends that the dose equivalent limit or effective dose equivalent replace MPD.
1980	ICRU adopts SI units for use with ionizing radiation.
1985	National Council of Radiation Protection (NCRP) adopts SI units for use.
1991	ICRP replaces effective equivalent dose with the term *effective dose (EfD)*.

History of Terminology Used to Determine Radiation Dose Limitation

1900-1930	Skin erythema dose (SED)
1930-1950	Tolerance dose (TD)
1950-1977	Maximum permissible dose (MPD)
1977-1991	Effective dose equivalent
1991-present	Effective dose (EfD)

exposure rates at various points near linear radium sources (tubes).

RADIATION QUANTITIES AND THEIR UNITS OF MEASURE

Diagnostic imaging professionals need to understand the following basic radiation quantities: exposure (X), absorbed dose (D), equivalent dose (EqD), and effective dose (EfD). In a simplified sense, exposure may be described as the amount of ionizing radiation that may strike an object such as the human body when in the vicinity of a radiation source. Absorbed dose is the deposition of energy per unit mass by ionizing radiation in the patient's body tissue. Equivalent dose also attempts to take into account the variation in biologic harm that is produced by different types of radiation. Both the type and the energy of the radiation of concern are considered. This quantity is used for radiation protection purposes. Effective dose is another radiation quantity utilized for radiation protection purposes. It begins with equivalent dose and, by applying modifying factors, attempts to take into account the part of the body that is being irradiated to arrive at an index of overall harm to a human. Effective dose is the quantity that attempts to summarize the overall potential for biologic damage to a human due to exposure to ionizing radiation (Box 3-3). Each radiation quantity has its own special unit of measure. These units are discussed in detail in the following section.

BOX 3-3

Difference between "Equivalent Dose" and "Effective Dose"

The quantity *equivalent dose* uses radiation weighting factors (W_R) to adjust the quantity, absorbed dose, so as to reflect the difference in biologic harm produced by different types and energies of ionizing radiation.

The quantity *effective dose* uses tissue weighting factors (W_T) to adjust the quantity, equivalent dose, so as to reflect the difference in harm to the person as a whole depending on the tissues and organs that have been irradiated.

Exposure (X)

When a volume of air is irradiated with x-rays or with gamma rays, the interaction that occurs between the radiation and neutral atoms in the air results in some electrons being liberated from those air atoms as they are ionized. Consequently, the ionized air can function as a conductor and carry electricity because of the negatively charged free electrons and positively charged ions that have been created. As the intensity of x-ray exposure of the air volume increases, the number of electron-ion pairs produced also increases. Thus the amount of radiation responsible for the ionization of a well-defined volume of air may be determined by measuring the number of electron-ion pairs or charged particles in that volume of air. This radiation ionization in the air is termed *exposure*.

Exposure (X) may be defined as the total electrical charge (of one sign, either all pluses or all minuses) per unit mass that x-ray and gamma ray photons with energies up to 3 million electron volts (MeV) generate in dry (i.e., nonhumid) air at standard temperature and pressure defined as 760 mm Hg or 1 atmosphere at sea level and 22° C.

For precise measurement of radiation exposure in radiography, the total amount of ionization an x-ray beam produces in a known mass of air must be obtained. This type of direct measurement is accomplished in an accredited calibration laboratory by using a standard or free-air ionization chamber (Fig. 3-6). The chamber contains a known quantity of air with precisely measured temperature, pressure, and humidity. If in that specified volume of dry air the total charge of all the ions of one sign (either all pluses or all minuses) produced are collected and measured, the total amount of radiation exposure may be accurately determined. The chamber response is modified to correspond to standard temperature and pressure of dry air.

Such an instrument, however, is not a practical device at locations other than a standardization laboratory. As a result, much smaller and less complicated instruments have been developed for use away from the laboratory. Although very convenient, these instruments must be periodically recalibrated in a standardization laboratory against a free-air chamber.

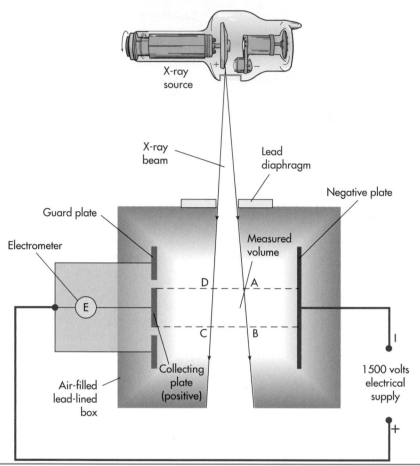

FIG. 3-6. This device determines radiation exposure by measuring the amount of ionization an x-ray beam produces within its air collection volume. The instrument consists of a box containing a known quantity of air, two oppositely charged metal plates, and an electrometer, an instrument that measures the total amount of charge collected on the positively charged metal plate. The chamber measures the total amount of electrical charge of all the electrons produced during the ionization of a specific volume of air at standard atmospheric pressure and temperature. The electrical charge is measured in units called *coulombs (C)* (charge of an electron = -1.6×10^{-19} C). A collected electrical charge of 2.58×10^{-4} C/kg of irradiated air constitutes an exposure of 1 roentgen (R).

The **coulomb (C)** is the basic unit of electrical charge. It represents the quantity of electrical charge flowing past a point in a circuit in 1 second when an electrical current of 1 ampere is used. The ampere is the SI unit of electrical current. In the International System, the exposure unit is measured in **coulombs per kilogram (C/kg).** No special name for this SI quantity has been assigned. This exposure unit is simply equal to an electrical charge of 1 C produced in a kilogram of dry air by ionizing radiation. The roentgen, however, is precisely defined as the photon (either x-ray or gamma ray) exposure that under standard conditions of pressure and temperature produces a total positive or negative ion charge of 2.58×10^{-4} C/kg of dry air. An exposure of 1 C/kg equals $[1/(2.58 \times 10^{-4})]$ R, or 3.88×10^{3} R. Therefore, conversion from roentgens (the traditional unit of exposure) to coulombs per kilogram (the SI unit) may be accomplished by multiplying the number of roentgens by 2.58×10^{-4}.

Example: To convert 100 R to C/kg:

1. Set up the equation: $100 \, R \times 2.58(10)^{-4} \dfrac{C/kg}{R}$

2. Cancel R: $100 \, \cancel{R} \times 2.58(10)^{-4} \dfrac{C/kg}{\cancel{R}}$

3. Obtain answer: 0.0258 C/kg
4. Write answer in standard scientific notation: $2.58(10)^{-2}$ (C/kg)

Conversion of coulombs per kilogram (C/kg) to roentgens (R) may be accomplished by dividing by $2.58(10)^{-4}$.

EXAMPLE: To convert 100 C/kg to R:

1. Set up the equation: $100 \, C/kg \div 2.58(10)^{-4} \dfrac{C/kg}{R}$

   or $\dfrac{100 \, C/kg}{2.58(10)^{-4} \dfrac{C/kg}{R}}$

2. Cancel C/kg: $100 \, \cancel{C/kg} \div 2.58 \, (10)^{-4} \, \cancel{C/kg}/R$
3. Obtain answer: $39(10)^4$ R or 390,000 roentgens (an enormous radiation exposure)

The coulomb per kilogram (roentgen) unit is used for x-ray equipment calibration because x-ray output is measured directly with an ionization chamber. It also is used to calibrate radiation survey instruments (refer to Chapter 10 for further information).

Absorbed Dose (D)

As ionizing radiation passes through an object, some of the energy of that radiation is transferred to that medium. It is actually absorbed by the object and stays within it. The quantity, **absorbed dose (D),** is defined as the amount of energy per unit mass absorbed by the irradiated object. This absorbed energy is responsible for any biologic damage resulting from the tissues being exposed to radiation.

Anatomic structures in the body possess different absorption properties; some structures can absorb more radiant energy than others. The amount of energy absorbed by a structure depends on the atomic number (Z) (number of protons contained within the nucleus of an atom) of the tissues composing the structure, the mass density of the tissue (measured in kg/m^3), and the energy of the incident photon; absorption increases as

atomic number and mass density increase and photon energy decreases. In other words, low-energy photons are generally more easily absorbed in a material such as biologic tissue than are high-energy photons.

The effective atomic number (Zeff) of a given tissue is a "composite," or weighted average, of the atomic numbers of the many chemical elements composing the tissue. Bone has a higher effective atomic number (Zeff = 13.8) than does soft tissue (Zeff = 7.4) because bone contains calcium (Z = 20) and phosphorus (Z = 15), whereas soft tissue is composed mostly of fat (Zeff = 5.9) and structures with atomic numbers close to that of water (Zeff = 7.4). Bone absorbs more ionizing radiation than does soft tissue in the diagnostic energy range (which includes mammography) of 23 to 150 kilovolts peak (kVp) because the photoelectric process for bone is the dominant mode of energy absorption within this range. The probability of photoelectric interaction strongly depends on the atomic number of the irradiated material. The higher the atomic number of the material, the greater the amount of energy absorbed by that material.

In the therapeutic energy range of 100 keV and above, however, the difference in absorption between bone and soft tissue gradually lessens (Fig. 3-7). This

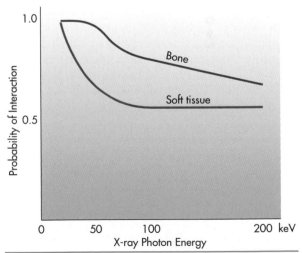

FIG. 3-7. Probability of interaction of x-rays when a 5-cm-thick layer of soft tissue or bone is encountered. The probability is greater at lower energies and is greater for bone than soft tissue, particularly at low energies.

is because the amount of photoelectric absorption decreases and the amount of Compton scattering relative to the photoelectric interaction increases as the energy of the x-ray beam increases; the amount of Compton scattering in a material does not depend on the atomic number of the material. Hence, as energy increases, the difference in amount of absorption between any two tissues of different atomic number decreases. Because the process of absorption is responsible for biologic damage and absorption properties vary with the quality of the radiation and the type of tissue irradiated, irradiation of tissues in therapeutic radiology is generally specified in terms of absorbed dose rather than in terms of exposure. However, at all energies mass density always has an effect on absorption. This effect is linear and directly proportional. Therefore, a material that is twice as dense as another will absorb twice as much energy from the same photon beam.

The SI unit of absorbed dose is the gray (Gy) and is defined as an energy absorption of 1 joule (J) per kilogram of matter in the irradiated object. One gray is therefore determined by the following simple equation:

$$1\,Gy = 1\,J/kg$$

A joule (a unit of energy) may be defined as the work done or energy expended when a force of 1 newton acts on an object along a distance of 1 meter. A single joule does not correspond to a large amount of energy. A typical microwave oven, for example, imparts 750 joules per second to the food it is heating.

Traditionally the rad has been used as the unit of absorbed dose. **Rad** stands for *radiation absorbed dose*. This unit has been used to indicate the amount of radiant energy transferred to an irradiated object by any type of ionizing radiation. The rad is equivalent to an energy transfer of 100 erg (another unit of energy and work) per gram of irradiated object. One rad may be expressed mathematically as follows:

$$1\,rad = 100\,erg/g$$

or

$$1\,rad = 1/100\,j/kg = 1/100\,Gy$$

Thus, gray and rad units are easily translated to compare absorbed dose values. If the absorbed dose is stated in rads, the equivalent number of gray may be determined by dividing by 100:

RULE: number of rads ÷ 100 = number of gray

EXAMPLE 1: 5000 rads = 5000 ÷ 100 rads per Gy = 50 Gy

EXAMPLE 2: 5 rads = 5 ÷ 100 rads per Gy = 0.05 Gy

If the absorbed dose is stated in gray, the number of rads may be determined by multiplying by 100:

RULE: number of gray × 100 = number of rads

EXAMPLE 1: 15 Gy = 15 × 100 rads per Gy = 1500 rads

EXAMPLE 2: 50 Gy = 50 × 100 rads per Gy = 5000 rads

SI subunits facilitate conversion from rads to gray. In therapeutic radiology, for example, the centigray (cGy) is replacing the rad for recording of absorbed dose. The following example of the subunit conversion of centigray to rads provides an example applicable to therapeutic radiology:

$$10\,cGy = 10\,rads$$

Equivalence of Radiation-Produced Damage from Different Sources of Ionizing Radiation

Equal absorbed doses of different types of radiation produce different amounts of biologic damage in body tissue. For example, a 1-Gy (100 rads) absorbed dose of fast neutrons causes more biologic damage than a 1-Gy absorbed dose of x-rays. A 1-Gy dose of neutrons would kill a laboratory rat, but a 1-Gy dose of x-rays would not. The concept of dose equivalence takes this biologic impact into consideration by using a specific modifying, or quality factor (Q), to adjust the absorbed dose value. Quality factor (Q) is an adjustment multiplier that was used in the calculation of dose equivalence to specify the ability of a dose of any kind of ionizing radiation to cause biologic damage.

X-rays, beta particles (high-speed electrons), and gamma rays produce virtually the same biologic effect in body tissue for equal absorbed doses. In terms of

TABLE 3-1

Quality Factors for Different Types of Ionizing Radiations

Type of Ionizing Radiation	Quality Factor*
X-ray photons	1
Beta particles	1
Gamma photons	1
Thermal neutrons	5
Fast neutrons	20
High-energy external protons	1
Low-energy internal protons[†]	2
Alpha particles	20
Multiple charged particles of unknown energy	20

*Data from National Council of Radiation Protection and Measurements (NCRP): *Report No. 116, limitation of exposure to ionizing radiation*, Bethesda, MD, 1993, NCRP.
[†]Protons produced as a result of neutrons interacting with the nuclei of tissue molecules.

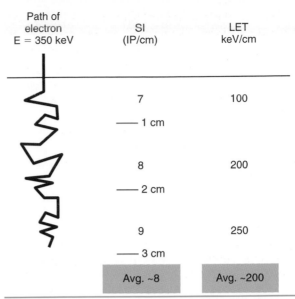

FIG. 3-8. An electron having energy E = 350 keV interacts in a tissue-like material. Its actual path is tortuous, changing direction a number of times, as the electron interacts with atoms of the material via excitations and ionizations. As interactions reduce the energy of the electron through excitation and ionization the electron's energy is transferred to the material. The interactions that take place along the path of the particle may be summarized as specific ionization (SI, ion pairs/cm) or as linear energy transfer (LET, keV/cm) along the straight line continuation of the particle's trajectory beyond its point of entry. (From Hendee WR and Ritenour ER: *Medical imaging physics,* ed 4, Chicago, 2002, John Wiley & Sons.)

quality factor, these radiations have been given a numeric adjustment value of 1 and are the base or standard against which to compare the effectiveness or efficiency of other types of ionizing radiation in producing biologic damage. The quality factors of different kinds of ionizing radiations are listed in Table 3-1. The concept of **linear energy transfer (LET)** helps explain the need for a quality, or modifying, factor. LET (Fig. 3-8) is the amount of energy transferred on average by incident radiation to an object per unit length of track through the object and is expressed in units of keV/μm (see Appendix E).

Radiation with a high LET transfers a large amount of energy into a small area and can therefore do more biologic damage than radiation with a low LET. Thus, a high-LET radiation has a quality factor that is greater than the quality factor for a low-LET radiation. LET and its relationship to biologic damage are discussed again in Chapter 5.

Equivalent Dose (EqD)

Equivalent dose (EqD) is the product of the average absorbed dose in a tissue or organ in the human body and its associated **radiation weighting factor (W_R)**

chosen for the type and energy of the radiation in question. Stochastic effects are nonthreshold, randomly occurring biologic effects of ionizing radiation such as cancer and genetic abnormalities. The probability of occurrence of these effects depends on the radiation dose and the type and energy of the radiation. What this means is that some radiations are more biologically efficient for causing damage than others for a given dose (see Chapter 7 for a more detailed discussion of stochastic and nonstochastic effects). The radiation weighting factor (W_R) takes this into account. The radiation weighting factors are selected by national and international scientific advisory bodies (NCRP, ICRP) and are based on quality factors and linear energy transfer. The NCRP, in Report #116, describes the radiation weighting factor as "a dimen-

Radiation Weighting Factors for Different Types and Energies of Ionizing Radiation

Radiation Type and Energy Range	Radiation Weighting Factor (W_R)
X-ray and gamma ray photons electrons (every energy)	1
Neutrons, energy <10 keV	5
10 keV to 100 keV	10
>100 keV to 2 MeV	20
>2 MeV to 20 MeV	10
>20 MeV	5
Protons	2
Alpha particles	20

Data adapted from International Commission on Radiological Protection (ICRP): *Recommendations, ICRP publication No. 60,* New York, 1991, Pergamon Press.

sionless factor" (a multiplier) that was chosen for radiation protection purposes to account for differences in biologic impact between various types of ionizing radiations.[1] This factor places risks associated with biologic effects on a common scale. Each type and energy of radiation has a specific radiation weighting factor, the numeric value of which may be found in Table 3-2. The radiation weighting factor actually has the same numeric value as the quality factor that was previously used for determining dose equivalence.

Equivalent dose (EqD) is used for radiation protection purposes when a person receives exposure from various types of ionizing radiation. Equivalent dose for measuring biologic effects may be determined and expressed in sieverts (SI units) or in rems (traditional units). It is obtained by multiplying the absorbed dose (D) by the radiation weighting factor (W_R) as follows:

$$EqD = D \times W_R$$

$$(Sv) = (Gy) \times W_R$$

EXAMPLE (using gray and sievert): An individual received the following absorbed doses: 0.1 Gy of x-radiation, 0.05 Gy of fast neutrons, and 0.2 Gy of alpha particles. What is the *total* equivalent dose?

$$EqD = (D \times W_R)_1 + (D \times W_R)_2 + (D \times W_R)_3$$

(The radiation weighting factor for each radiation in question may be obtained from Table 3-2.)

ANSWER:

RADIATION TYPE	D	×	W_R	=	EqD
X-radiation	0.1 Gy	×	1	=	0.1 Sv
Fast neutrons	0.05 Gy	×	20	=	1.0 Sv
Alpha particles	0.2 Gy	×	20	=	4.0 Sv
	Total EqD			=	5.1 Sv

EXAMPLE (using rad and rem): An individual received the following absorbed doses: 10 rads of x-radiation, 5 rads of fast neutrons, and 20 rads of alpha particles. What is the *total* equivalent dose?

$$EqD = (D \times W_R)_1 + (D \times W_R)_2 + (D \times W_R)_3$$

(The radiation weighting factor for each radiation in question may be obtained from Table 3-2.)

ANSWER:

RADIATION TYPE	D	×	W_R	=	EqD
X-radiation	10 rads	×	1	=	10 rem
Fast neutrons	5 rads	×	20	=	100 rem
Alpha particles	20 rads	×	20	=	400 rem
	Total EqD			=	510 rem

Effective Dose (EfD)

Effective dose (EfD) provides a measure of the overall risk of exposure to ionizing radiation. The NCRP, in Report #116, defines it as "the sum of the weighted equivalent doses for all irradiated tissues or organs."[1] Effective dose incorporates both the effect of the type of radiation used (x-radiation, gamma, neutron, etc.) and the radiosensitivity of the organ or body part irradiated through the utilization of appropriate weighting factors. These factors determine the overall harm to those biologic components for developing a radiation-induced cancer, or for the reproductive organs, the risk of genetic damage. The weighting factor that takes into account the relative detriment to each organ and tissue is called the **tissue weighting factor (W_T).** The tissue weighting factor is a conceptual measure for the relative risk associated with irradiation of different body tissues (see Chapter 7).

The tissue weighting factor (Table 3-3), more precisely, is a value that denotes the percentage of the summed stochastic (cancer plus genetic) risk stemming from irradiation of tissue (T) to the all-inclusive risk, when the entire body is irradiated in a uniform fashion. W_T accounts for the risk to the entire organism brought on by irradiation of individual tissues and organs. The ICRP originally introduced the tissue weighting factor concept because uniform, whole-body irradiation seldom occurs and some organs and body tissues vary considerably in the absorbed dose received and their sensitivity to random radiation-induced responses.

To determine effective dose (EfD), an absorbed dose (D) is multiplied by a radiation weighting factor (W_R) to obtain equivalent dose (EqD) and by a tissue weighting factor (W_T) to obtain effective dose. Effective dose may be expressed in sievert (SI unit) or in rem (traditional unit).

$$EfD = D \times W_R \times W_T$$

Effective dose can be used to compare the average amount of radiation received by the entire body from a specific radiologic examination with that from natural background radiation (see Table 1-1). By using the background equivalent radiation time (BERT) method as discussed in Chapter 1, it is possible to describe the examination radiation dose in terms of the length of time it would take to acquire a comparable effective dose from environmental sources.

Table 3-4 gives some typical values for radiation doses that are associated with a radiographic examination of the lumbar spine, and it illustrates some of the principles of the different ways to specify radiation dose. The dose to the patient is highest at the "entrance skin surface," the surface of the patient that

TABLE 3-3

Organ or Tissue Weighting Factors

Organ or Tissue	Weighting Factor (W_T)*
Gonads	0.20
Red bone marrow	0.12
Colon	0.12
Lung	0.12
Stomach	0.12
Bladder	0.05
Breast	0.05
Liver	0.05
Esophagus	0.05
Thyroid	0.05
Skin	0.01
Bone surface	0.01
Remainder[†,‡]	0.05

*Data from National Council on Radiation Protection and Measurements (NCRP): *Report #116, limitation of exposure to ionizing radiation*, Bethesda, MD, 1993, NCRP.
[†]The remainder takes into account the following additional tissues and organs: adrenals, brain, small intestine, large intestine, kidney, muscle, pancreas, spleen, thymus, and uterus.
[‡]In extraordinary circumstances in which one of the remainder tissues or organs receives an equivalent dose in excess of the highest dose in any of the 12 organs for which a weighting factor (W_T) is specified, a W_T of 0.025 should be applied to that tissue or organ and a W_T of 0.025 to the average dose in the other remainder tissues or organs.

TABLE 3-4

Typical Values for Radiation Doses Associated with an AP Lumbar Spine Examination

Absorbed Dose to Skin at Entrance Surface	6.4 mGy
Absorbed Dose to Bone Marrow	0.6 mGy
Absorbed Dose to a Fetus	3.5 mGy
Equivalent Dose to a Fetus	3.5 mSv
Effective Dose	3.3 mSv

is toward the x-ray tube. This surface will be exposed to the unattenuated primary beam of x-rays. Absorbed doses to various organs may be calculated from standard tables. Two organ absorbed doses are given in Table 3-4, bone marrow and fetus. The equivalent dose to the fetus is also given and is the same as the absorbed dose to the fetus because the radiation weighting factor is 1. Finally, the effective dose is given. It was calculated from the various tissue weighting factors and organ absorbed doses for organs in the field of view of this examination.

Collective Effective Dose (ColEfD)

In addition to equivalent dose and effective dose, another dosimetric quantity has been derived and implemented for use in radiation protection to describe internal and external dose measurements. The quantity, **collective effective dose (ColEfD),** is used to describe radiation exposure of a population or group from low doses of different sources of ionizing radiation. It is determined as the product of the average effective dose for an individual belonging to the exposed population or group and the number of persons exposed. The radiation unit for this quantity is *person-sievert* (previously referred to as *man-rem*). The following is an example using the unit:

EXAMPLE: If 200 people receive an average effective dose of 0.25 Sv (25 rem), the collective effective dose is $200 \times 0.25 = 50$ person-sieverts (5000 man-rem).

Tables 3-5 and 3-6 summarize radiation quantities, units, and equivalents.

TABLE 3-5

SI and Traditional Unit Equivalents

1 SI exposure unit equals	1. $C/kg = \dfrac{1}{2.58 \times 10^{-4}} R$
1 coulomb equals	1. 1 ampere-second
1 coulomb per kilogram of air equals	1. 1 SI unit of exposure
	2. $\dfrac{1}{2.58 \times 10^{-4}} R$
1 gray equals	1. 1 J/kg
	2. 100 rads
	3. 100 cGy
	4. 1000 mGy
1 sievert equals	1. 1 J/kg (for x-radiation, Q = 1)
	2. 100 rem
	3. 100 cSv
	4. 1000 mSv
1 erg equals	1. 10^{-7} J
1 joule equals	1. 10^7 erg
	2. 1 newton-meter
	3. 6.24×10^{18} eV
1 roentgen (R) equals	1. 2.58×10^{-4} C/kg of air
1 milliroentgen (mR) equals	1. 1/1000 R or 10^{-3} R
1 rad equals	1. 100 erg/g
	2. 1/100 J/kg
	3. 1/100 Gy
	4. 1 cGy
1 millirad equals	1. 1/1000 rad
1 rem equals	1. 1/100 J/kg (for x-radiation, Q = 1)
	2. 1/100 Sv
	3. 1 centisievert (cSv)
	4. 10 mSv
1 millirem equals	1. 1/1000 rem

TABLE 3-6

Summary of Radiation Quantities and Units

Type of Radiation	Quantity	SI Unit	Traditional Unit	Measuring Medium	Radiation Effect Measured
X-radiation or gamma	Exposure (X)	Coulomb per kilogram (C/kg)	Roentgen (R)	Air	Ionization of air radiation
All ionizing radiations	Absorbed dose (D)	Gray (Gy)	Rad	Any object	Amount of energy per unit mass absorbed by object
All ionizing radiations	Equivalent dose (EqD)	Sievert (Sv)	Rem	Body tissue	Biologic effects
All ionizing radiations	Effective dose (EfD)	Sievert (Sv)	Rem	Body tissue	Biologic effects

SUMMARY

➤ Radiation units can be expressed in the International System (SI) or the traditional system.

➤ Coulomb per kilogram (C/kg) or roentgen (R) is used for exposure in air only.

➤ The gray (Gy) or rad is used for absorbed dose (D) measurement.

➤ Equivalent dose (EqD) and effective dose (EfD) are the quantities of choice for measuring biologic effects when all types of radiation must be considered.

➤ Equivalent dose specifies how biologic damage from different types and doses of radiation will be equivalent if correct weighting factors are included.

➤ Effective dose describes the way the same effective amount of damage can be attained by giving different equivalent doses to different organs.

➤ Sievert (Sv) and rem are units used when calculating the radiation quantities, equivalent dose and effective dose.

➤ Collective effective dose (ColEfD) is used when calculating group/population radiation exposure from low doses of different sources of ionizing radiation.

➤ Person-sievert is the unit used to calculate the radiation quantity, collective effective dose.

➤ To calculate equivalent dose: $EqD = D \times W_R$.

➤ To calculate effective dose: $EfD = D \times W_R \times W_T$.

Reference

1. National Council on Radiation Protection and Measurements (NCRP): *Report #116, limitation of exposure to ionizing radiation*, Bethesda, MD, 1993, NCRP.

GENERAL DISCUSSION QUESTIONS

1. Why should diagnostic imaging personnel be familiar with standardized radiation quantities and units?

2. When, where, and how did Wilhelm Conrad Roentgen discover x-rays?

3. What type of medical problems did early radiation workers develop as a consequence of their occupational exposure?

4. What is the benefit of using the International System of Units of measurement for ionizing radiation?

5. What is a threshold dose?

6. In 1991, the ICRP revised tissue weighting factors. What data were this revision based on?

7. What radiation quantities are currently in use, and what SI and traditional units are used to relate these quantities?

8. How is the conversion of the roentgen to coulombs per kilogram accomplished?

9. What factors determine the amount of x-ray energy absorbed by a human anatomic structure?

10. When a person receives exposure from various types of ionizing radiation, what radiation quantity and what SI and traditional unit can be used for radiation protection purposes?

REVIEW QUESTIONS

1. **Which of the following was used as the *first* measure of exposure for ionizing radiation?**
   A. Roentgen
   B. Skin erythema
   C. Sievert
   D. Rad

2. **A radiation weighting factor (W_R) has been established for each of the following ionizing radiations: x-rays ($W_R = 1$), fast neutrons ($W_R = 20$), and alpha particles ($W_R = 20$). What is the *total* equivalent dose (EqD) in sievert for a person who has received the following exposures: 0.2 Gy of x-rays, 0.07 Gy of fast neutrons, and 0.3 Gy of alpha particles?**
   A. 9.4 Sv
   B. 7.6 Sv
   C. 4.3 Sv
   D. 1.9 Sv

3. **Which of the following is the unit of collective effective dose (ColEfD)?**
   A. Coulomb per kilogram-sievert
   B. Gray-sievert
   C. Person-sievert
   D. Rad-sievert

4. **The concept of tissue weighting factor (W_T) is used to do which of the following?**
   A. Account for the risk to the entire organism brought on by irradiation of individual tissues and organs
   B. Eliminate the need for determining effective dose
   C. Measure absorbed dose from all different types of ionizing radiations
   D. Modify the radiation weighting factor for different types of ionizing radiations

5. **If the absorbed dose is stated in rads, gray may be determined by performing which of the following operations?**
   A. Adding 100
   B. Dividing by 100
   C. Multiplying by 100
   D. Subtracting 100

6. **What does the traditional radiation unit, the roentgen, measure?**
   A. Equivalent dose
   B. Absorbed dose in biologic tissue
   C. Radiation exposure in air only
   D. Speed at which x-ray photons travel

7. **Which of the following radiation quantities accounts for some biologic tissues being *more* sensitive to radiation damage than other tissues?**
   A. Absorbed dose
   B. Exposure
   C. Equivalent dose
   D. Effective dose

8. **The radiation weighting factor for alpha particles is 20, and the tissue weighting factor for the lungs is 0.12. If the lungs receive an absorbed dose of 0.2 Gy from exposure to alpha particles, what is the effective dose in sievert?**
   A. 0.48 Sv
   B. 4.8 Sv
   C. 48.0 Sv
   D. 480.0 Sv

9. **If 100 people received an average effective dose of 0.35 Sv (35 rem), what is the collective effective dose?**
   A. 17.5 person-sievert (1750 man-rem)
   B. 35 person-sievert (3500 man-rem)
   C. 70 person-sievert (7000 man-rem)
   D. 285 person-sievert (28,000 man-rem)

10. **Which of the following is determined by dividing the number of rads by 100?**
    A. Number of coulombs per kilogram
    B. Number of ergs per gram
    C. Number of gray
    D. Number of sievert

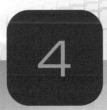

Overview of Cell Biology

KEY TERMS

anaphase
carbohydrates (saccharides)
cell division
cell membrane
chromosomes
cytoplasm
cytoplasmic organelles
deoxyribonucleic acid (DNA)
endoplasmic reticulum (ER)
genes

human genome
inorganic compounds
interphase
lipids (fats)
meiosis
messenger RNA (mRNA)
metaphase
mitochondria
mitosis (M)
nucleic acids

nucleus
organic compounds
prophase
protein synthesis
proteins
protoplasm
ribonucleic acid (RNA)
ribosomes
telophase
transfer RNA (tRNA)

OBJECTIVES

After completing this chapter, the reader will be able to perform the following:

- State the purpose for acquiring a basic knowledge of cell structure, composition, and function as a foundation for radiation biology.
- Identify and describe some important functions of the major classes of organic and inorganic compounds that exist in the cell.
- List the essential functions of water in the human body.
- Name and describe a landmark event pertaining to the human genome that occurred in 2001.
- Describe the molecular structure of deoxyribonucleic acid and explain the way it functions in the cell.
- List the various cellular components and identify their physical characteristics and functions.
- Distinguish between the two types of cell division, mitosis and meiosis, and describe each process.

Biology is a science that explores living things and life processes. Cells are the basic units of all living matter and are essential for life. The cell is the fundamental component of structure, development, growth, and life processes in the human body. Before imaging professionals can understand the effects of ionizing radiation on the human body, they must acquire a basic knowledge of cell structure, composition, and function. This chapter provides a foundation for radiation biology.

THE CELL

The human body is composed of trillions of cells. These cells exist in a multitude of different forms and perform many diverse functions for the body such as conduction of nerve impulses, contraction of muscles, support of various organs, and transportation of body fluids such as blood. Some cells are free-moving, independent units (e.g., leukocytes), and some remain in one position as part of the tissues of larger organisms throughout their lifetimes (e.g., bone marrow cells). Every mature human cell is highly specialized and has predetermined tasks to perform in support of the body. Cells move, grow, react, protect themselves and repair damage, regulate life processes, and reproduce. To ensure efficient cell operation, the body must provide food as a source of raw material for the release of energy, supply oxygen to help break down the food, and have enough water to transport inorganic substances such as calcium and sodium into and out of the cell. In turn, proper cell function enables the body to maintain homeostasis or equilibrium, which is the ability to function in a normal manner despite any changes the body may undergo due to outside influences such as stress, exercise, injury, or disease.

In summary, cells are engaged in an ongoing process of obtaining energy and converting it to support their vital functions. They absorb molecular nutrients through the cell membrane and use these nutrients to produce energy and synthesize molecules. If exposure to outside influences such as ionizing radiation damages the components involved in molecular synthesis beyond repair, then cells either behave abnormally or die.

CELL CHEMICAL COMPOSITION

Protoplasm

Cells are made of **protoplasm,** the chemical building material for all living things. This substance carries on the complex process of metabolism, the reception and processing of food and oxygen, and the elimination of waste products. Metabolism enables the cell to perform the vital functions of synthesizing proteins and producing energy.

Protoplasm consists of organic compounds (those compounds that contain carbon) and inorganic materials (compounds that do not contain carbon) either dissolved or suspended in water. The biomolecules that compose protoplasm are formed from 24 elements, with the four primary elements involved being carbon, hydrogen, oxygen, and nitrogen. When combined with phosphorus and sulfur, they compose the essential major organic compounds: proteins, carbohydrates, lipids, and nucleic acids. These compounds are discussed later in this chapter.

The most important inorganic substances are water and mineral salts (electrolytes). Water aids in sustaining life and is the most abundant inorganic compound in the body. The essential functions of water are listed in Box 4-1. These functions are also discussed later in

---

BOX 4-1

Life-Sustaining Role of Water in the Human Body

- Acts as the medium in which acids, bases, and salts are dissolved
- Functions as a solvent by dissolving chemical substances in the cell
- Functions as a transport vehicle for material the cell uses or eliminates
- Maintains a constant body core temperature of 98.6° F (37° C)
- Provides a cushion for vital organs such as the brain and lungs
- Regulates concentration of dissolved substances
- Lubricates the digestive system
- Lubricates skeletal articulations (joints)

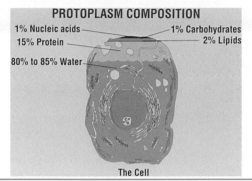

FIG. 4-1. Depending on cell type, water normally accounts for 80% to 85% of protoplasm. (From *Mosby's radiographic instructional series,* St. Louis, 1999, Mosby.)

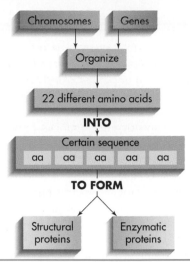

FIG. 4-2. Chromosomes and genes organize the 22 different amino acids into certain sequences to form the different structural and enzymatic proteins.

this chapter. Depending on cell type, water normally accounts for 80% to 85% of protoplasm (Fig. 4-1). Mineral salts exist in smaller quantities and also are of vital importance in sustaining cell life.

Organic Compounds

The four major classes of **organic compounds** (proteins, carbohydrates, lipids [fats], and nucleic acids) all contain carbon (Box 4-2). Carbon is the basic constituent of all organic matter. By combining with hydrogen, nitrogen, and oxygen, it makes life possible. Of all the organic compounds, protein contains the most carbon.

Proteins

Proteins constitute about 15% of cell content (see Fig. 4-1). They are essential for growth, the construction of new body tissue (including acellular tissue such as hair and nails), and the repair of injured or debilitated tissue. Proteins are formed when amino acids combine into long, chainlike molecular complexes. In these

complexes, a chemical link called a peptide bond connects each amino acid. Protein production, or **protein synthesis,** involves 22 different amino acids. The order of arrangement of these amino acids determines the precise function of each protein molecule, and the types of protein molecules that any given cell contains determine the characteristics of that cell. Chromosomes and genes organize the amino acids into different orderings to make different types of proteins (Fig. 4-2).

Structural and Enzymatic Proteins Structural proteins such as those found in muscle provide the body with its shape and form and are a source of heat and energy. Enzymatic proteins function as organic catalysts, agents that affect the rate or speed of chemical reactions without being altered themselves. Enzymatic proteins (sometimes just called "enzymes") control the cell's various physiologic activities. Enzymes cause an increase in cellular activity that in turn causes biochemical reactions to occur more rapidly to meet the needs of the cell. Hence, proper cell functioning depends on enzymes.

Repair Enzymes Many of the proteins produced in the ribosome are enzymes, which cause vital chemical reactions to take place within the cell at the appropriate time. Some of the enzymes produced are called

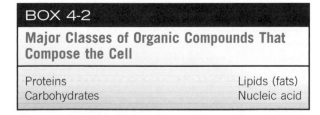

BOX 4-2	
Major Classes of Organic Compounds That Compose the Cell	
Proteins	Lipids (fats)
Carbohydrates	Nucleic acid

repair enzymes. These enzymes can mend damaged molecules and are therefore capable of helping the cell to recover from a small amount of radiation-induced damage. Both the catalytic and repair capabilities of enzymes are of vital importance to the survival of the cell.

Repair enzymes work effectively in both the diagnostic and therapeutic energy ranges. However, if the radiation damage is excessive because of the delivered equivalent dose, the damage will be too severe for repair enzymes to have a positive effect. When ionizing radiation is used for therapeutic purposes to destroy malignant cells, an attempt is also made to spare healthy surrounding tissue. In radiation therapy this concept is referred to as a "therapeutic ratio," wherein there is an attempt to deliver enough radiation to kill cancerous cells (i.e., make them not repairable by repair enzymes) while delivering a less than cell-killing, and therefore repairable, equivalent dose to surrounding noncancerous tissue structure.

Hormones and Antibodies In addition to providing structure and support for the body, proteins also may function as hormones and antibodies. Hormones are chemical secretions manufactured by various endocrine glands and carried by the bloodstream to influence the activities of other parts of the body. For example, hormones produced by the thyroid gland located in the neck control metabolism throughout the body. Hormones also regulate body functions such as growth and development.

Antibodies are protein molecules produced by specialized cells in the bone marrow called B lymphocytes. Lymphocytes are white blood cells involved in the body's immune reactions. Antibodies are produced when other lymphocytes in the body, known as T lymphocytes, detect the presence of molecules that do not belong to the body. These foreign objects (e.g., bacteria, flu viruses) are called antigens. Although the skin of the body is the initial barrier to any outside invasion by pathogens or the like, once it has been penetrated, the body's primary defense mechanism against infection and disease are the antibodies that chemically attack any foreign invaders or antigens.

Carbohydrates

Carbohydrates, also referred to as **saccharides,** make up about 1% of cell content (see Fig. 4-1). They

---

BOX 4-3

Simple to Complex Carbohydrates

Monosaccharides

$C_6H_{12}O_6$

Disaccharides

$C_6H_{12}O_6 + C_6H_{12}O_6$

Polysaccharides

$C_6H_{12}O_6 + C_6H_{12}O_6 + C_6H_{12}O_6 + C_6H_{12}O_6$

---

include starches and various sugars. Carbohydrates range from simple to complex compounds (Box 4-3), even though they are composed of only carbon, hydrogen, and oxygen. Simple sugars such as glucose, fructose, and galactose have six carbon atoms and six molecules of water (e.g., glucose has the chemical formula $C_6H_{12}O_6$). Glucose is the primary energy source for the cell. Because it is a simple sugar, it is called a monosaccharide. Other sugars that have two units of a simple sugar linked together are called disaccharides. Sucrose (cane sugar) is an example of a disaccharide. Both monosaccharides and disaccharides are relatively small molecules. Polysaccharides contain several or many molecules of simple sugar. Plant starches and animal glycogen are the two most important polysaccharides. Through the process of metabolism, the body breaks these down into simpler sugars for energy.

Carbohydrates, simply described as chains of sugar molecules, function as short-term energy warehouses for the body. Their primary purpose is to provide fuel for cell metabolism. Although carbohydrates are found throughout the human body, they are most abundant in the liver and in muscle tissue. They also are important structural parts of cell walls and intercellular materials.

Lipids

Lipids, also referred to as **fats** or fatlike substances, constitute about 2% of cell content (see Fig. 4-1). They are made up of a molecule of glycerin (Box 4-4) and three molecules of fatty acid. When glucose is broken down in the body during respiration, fats are among the generated intermediate products. When

SUGARS

D-ribose   D-2-deoxyribose

PURINES

Adenine (A)   Guanine (G)

PYRIMIDINES

Cytosine (C)   Uracil (U)   Thymine (T)

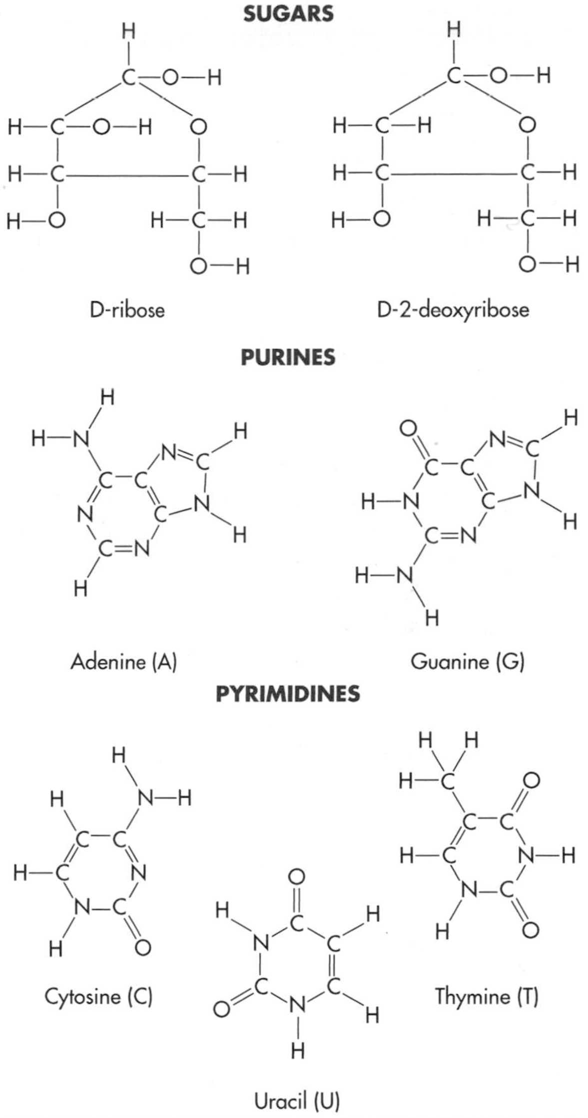

FIG. 4-3. The components of nucleic acid (H = hydrogen, C = carbon, N = nitrogen, O = oxygen). Sugars are strung together with phosphate groups, and a base is attached to each sugar. DNA uses D-2-deoxyribose sugar, and RNA uses D-ribose. Both nucleic acids use the same two purines, but thymine (T) in DNA is replaced by uracil (U) in RNA.

BOX 4-4

Lipid Formation

Fats or lipids
↑
1 molecule of glycerin + 3 molecules of fatty acid
↑
Carbon, oxygen, hydrogen

---

some of these fats combine with an acidic group of atoms (e.g., the carboxyl group, COOH), a fatty acid is formed. An example of a fatty acid is CH_3COOH, which is commonly known as acetic acid. Fatty acids are constituents of amino acids from which proteins are built. Lipids are organic macromolecules, large molecules built from smaller chemical structures. They are the structural parts of cell membranes. Lipids are present in all body tissue and perform the following functions for the body: (1) act as reservoirs for the long-term storage of energy, (2) insulate and guard the body against the environment, (3) support and protect organs such as the eyes and kidneys, (4) provide essential substances necessary for growth and development, (5) lubricate the joints, and (6) assist in the digestive process.

Nucleic Acids

Nucleic acids, which compose about 1% of the cell (see Fig. 4-1), are very large, complex macromolecules (Fig. 4-3). The much smaller structures that make up nucleic acids are called nucleotides. Each nucleotide is a unit formed from a nitrogen-containing organic base, a five-carbon sugar molecule (deoxyribose), and a phosphate molecule.

Deoxyribonucleic Acid (DNA) and Ribonucleic Acid (RNA) Cells contain two types of nucleic acids that are important to human metabolism: **deoxyribonucleic acid (DNA)** and **ribonucleic acid (RNA).** The DNA macromolecule is composed of two long sugar-phosphate chains, which twist around each other in a double-helix configuration and are linked by pairs of nitrogenous organic bases at the sugar molecules of the chain to form a tightly coiled structure resembling a twisted ladder or spiral staircase. The sugar-phosphate compounds are the rails, and the pairs

of nitrogenous bases, which consist of complementary chemicals, are the steps or rungs of the DNA ladder-like structure (Fig. 4-4). Hydrogen bonds attach the bases to each other, joining the two side rails of the DNA ladder.

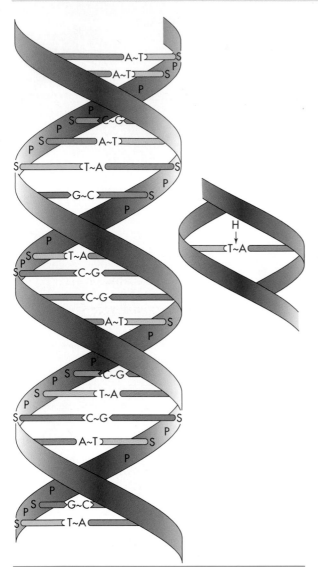

FIG. 4-4. Diagram of a DNA macromolecule that illustrates its twisted ladderlike or spiral-staircase-like configuration. Alternating sugar and phosphate molecules form the side rails of the ladder, and the nitrogenous organic bases, which consist of the complementary chemicals adenine *(A),* thymine *(T),* guanine *(G),* and cytosine *(C),* form the rungs or steps. A hydrogen bond joins the bases together.

Nitrogenous organic bases in DNA The

four nitrogenous organic bases in DNA macromolecules are adenine (A), cytosine (C), guanine (G), and thymine (T). Adenine and guanine are compounds called *purines*, and the compounds cytosine and

thymine are classified as *pyrimidines*. A significant characteristic of the organic bases is that purines only link with pyrimidines in certain specific combinations; more precisely, adenine always bonds only with thymine and cytosine bonds only with guanine. This characteristic is the reason the two strands of DNA are described as complementary.

DNA, the master chemical DNA, is sometimes referred to as the master chemical, because it contains all the information the cell needs to function. It carries the genetic information necessary for cell replication and regulates all cellular activity to direct protein synthesis. DNA determines a person's characteristics by regulating the sequence of amino acids in the person's constituent proteins during the synthesis of these proteins. These sequences of amino acids are determined by the order of adenine-thymine and cytosine-guanine base pairs in the DNA macromolecules. Therefore, it is the sequence of nitrogenous base pairs in the DNA molecule that constitutes the *genetic code*. Different sequences of amino acids produce proteins with different functions. Protein characteristics determine cell characteristics, and cell characteristics ultimately determine the characteristics of the entire individual. All the information necessary to construct and maintain a living organism is written in the "genetic code book" of DNA—the letters, words, and sentences are composed of the nitrogenous organic bases. What makes one person's DNA different from another's? Differences in base pair arrangements, which result in the production of different types of proteins to be made in different amounts at different times.

Messenger RNA (mRNA) Because DNA is found mostly in the cell nucleus, it cannot directly influence cellular activity such as growth and differentiation, which occur in the cytoplasm (the part of the cell that lies outside the nucleus). Instead, DNA regulates cellular activity indirectly, transmitting its genetic information outside the cell nucleus by reproducing itself in the form of **messenger RNA (mRNA),** which can leave the cell nucleus and, once in the cytoplasm, directs the process of making proteins out of amino acids.

DNA serves as a prototype for mRNA. Messenger RNA differs from DNA in two important ways: (1) Messenger RNA contains in its backbone the sugar molecule, ribose, which differs only in the presence of an extra "O-H" bond from the sugar molecule, deoxyribose, found in the backbone of DNA. (2) In mRNA a pyrimidine base called uracil (U) replaces the thymine that is found in DNA. An mRNA macromolecule resembles one half of a DNA macromolecule. It appears as a single strand of the DNA ladderlike configuration, the ladder being severed in half lengthwise (Fig. 4-5).

Transfer RNA (tRNA) Macromolecules of mRNA carry their genetic codes in their sequences of nitrogenous organic bases (e.g., U, U, C, C, A, U, G) from the cell nucleus to the ribosomes where proteins are manufactured. Here the mRNA transfers its genetic code to another kind of RNA molecule called the **transfer RNA (tRNA).** This tRNA combines with individual amino acids from different areas of the cell and attaches them to the ribosomes, where the amino acids are arranged in specific orders to form chainlike protein molecules. Each tRNA molecule is coded for a particular amino acid. Because each of the 22 different amino acids has an associated tRNA, at least 22 different types of tRNA exist. The ribosomes travel along the mRNA, linking tRNA and its corresponding amino acids in the correct order so that the proteins necessary to provide for the needs of the cell are produced (Fig. 4-6).

Chromosomes and genes Chromosomes are tiny rod-shaped bodies, which under a microscope appear to be long threadlike structures that become visible in dividing cells. Chromosomes are composed of DNA. A normal human being has 46 different chromosomes (23 pairs) in each somatic (nonreproductive) cell. Individual male and female reproductive cells also known as germ cells exist singly. Thus, each of these germ cells has only 23 chromosomes, which pair up to form a full set of 46 chromosomes when a sperm fertilizes an egg cell. The DNA that makes up every chromosome is divided into hundreds of segments called **genes.** Each gene, because of the ordering of its nitrogenous base pairs, contains information responsible for directing cytoplasmic activities, controlling growth and development of the cell, and transmitting hereditary information. Thus, genes are the basic units of heredity (Fig. 4-7). They control the formation of proteins in every cell through the intricate process of genetic coding.

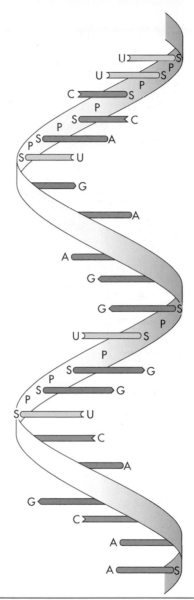

FIG. 4-5. Messenger RNA *(mRNA)* resembles one half of a DNA macromolecule. It appears as a single strand (one side rail) of the DNA ladderlike configuration, the ladder being severed in half lengthwise. Uracil *(U)* replaces thymine *(T)* as one of the nitrogenous organic bases in the mRNA molecule.

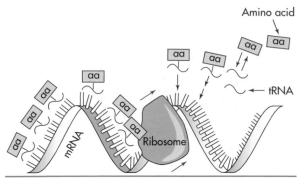

FIG. 4-6. Ribosomes, the cell's protein factories, travel along the mRNA rails, linking tRNA and its corresponding amino acids in the proper sequences to produce the proteins appropriate for the needs of the cell.

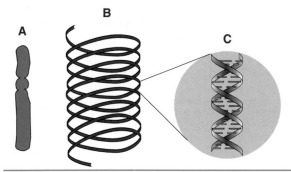

FIG. 4-7. A chromosome viewed under a microscope appears rod shaped **(A)**; when further magnified, a chromosome appears as a tightly wound spiral structure **(B)** composed of hundreds of genes, which is a segment of the DNA macromolecule **(C)**.

The human genome The total amount of genetic material (DNA) contained within the chromosomes of a human being is called the **human genome.** The process of locating and identifying the genes in the genome is called *mapping.* A landmark event occurred in 2001 when after years of intense effort two rival groups succeeded in deciphering the human genome. Essentially, they uncovered the entire sequence of DNA base pairs (i.e., all of the "rungs" of the DNA ladder structure) on all 46 chromosomes. This major milestone in biology and medicine was accomplished by Celera Genomics (a private company in Rockville, Maryland) and the Inter-

national Human Genome Sequencing Consortium, a group of academic centers funded mostly by the National Institutes of Health and the Wellcome Trust of London.[1]

The groups found that there are 2.9 billion base pairs in the human genome and that these base pairs are arranged into approximately 30,000 genes. It is estimated that these genes are capable of producing at least 90,000 different proteins.

As amazing as the accomplishment is, it remains only the first step toward a complete understanding of the biochemical processes that occur in health and disease. The challenge in interpreting the map of the human genome is similar to that of a building contractor finding a list of all the things that are needed to build a house but not having a blueprint that shows how often or in what order to do things. Over the next few decades, the great challenge will be to answer questions such as the following:

1. What determines when genes will produce proteins and when genes will not?
2. In what order are various proteins produced during development and throughout life?
3. What genes cause some individuals to be susceptible to a certain disease?
4. Is it possible to learn how to deactivate those genes and turn on other genes that provide resistance?
5. Are there genes that make some people more or less sensitive to the effects of ionizing radiation?
6. Can we use our new insight into the human genome to both detect and properly correct the defective genes that are the root of genetically transmitted disease?

The Human Genome Project has given us data that allow us to work on problems in molecular biology such as those listed here. It is surprising, then, to realize that the primary stimulus for initiating the project[2] can be traced to an urgency to attack radiobiologic questions that were raised during a scientific conference held in March of 1984 at Hiroshima, Japan. At this conference, participants repeatedly stressed the need to use molecular DNA tools to be able to directly detect radiation exposure–induced mutations that could be inherited from the survivors of the atomic bomb blasts. Another conference was held some 9 months later in Alta, Utah. At this meeting, it was concluded that available knowledge was still insufficient to detect such mutations, which could be as few as 30 per individual genome per generation, and that only a massive effort, designed to improve the technology by orders of magnitude, would suffice for unraveling the human genome to the required degree. The intense discussions and ideas put forth at this meeting by the attendees were what ultimately led to the establishment of the Human Genome Project.

Inorganic Compounds

Inorganic compounds are compounds that do not contain carbon. The inorganic compounds found in the body occur in nature independent of living things; they are acids, bases, and salts (electrolytes). Acids are hydrogen-containing compounds such as HNO_3 (nitric acid) that can attack and dissolve metal. Bases are alkali or alkaline earth OH compounds such as $Mg(OH)_2$ (otherwise known as milk of magnesia) that can neutralize acids. Salts are chemical compounds resulting from the action of an acid and a base on one another. Salts are sometimes referred to as electrolytes. Water is the primary inorganic substance contained in the human body; it comprises approximately 80% to 85% of the body's weight (Fig. 4-8).

Function of Water Within and Outside of the Cell

Within the cell, water is indispensable for metabolic activities because it is the medium in which the chemical reactions that are the basis of these activities occur. It also acts as a solvent, keeping compounds dissolved where they can more easily interact and where their concentration may be regulated. Outside the cell, water functions as a transport vehicle for materials the cell uses or eliminates. In addition, water is responsible for maintaining a constant body core temperature of 98.6° F (37° C) (Fig. 4-9) while at the same time serving to lubricate both the digestive system and skeletal articulations (joints). Organs such as the brain and lungs are also protected by a cushion of water.

Function of Mineral Salts Within the Cell

Salts such as sodium (Na) and potassium (K) keep the correct proportion of water in the cell. Mineral salts are necessary for proper cell performance, the creation of energy, and the conduction of impulses along nerves. The constituents of salts exist as ions (particles carrying a positive or negative electric charge) in the cell. These ions via chemical reactions cause materials to be altered, broken down, and recombined to form new substances. Potassium (K) contributes most of the positive ions (cations) present in cells, whereas phosphorus (P) contributes the majority of negative ions (anions). Potassium is of primary importance in

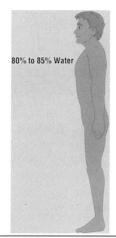

80% to 85% Water

FIG. 4-8. Water constitutes approximately 80% to 85% of the body's weight. (From *Mosby's radiographic instructional series,* St Louis, 1999, Mosby.)

As a transportation system to and from cells

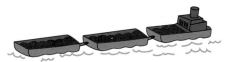

As a medium to dissolve and regulate acids, bases, and salts

As a means of maintaining a constant body temperature

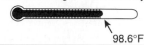

98.6°F

FIG. 4-9. Water's role outside the cell. (From *Mosby's radiographic instructional series,* St Louis, 1999, Mosby.)

maintaining adequate amounts of intracellular fluid. Water tends to move across cell surfaces or membranes into areas in which a high concentration of ions is present. This motion is referred to as osmosis. Thus, by balancing the concentration of potassium ions (as well as sodium [Na] and chloride [Cl] ions), the cell regulates the amount of fluid it contains. By maintaining the correct proportion of water in the cell, osmotic pressure is maintained. Potassium also aids in maintaining acid-base balance, a state of equilibrium or stability between acids and bases.

CELL STRUCTURE

The normal cell (Fig. 4-10) has a number of components:
1. Cell membrane
2. Cytoplasm
3. Cytoplasmic organelles
   a. Endoplasmic reticulum
   b. Golgi apparatus or complex
   c. Mitochondria

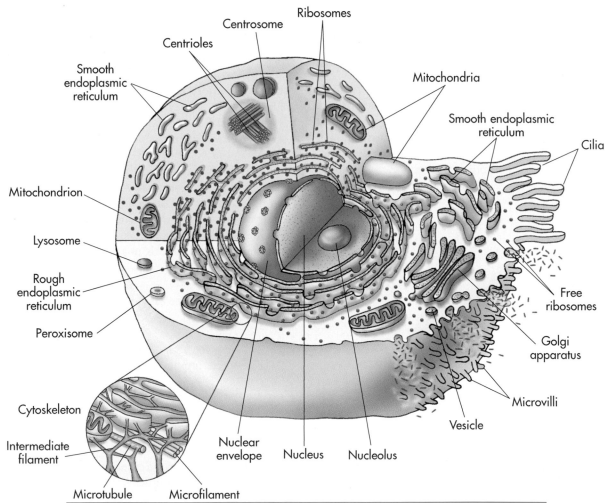

FIG. 4-10. Diagram of a typical cell, demonstrating its basic components. (From Thibodeau A: *Anatomy and physiology,* ed 5, St Louis, 2003, Mosby.)

d. Lysosomes
e. Ribosomes
f. Centrosomes
4. Nucleus

3. Packages substances for distribution to other areas of the cell or to various sites in the body through the circulation
4. Eliminates waste products

Cell Membrane

The **cell membrane** is a frail, semipermeable structure encasing and surrounding the human cell. It functions as a barricade to protect cellular contents from the outside environment and controls the passage of water and other materials into and out of the cell. Because the cell membrane allows penetration only by certain types of substances and regulates the speed at which these substances travel within the cell, it plays a primary role in the cell's transport system. When a substance moves through the cell membrane by osmosis, the transport system is classified as passive because the cell uses no energy to maintain the concentration. When the movement of a substance across a cell membrane is controlled more by the properties and powers of the cell membrane than it is by the relative concentrations of particles in fluid, the transport system is classified as active. In active transport, the cell must expend energy to pump substances into and out of it.

Cytoplasm

Cytoplasm is the protoplasm that exists outside the cell's nucleus. It is primarily composed of water but also contains proteins, carbohydrates, lipids, salts, and minerals. The cytoplasm makes up the majority of the cell and contains large amounts of all the cell's molecular components with the exception of DNA. All cellular metabolic functions occur in the cytoplasm. Functioning like a factory, it performs the following major functions:

1. Accepts and builds up unrefined materials and assembles from these materials new substances such as carbohydrates, lipids, and proteins; the assembly of larger molecules from smaller ones is known as anabolism
2. Breaks down organic materials to produce energy (catabolism)

Cytoplasmic Organelles

The cytoplasm contains all the miniature cellular components that enable the cell to function in a highly organized manner. These little organs of the cell are collectively referred to as **cytoplasmic organelles.** They consist of tiny tubules (small tubes), vesicles (small cavities or sacs containing liquid), granules (small insoluble nonmembranous particles found in cytoplasm), and fibrils (minute fibers or strands that are frequently part of a compound fiber). Together these structures perform the major functions of the cell in a systematized way. DNA, which is located in the cell nucleus, separated from the cytoplasm, determines the function of each cytoplasmic organelle. Messenger ribonucleic acid (mRNA) carries the DNA code from the nucleus into the cytoplasm.

Endoplasmic Reticulum

The **endoplasmic reticulum (ER)** is a vast irregular network of tubules and vesicles spreading and interconnecting in all directions throughout the cytoplasm. It enables the cell to communicate with the extracellular environment and transfer food and molecules from one part of the cell to another. Thus, the ER functions as the highway system of the cell. For example, mRNA travels from the nucleus to different locations in the cytoplasm through the ER.

Cells have two types of ER: rough surfaced (granular) and smooth (agranular). If numerous ribosomes (the small, spherical organelles that are the sites where mRNA and tRNA assemble amino acids into proteins) are present on the surface of the ER, the surface is rough or granular. If they are not present, the surface is smooth or agranular. The "smooth" or "rough" distinction refers to the ER's appearance when viewed with an electron microscope. The cell type determines the type of ER. For example, cells that actively manufacture proteins for export, such as the pancreatic cells, which produce insulin, need more ribosomes and therefore have a lot of rough or granular ER. A lesser amount of rough or granular ER is found in cells that synthesize proteins mainly for their own use.

Golgi Apparatus or Complex

The Golgi apparatus or complex extends from the nucleus to the cell membrane and consists of tubes and a tiny sac located near the nucleus. It unites large carbohydrate molecules and then combines them with proteins to form glycoproteins. When the cell manufactures enzymes and hormones, the Golgi apparatus concentrates, packages, and transports them through the cell membrane so that they can exit the cell, enter the bloodstream, and be carried to the areas of the body where they are required.

Mitochondria

Large, double-membranous, oval or bean-shaped structures called **mitochondria** function as the "powerhouses" of the cell. They contain highly organized enzymes in their inner membranes that produce energy for cellular activity by breaking down nutrients such as carbohydrates, fats, and proteins through the process of oxidative metabolism. Oxidation is any chemical reaction in which an atom loses electrons. The substance that loses electrons is said to have been oxidized. The oxidation of iron produces iron oxide, commonly known as rust. Metabolism is the breaking down of large molecules into smaller ones. So oxidative metabolism is the breaking down of large molecules into smaller ones through the process of oxidation. Some of the enzymes contained within the mitochondria are essential in the production of adenosine triphosphate (ATP), an energy-releasing phosphate compound essential for sustaining life. This compound plays a role in active transport within the cell. In active transport, molecules are moved through cell membranes regardless of the relative concentrations of particles. This requires energy, which is supplied by ATP. The number of mitochondria in cells varies from a few hundred to several thousand. The greatest number is found in cells exhibiting the greatest activity.

Lysosomes

Lysosomes are small pealike sacs or spherical bodies that are of great importance for digestion within the cytoplasm. They contain a group of different digestive enzymes, and their primary function appears to be the breaking down of unwanted large molecules that either penetrate into the cell through microscopic channels or are drawn in by the cell membrane itself. If lysosomes fail in their cellular "garbage disposal" tasks, the resulting accumulation of large molecules may ultimately obstruct normal functions in organs. Lysosomes are sometimes referred to as "suicide bags," because the enzymes they contain can break down and digest not only proteins and certain carbohydrates, but also the cell itself should the lysosome's surrounding membrane break. Exposure to radiation may induce such a rupture. When this occurs, the cell is likely to die.

Ribosomes

Ribosomes are small spherical organelles that attach to the ER. They consist of two-thirds RNA and one-third protein. Ribosomes are commonly referred to as the cell's "protein factories," because their job is to manufacture (synthesize) the various proteins that cells require using the blueprints provided by mRNA. Their role in the assembly of amino acids into proteins was described earlier in this chapter.

Centrosomes

Centrosomes are located in the center of the cell near the nucleus. They contain the centrioles, which are pairs of small, hollow, cylindrical structures believed to play a part in the formation of the mitotic spindle during cell division. Cell division is discussed later in this chapter.

Nucleus

Separated from the other parts of the cell by a double-walled membrane (nuclear envelope), the **nucleus** forms the heart of the living cell. It is a spherical mass of protoplasm containing the genetic material, DNA, and protein. These two nuclear components are arranged in long threads called chromatin. When a cell divides, this genetic-containing material contracts into tiny rod-shaped bodies called chromosomes.

The nucleus also contains at least one rounded body called the *nucleolus*, which manufactures and

TABLE 4-1

Summary of Cell Components

Title	Site	Activity
Cell membrane	Cytoplasm	Functions as a barricade to protect cellular contents from their environment and controls the passage of water and other materials into and out of the cell; performs many additional functions such as elimination of wastes and refining of material for energy through breakdown of the materials
Endoplasmic reticulum	Cytoplasm	Enables the cell to communicate with the extracellular environment and transfers food from one part of the cell to another
Golgi apparatus	Cytoplasm	Unites large carbohydrate molecules and combines them with proteins to form glycoproteins and transports enzymes and hormones through the cell membrane so that they can exit the cell, enter the bloodstream, and be carried to areas of the body in which they are required
Mitochondria	Cytoplasm	Produce energy for cellular activity by breaking down nutrients through a process of oxidation
Lysosomes	Cytoplasm	Dispose of large particles such as bacteria and food as well as smaller particles; also contain hydrolytic enzymes that can break down and digest proteins, certain carbohydrates, and the cell itself if the lysosome's surrounding membrane breaks
Ribosomes	Cytoplasm	Manufacture the various proteins that cells require
Centrosomes	Cytoplasm	Believed to play some part in the formation of the mitotic spindle during cell division
DNA	Nucleus	Contains the genetic material, controls cell division and multiplication and also biochemical reactions that occur within the living cell
Nucleolus	Nucleus	Holds a large amount of RNA

holds a large amount of RNA and protein. The nucleus controls cell division and multiplication and the biochemical reactions that occur within the cell. By directing protein synthesis, the nucleus plays an essential role in active transport, metabolism, growth, and heredity. A summary of cell components is presented in Table 4-1.

CELL DIVISION

Cell division is the multiplication process whereby one cell divides to form two or more cells (Fig. 4-11). Mitosis (M) and meiosis are the two types of cell division that occur in the body. When somatic cells (all cells in the human body except the germ cells) divide, they undergo mitosis. Genetic cells (the oogonium, or female germ cell, and the spermatogonium, or male germ cell) undergo meiosis.

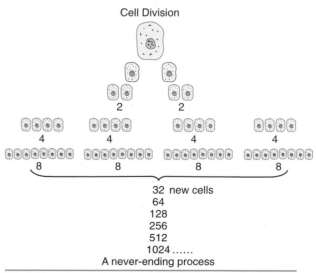

FIG. 4-11. Cell division is the multiplication process whereby one cell divides to form two or more cells. (From *Mosby's radiographic instructional series,* St Louis, 1999, Mosby.)

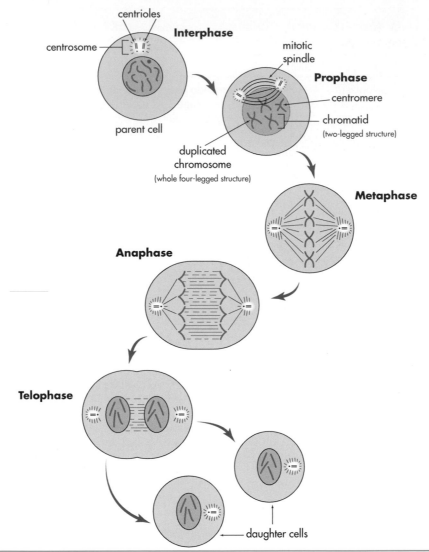

FIG. 4-12. Diagram of mitosis. An animal cell with four chromosomes first multiplies (duplicates its DNA) and then divides, forming two new daughter cells, each of which contains exactly the same genetic material as the parent cell.

Mitosis

Through the process of **mitosis (M)** (Fig. 4-12), a parent cell divides to form two daughter cells identical to the parent cell. This process results in an approximately equal distribution of all cellular material between the two daughter cells. The cellular life cycle may be pictured as in Fig. 4-13. Different phases of cell growth, maturation, and division occur in each cell cycle. Four distinct phases of the cellular life cycle are identifiable: M (mitosis phase), G_1 (pre-DNA synthesis phase), S (synthesis phase), and G_2 (post-DNA synthesis phase). Additionally, mitosis (M) can be divided into four subphases: prophase, metaphase, anaphase, and telophase.

Mitosis is the division phase of the cellular life cycle. It is actually the last phase of the cycle. After it has commenced, it takes only about 1 hour to complete in

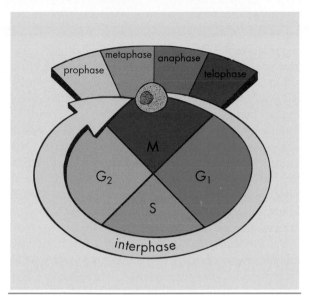

FIG. 4-13. The cellular life cycle may be pictured as four distinct, identifiable phases: M, G₁, S, and G₂. M may be divided into four subphases: prophase, metaphase, anaphase, and telophase. (From Bushong SC: *Radiologic science for technologists: physics, biology and protection,* ed 8, St Louis, 2004, Mosby.)

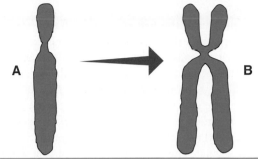

FIG. 4-14. While the S phase is taking place, the chromosome changes in shape from a figure with two chromatids connected to a centromere to a figure with four chromatids connected to a centromere. **A,** Two-chromatid figure. **B,** Four-chromatid figure.

all cells. Interphase, the period of cell growth that occurs before actual mitosis, consists of three intervals: G_1, S, and G_2. G_1, the earliest, is the phase between reproductive events. It is the gap in the growth of the cell that occurs between mitosis and DNA synthesis. Depending on the type of cells involved, this interval may take just a few minutes or it may take several hours. G_1 is designated as the pre-DNA-synthesis phase. During G_1 a form of RNA is synthesized in the cells that are to reproduce. This RNA is needed before actual DNA synthesis can efficiently begin. S is the actual DNA synthesis period. While in S phase, each DNA molecule is copied and then divided (replicated) into corresponding daughter DNA molecules. The chromosome changes in shape from a figure with two chromatids (highly coiled duplicate strands of DNA) connected to a centromere (region on a chromosome serving as a junction point) to a figure with four chromatids connected to a centromere (Fig. 4-14). Two pairs of chromatids with exactly the same DNA substance and form result. When compared with G_1 and G_2, the S phase is relatively long. It can take up to 15

hours. G_2 is the post-DNA-manufacturing interval in the cellular life cycle. It is a relatively short period occupying approximately 1 to 5 hours of the whole cycle. During this phase, cells manufacture certain proteins and RNA molecules needed to enter and complete the next mitosis. When G_2 is complete, cells enter the first phase of mitosis, the prophase, and the process of division commences.

Interphase

Interphase is the period of cell growth that occurs before actual mitosis. As previously stated, G_1, S, and G_2 are the phases of the cell cycle that compose interphase. Cells are not yet undergoing division during this phase. If a cell is viewed through a microscope during interphase, the nucleus looks somewhat odd. DNA may be visualized by using a specific stain designed to make it visible; it appears as clumps of material shaped in different patterns. These patterns are seen throughout the nucleus. Individual chromosomes are not visible during interphase. During the synthesis portion of interphase (S), each chromosome reproduces itself and splits longitudinally, forming two chromatids attached to each other at the centromere. Hence, the cell's DNA molecules have duplicated in preparation for cell division. Genetic information also is transcribed into different kinds of RNA molecules such as mRNA and tRNA, which, after passing into the cytoplasm, translate the genetic information by promoting the synthesis of specific proteins.

Prophase

During **prophase,** the first phase of cell division, the nucleus enlarges, the DNA complex (the chromatid network of threads) coils up more tightly, and the chromatids become more visible on stained microscopic slides. Chromosomes enlarge, and the DNA begins to take structural form. The nuclear membrane disappears, and the centrioles (small hollow cylindrical structures) migrate to opposite sides of the cell and begin to regulate the formation of the mitotic spindle, the delicate fibers that are attached to the centrioles and extend from one side of the cell to the other across the equator of the cell.

Metaphase

As **metaphase** begins, the fibers collectively referred to as the mitotic spindle form between the centrioles. Each chromosome (which now consists of two chromatids) lines up in the center or equator of the cell attached by its centromere to the mitotic spindle. This forms the equatorial plate. The centromeres then duplicate, and each chromatid attaches itself individually to the spindle. At the end of metaphase, the chromatids are strung out along the mitotic spindle much like laundry hung on a clothesline. During metaphase, cell division can be stopped and visible chromosomes can be examined under a microscope. Chromosome damage caused by radiation can then be evaluated.

Anaphase

During **anaphase,** the duplicate centromeres migrate in opposite directions along the mitotic spindle, carrying the chromatids to opposite sides of the cell. The cell is now ready to begin the last phase of division.

Telophase

During **telophase,** the chromatids undergo changes in appearance by uncoiling and becoming long, loosely spiraled threads. Simultaneously the nuclear membrane re-forms, and two nuclei (one for each new daughter cell) appear. The cytoplasm also divides (cytokinesis) near the equator of the cell to surround each new nucleus. After this cell division completes, each daughter cell has a complete cell membrane and contains exactly the same amount of genetic material (46 chromosomes) as the parent cell.

Meiosis

Meiosis (Fig. 4-15) is a special type of cell division that reduces the number of chromosomes in each daughter cell to half the number of chromosomes in the parent cell. Male and female germ cells, or sperm and ova, of sexually mature individuals each begin meiosis with 46 chromosomes. However, before the male and female germ cells unite to produce a new organism, the number of chromosomes in each must be reduced by one half to ensure that the daughter cells (zygotes) formed when they unite will contain only the normal number of 46 chromosomes. Hence, meiosis is really a process of reduction division (Fig. 4-16).

Paradoxically, meiosis begins with a doubling of the amount of genetic material; as in mitosis, DNA replication occurs during interphase. As a result of DNA replication, each one-chromatid chromosome duplicates, forming a two-chromatid chromosome. This means that sperm and egg cells begin meiosis with twice the amount of genetic material as the original parent cell. Thus, at the beginning of meiosis, the number of chromosomes increases from $2n$ to $4n$ ($n = 23$).

The various phases of meiosis are similar to those occurring in mitosis. The major difference between the two types of cell division begins at the end of telophase. In meiosis, after the parent germ cell has formed two daughter cells, each of which (in human beings) contains 46 chromosomes, the daughter cells divide without DNA replication; chromosome duplication does not occur at this phase of division. These two successive divisions result in the formation of four granddaughter cells, each of which contains only 23 chromosomes. This means that the proper number of 46 chromosomes will be produced when a female ovum containing 23 chromosomes is fertilized by a male sperm containing 23 chromosomes.

During meiosis, the sister chromatids exchange some chromosomal material (genes). This process, called cross over, results in changes in genetic composition and traits that can be passed on to future generations.

Multiple Births

There are two ways that multiple births can occur during one pregnancy. One way is if a fertilized ovum

MEIOSES

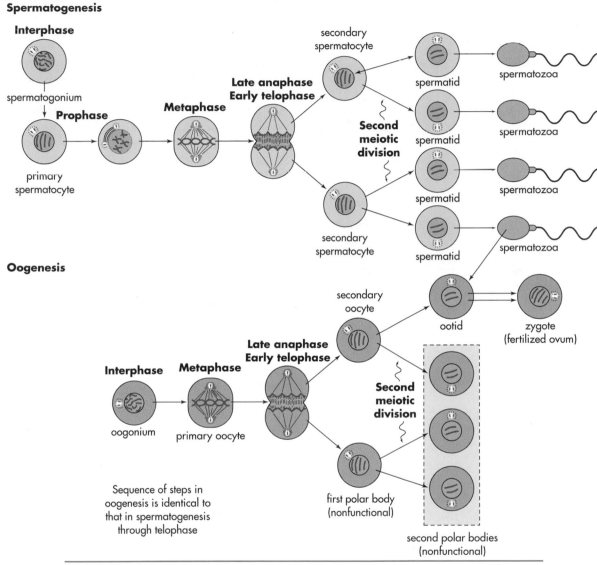

FIG. 4-15. Diagram of meiosis. Four cells result from one germ cell. In spermatogenesis, four spermatids become mature spermatozoa. In oogenesis, one ootid may be fertilized, and three second polar bodies remain nonfunctional.

(zygote) splits after fertilization and two separate offspring develop. The two offspring would be referred to as monozygotic (coming from one zygote) twins. Monozygotic twins are also known as identical twins because they contain exact replicas of genetic material. Another way to achieve a multiple birth is if more than one ootid is available for fertilization and the separate ootids are fertilized by separate spermatozoa. In this case, the offspring would have no more resemblance to each other than other offspring born

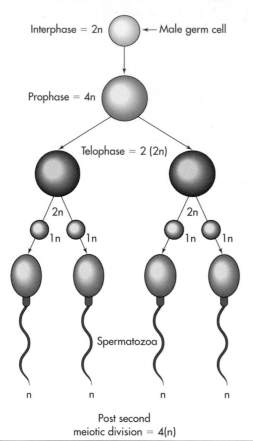

Interphase = 2n ← Male germ cell

Prophase = 4n

Telophase = 2 (2n)

2n   2n

1n   1n   1n   1n

Spermatozoa

n   n   n   n

Post second
meiotic division = 4(n)

FIG. 4-16. This figure indicates the total amount of genetic material at different stages of meiosis of a male germ cell. Twenty-three chromosomes, half the amount needed to produce a new human organism, are needed in the spermatozoa. If we refer to 23 chromosomes as an amount of genetic material n, then before meiosis (during interphase) the germ cell has 2n. During prophase, this number doubles to 4n. There then follows two reduction divisions to form the final 1n (23 chromosomes) in the spermatozoa. An egg cell undergoes a similar process, but only one of the four resulting germ cells at the end of the process is functional.

at different times from the same parents. Such dizygotic twins are also known as fraternal twins. More than two such twins would be known as polyzygotic siblings. Fraternal twins or multiple siblings, as with siblings born in different pregnancies, sometimes bear a striking resemblance to one another. However, unless they were monozygotic, they are not identical twins and do not have exact copies of all of their chromosomes.

SUMMARY

➤ Cells are made of protoplasm, which consists of proteins, carbohydrates, lipids, nucleic acids, water, and mineral salts (electrolytes).
 ■ Proteins are essential to growth, construction, and repair of tissue; they may function as hormones and antibodies.
 ■ Carbohydrates provide fuel for cell metabolism.
 ■ Lipids act as a reservoir for long-term storage of energy, guard the body against the environment, and protect organs.
 ■ Nucleic acids (DNA, RNA) carry genetic information necessary for cell replication.
 ■ Water constitutes the bulk of body weight, is essential to sustaining life, and serves as the transport medium for material the cell uses and eliminates.
 ■ Mineral salts maintain the correct portion of water in the cell and support cell function and conduction of nerve impulses.
➤ Cells have several components:
 ■ The cell membrane surrounds the cell, functions as a barricade, and controls passage of water and other materials in and out of the cell.
 ■ Cytoplasm is the portion of a cell outside the nucleus in which all metabolic activity occurs.
 ■ The ER transports food and molecules from one part of the cell to another.
 ■ The Golgi apparatus unites large carbohydrate molecules with proteins to form glycoproteins.
 ■ Mitochondria contain enzymes that produce energy for cellular activity.
 ■ Lysosomes break down unwanted large molecules; they may rupture when exposed to radiation, resulting in cell death.
 ■ Ribosomes synthesize the various proteins that cells require.
 ■ The nucleus controls cell division, multiplication, and biochemical reactions.
➤ Somatic cells divide through the process of mitosis:
 ■ The cellular life cycle has four distinct phases of mitosis: pre-DNA synthesis, actual DNA synthesis, post-DNA manufacturing, and division.
 ■ Mitosis has four subphases: prophase, metaphase, anaphase, and telophase.

➤ Genetic cells divide through meiosis:
  ■ Meiosis is similar to mitosis except no DNA replication occurs in telophase; the number of chromosomes in the daughter cell is reduced to half the number of chromosomes in the parent cell.
➤ The Human Genome Project has mapped the entire sequence of DNA base pairs on all 46 chromosomes.
  ■ There are 2.9 billion base pairs arranged into about 30,000 genes.

References

1. Ventner JC: The sequence of the human genome, *Science* 291:1304-1351, 2001.
2. Lee TF: *The Human Genome Project: cracking the genetic code of life,* New York, 1991, Plenum Press.

GENERAL DISCUSSION QUESTIONS

1. What are the essential functions of water in the human body?
2. What role do antibodies fulfill for the human body?
3. Describe the structure of a DNA (deoxyribonucleic) macromolecule.
4. Name the four nitrogenous base pairs in DNA (deoxyribose) macromolecule.
5. How do genes control the formation of proteins in every cell?
6. Describe the Human Genome Project.
7. Why is potassium of primary importance to the human body?
8. List the components of the normal cell, and explain their function.
9. Describe the processes of mitosis and meiosis.
10. How can multiple births occur from one pregnancy?

REVIEW QUESTIONS

1. In a DNA macromolecule, the sequence of _____ determines the characteristics of every living thing.
   A. Sugars
   B. Phosphates
   C. Nitrogenous organic bases
   D. Hydrogen bonds

2. How many base pairs are there in the human genome?
   A. 2.58×10^4
   B. 2.58×10^{-4}
   C. 2.9×10^9
   D. 2.9×10^{-9}

3. Radiation-induced chromosome damage may be evaluated during which of the following processes?
   A. Prophase
   B. Metaphase
   C. Anaphase
   D. Telophase

4. If exposure to ionizing radiation damages the components involved in molecular synthesis beyond repair, cells do which of the following?
   A. Continue to function normally
   B. Function abnormally or die
   C. Repair themselves immediately because of the enzymatic proteins they contain
   D. Reproduce themselves in pairs

5. Which of the following produces antibodies?
   A. Erythrocytes
   B. Lymphocytes
   C. Thrombocytes
   D. Platelets

6. Water constitutes approximately _____ of the weight of the human body.
   A. 30% to 35%
   B. 50% to 55%
   C. 65% to 70%
   D. 80% to 85%

7. Which of the following must the human body provide to ensure efficient cell operation?
   1. Food as a source of raw material for the release of energy
   2. Oxygen to help break down food
   3. Water to transport inorganic substances into and out of the cell
   A. 1 and 2 only
   B. 1 and 3 only
   C. 2 and 3 only
   D. 1, 2, and 3

8. Which human cell component controls cell division and multiplication as well as biochemical reactions that occur within the cell?
   A. Endoplasmic reticulum
   B. Mitochondria
   C. Lysosomes
   D. Nucleus

9. What term is used to describe chemical secretions that are manufactured by various endocrine glands and carried by the bloodstream to influence the activities of other parts of the body?
   A. Amino acids
   B. Antibodies
   C. Hormones
   D. Disaccharides

10. Somatic cells divide through the process of:
    A. Meiosis
    B. Mitosis
    C. Mapping
    D. Metabolism

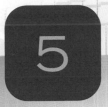

5 Molecular and Cellular Radiation Biology

KEY TERMS

apoptosis
cell survival curve
chromosome breakage
direct action
free radical
indirect action

Law of Bergonié and
  Tribondeau
linear energy transfer (LET)
mutation
oxygen enhancement ratio
  (OER)

point mutation
radiation weighting factor (W_R)
relative biologic effectiveness
  (RBE)
target theory

OBJECTIVES

After completing this chapter, the reader will be able to perform the following:

- List the three radiation energy transfer determinants and explain their individual concepts.
- Differentiate between the three levels of biologic damage that may occur in living systems as a result of exposure to ionizing radiation and describe how the process of direct and indirect action of ionizing radiation on the molecular structure of living systems occurs.

Continued

- Draw a diagram to illustrate the various effects of ionizing radiation on a DNA macromolecule and describe the effects of ionizing radiation on chromosomes, various types of cells, and ultimately the entire human body.
- Describe target theory.
- Explain the purpose for and function of survival curves for mammalian cells.
- List the factors that affect cell radiosensitivity.
- State and describe the law of Bergonié and Tribondeau.

Radiation biology is the branch of biology concerned with the effects of ionizing radiation on living systems. Areas of study included in this science are the sequence of events occurring after the absorption of energy from ionizing radiation, the action of the living system to make up for the consequences of this energy assimilation, and the injury to the living system that may be produced.

The human body is a living system composed of large numbers of various types of cells, most of which may be damaged by radiation. Because the potentially harmful effects of ionizing radiation on living systems occur primarily at the cellular level, those who administer radiation to humans for medical purposes should have a basic understanding of cell structure, composition, and function as well as the adverse effects on these by ionizing radiation. This chapter provides the reader with a basic knowledge of aspects of molecular and cellular radiation biology that are relevant to the subject of radiation protection. It also provides a foundation for radiation effects on organ systems that are covered in the next chapter.

IONIZING RADIATION

Ionizing radiation damages living systems by ionizing (removing electrons from) the atoms composing the molecular structures of these systems. X-ray and gamma-ray photons can impart energy to orbital electrons in atoms if the photons happen to pass near the electrons. High-energy charged particles such as alpha and beta particles and protons also may ionize atoms by interacting electromagnetically with orbital electrons. The alpha particle (see Chapter 1), which is composed of two protons and two neutrons and therefore carries an electric charge of plus two, strongly attracts the negatively charged electron as it passes by.

Biologic damage, then, begins with the ionization produced by various types of radiation. An ionized atom will not bond properly in molecules. If the molecule in question is necessary for the normal functioning of an organism, then the entire organism may be affected.

RADIATION ENERGY TRANSFER DETERMINANTS

Characteristics of ionizing radiation such as *charge*, *mass*, and *energy* vary among the different types of radiation. These attributes determine the extent to which different radiation modalities transfer energy into biologic tissue. To understand the way ionizing radiation causes injury and how the effects may vary in biologic tissue, three important concepts must be studied:

1. Linear energy transfer (LET)
2. Relative biologic effectiveness (RBE)
3. Oxygen enhancement ratio (OER)

Linear Energy Transfer

When passing through a medium, ionizing radiation may interact with it during its passage and, as a result,

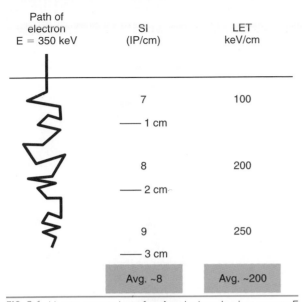

Path of electron E = 350 keV	SI (IP/cm)	LET keV/cm
	7	100
	— 1 cm	
	8	200
	— 2 cm	
	9	250
	— 3 cm	
	Avg. ~8	Avg. ~200

FIG. 5-1. Linear energy transfer. An electron having energy E = 350 keV interacts in a tissue-like material. Its actual path is tortuous, changing direction a number of times, as the electron interacts with atoms of the material via excitations and ionizations. As interactions reduce the energy of the electron through excitation and ionization the electron's energy is transferred to the material. The interactions that take place along the path of the particle may be summarized as specific ionization (SI; ion pairs/cm) or as linear energy transfer (LET; keV/cm) along the straight line continuation of the particle's trajectory beyond its point of entry. (From Hendee WR and Ritenour ER: *Medical imaging physics,* ed 4, Chicago, 2002, John Wiley & Sons.)

deposit energy along its path (called a *track*). The average energy deposited per unit length of track is called **linear energy transfer (LET)** (Fig. 5-1). The energy average is calculated by dividing the track into equal energy intervals and averaging the lengths of the tracks that contain that specific energy amount. LET is generally described in units of kiloelectron volts (keV) per micron (1 micron [μm] = 10^{-6} m). Because the amount of ionization produced in an irradiated object corresponds to the amount of energy it absorbs and because both chemical and biologic effects in tissue coincide with the degree of ionization experienced by the tissue, LET is an important factor in assessing potential tissue and organ damage from exposure to ionizing radiation.

Radiation Categories According to LET

Radiation may be divided into two general categories according to its LET: (1) low and (2) high (Box 5-1).

Low-LET Radiation Low-LET radiation is electromagnetic radiation such as x-rays and gamma rays (short-wavelength, high-energy waves emitted by the nuclei of radioactive substances). This penetrating electromagnetic radiation is sparsely ionizing and interacts randomly along the length of its track. It does not relinquish all of its energy quickly. When low-LET radiation interacts with biologic tissue, it causes damage primarily through an indirect action that involves the production of free radicals. Also, but much less likely, the radiation may directly induce single-strand breaks in the ladderlike deoxyribonucleic acid (DNA) structure. (Both free radicals and DNA are discussed in detail later in this chapter.) Because low-LET radiation generally causes sublethal damage to DNA, repair enzymes can usually reverse the cellular damage. Because of a property known as *wave-particle duality*, we can also refer to x-rays and gamma rays as streams of particles, each of which has no mass and no charge.

High-LET Radiation High-LET radiation includes particles that possess substantial mass and charge. These radiations cause dense ionization along their length of track. Some typical examples of high-LET radiations are alpha particles, ions of heavy nuclei, and charged particles released from interactions between neutrons and atoms. Low-energy neutrons, which carry no electrical charge, also are a form of high-LET radiation. All of these lose energy more rapidly than

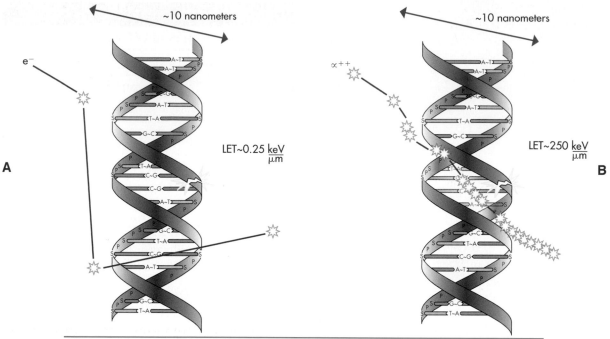

FIG. 5-2. Electron and alpha particle passing through nucleus of a cell near strand of DNA. **A,** For an electron, several interactions may occur in the vicinity of a DNA strand, creating a risk of damage to the DNA. **B,** Because so many interactions may occur in the vicinity of a DNA strand, some damage is likely.

low-LET radiations because they produce much more ionization per unit of distance traveled. As a result, they exhaust their energy in a shorter length of track and therefore cannot travel or penetrate as far. Because high-LET radiations deposit more energy per unit of biologic tissue traversed, they are more destructive to biologic matter than are low-LET radiations.

Risk of damage to DNA Fig. 5-2 shows an electron and an alpha particle passing through the nucleus of a cell in the vicinity of a strand of DNA. The size of the entire area is only about 10 nanometers (10 billionths of a meter, or 10 millionths of a millimeter). The electron represents either a Compton scattered electron or a photoelectron resulting from the interaction of a photon from a diagnostic x-ray beam. The alpha particle represents one of the particles ejected from the nucleus of an atom after radioactive decay of an element such as radon.

Probability of interaction with DNA As mentioned previously, the parameter that describes the

average energy deposited over small distances in the material is the LET. The presence of many more alpha particle interactions in the small region displayed is reflected in the fact that the LET for the alpha particle shown in this example is 1000 times the LET of the electron. Each time the particle interacts, it loses some energy and slows down in the cell. When enough interactions have occurred, the particle comes to a stop and no further interactions take place. Because it does not interact as often, the electron, however, can travel significantly farther than the alpha particle. A Compton scattered electron or photoelectron set in motion in a patient exposed to diagnostic x-rays may travel through thousands of cells (interacting in only some of them), with a low probability that a significant number of interactions will occur by chance in the DNA. On the other hand, an alpha particle such as the one shown may travel through only one or two cells but will have a high probability of interacting with the DNA of a cell it encounters.

High-LET radiation and internal contamination For radiation protection, high-LET radiation is of greatest concern when internal contamination is possible—that is, when a radionuclide has been implanted, ingested, injected, or inhaled. Then the potential exists for irreparable damage because, with high-LET radiation, multiple-strand breaks in DNA are possible. For example, with a double-strand break in the same rung of the DNA ladderlike structure, complete chromosome breakage occurs (see Fig. 5-8, A later in this chapter). Repair enzymes are not effective at undoing this damage, and hence cell death will probably occur.

Relative Biologic Effectiveness

Biologic damage produced by radiation escalates as the LET of radiation increases, because identical doses of radiations of various LETs do not render the same biologic effect. The **relative biologic effectiveness (RBE)** describes the relative capabilities of radiation with differing LETs to produce a particular biologic reaction. RBE of the type of radiation being used is the ratio of the dose of a reference radiation (conventionally 250-kVp x-rays) to the dose that is necessary to produce the same biologic reaction in a given experiment. The reaction is produced by a dose of the test radiation delivered under the same conditions. Box 5-2 demonstrates how RBE can be expressed mathematically.

Use of the RBE Concept for Specific Experiments

The concept of RBE is used to refer to specific experiments with specific cells or animal tissues (e.g., tumor cells in a Petri dish, skin of the left hind flank of a certain strain of laboratory rat). Because the various types of cells or tissues differ in their biologic response per unit quantity of absorbed dose, the concept of RBE is not practical for specifying radiation protection dose levels in humans. To overcome this limitation, a **radiation weighting factor (W_R)** is used to calculate equivalent dose (EqD) to determine the ability of a dose of any kind of ionizing radiation to cause biologic damage. The values of radiation weighting factors are similar to the values of RBE for any particular type of radiation. The radiation weighting factors for different

---

BOX 5-2

Mathematical Expression of Relative Biologic Effectiveness (RBE)

$$RBE = \frac{\text{Dose in Gy from 250-kVp x-rays}}{\text{Dose in Gy of test radiation}}$$

EXAMPLE: A biologic reaction is produced by 2 Gy of a test radiation. It takes 10 Gy of 250-kVp x-rays to produce the same biologic reaction. What is the RBE of the test radiation?

$$\frac{10}{2} = 5$$

The RBE is 5, which means that the test radiation is five times as effective in producing this biologic reaction as are 250-kVp x-rays.

BOX 5-3

Oxygen Enhancement Ratio (OER)

$$OER = \frac{\text{Radiation dose required to cause biologic response without } O_2}{\text{Radiation dose required to cause biologic response with } O_2}$$

---

types of ionizing radiations are listed in Table 3-2 of this text.

Oxygen Enhancement Ratio

The **oxygen enhancement ratio (OER)** is the ratio of the radiation dose required to cause a particular biologic response of cells or organisms in an oxygen-deprived environment to the radiation dose required to cause an identical response under normal oxygenated conditions. The OER formula is given in Box 5-3.

In general, x-rays and gamma rays, which are low-LET radiations, have an OER of about 3.0 when the radiation dose is high. The OER may be less (about 2.0) when radiation doses are below 2 Gy (200 rads). This surprising result exists because a 2-Gy dose is associated with the linear (i.e., straight-line) portion of the linear-quadratic dose-response relationship for cell killing (see Chapter 6), whereas higher doses can fall on the curved (i.e., quadratic) portion of the dose-response curve.[1] Because high-LET radiations such as alpha particles produce their biologic effects from direct action—namely, direct ionization and disruption of biomolecules—the presence or absence of oxygen is of no consequence. Therefore, the OER of high-LET radiation is approximately equal to 1. For low-LET radiation a significant fraction of bioeffects are caused by indirect actions in which a chemical species called a **free radical** is formed. A free radical is a solitary atom or most often a combination of atoms that behaves as an extremely reactive single entity as a result of the presence of an unpaired electron. Free radicals dramatically increase the amount of biologic damage. (Both the direct and indirect actions of radiation are discussed later in this chapter.) However, the presence of oxygen in biologic tissues makes the damage produced by these free radicals permanent because oxygen reacts with free radicals to produce organic peroxide compounds, which represent nonrestorable changes in the chemical composition of the target material. Without oxygen, damage produced by the indirect action of radiation on a biologic molecule may be repaired, but when damage occurs through an oxygen-mediated process, the end result is permanent, or fixed. This phenomenon has been called *the oxygen fixation hypothesis*.

MOLECULAR EFFECTS OF IRRADIATION

In living systems, biologic damage resulting from exposure to ionizing radiation may be observed on three levels: *molecular, cellular,* and *organic*. Any visible radiation-induced injuries of living systems at the cellular or organic level always begin with damage at the molecular level. Molecular damage results in the formation of structurally changed molecules that may impair cellular functioning.

Effects of Irradiation on Somatic and Genetic Cells

Cells of the human body are highly specialized, with each cell having a predetermined task to perform; each cell's function is determined and defined by the structures of its constituent molecules. Because exposure to ionizing radiation can alter these structures, such exposure may disturb the cell's chemical balance and ultimately the way it operates. When this occurs, the cell no longer performs its normal tasks. If a sufficient quantity of somatic cells (i.e., all cells in the body other than female and male germ cells) are affected, entire body processes may be disrupted. On the other hand, if radiation damages the germ (reproductive) cells, the damage may be passed on to future generations in the form of genetic mutations (changes in the genes). (More information pertaining to somatic and genetic effects is presented later in this chapter and in Chapter 6.)

Classification of Ionizing Radiation Interaction

When ionizing radiation interacts with a cell, ionizations and excitations (the addition of energy to a molecular system, transforming it from a ground state to an excited state) are produced either in vital biologic macromolecules (such as DNA), or in water (H_2O), the medium in which the cellular organelles are suspended. Based on the site of the interaction, the action of radiation on the cell is classified as either *direct* or *indirect* (Fig. 5-3). In **direct action,** biologic damage occurs as a result of ionization of atoms on master, or key, molecules (DNA), which can cause these molecules to become inactive or functionally altered. **Indirect action** refers to the effects produced by reactive free radicals that are created by the interaction of radiation with water (H_2O) molecules. These unstable, highly reactive agents have the potential to substantially disrupt master molecules, resulting in cell death.

Direct action may occur after exposure to any type of radiation. However, direct action is much more likely to happen after exposure to high-LET radiations such as alpha particles, which produce a very large number of ionizations in a very short distance of travel. This is in contrast to exposure to low-LET radiations such as x-rays, which are only sparsely ionizing.

Direct Action

When ionizing particles interact directly with vital biologic macromolecules such as DNA, ribonucleic

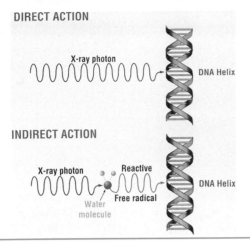

DIRECT ACTION

X-ray photon

DNA Helix

INDIRECT ACTION

X-ray photon   Reactive

DNA Helix

Water molecule   Free radical

FIG. 5-3. The action of radiation on the cell can be direct or indirect. It is direct when ionizing particles interact with a vital biologic macromolecule such as DNA. The action is indirect when ionizing particles interact with a water molecule, resulting in the creation of ions and reactive free radicals that eventually produce toxic substances that can create biologic damage. (From *Mosby's radiographic instructional series: radiobiology and radiation protection*, St. Louis, 1999, Mosby.)

acid (RNA), proteins, and enzymes, damage to these molecules occurs from absorption of energy through photoelectric and Compton interactions. The ionization or excitation of the atoms of the biologic macromolecules results in breakage of the macromolecules' chemical bonds, causing them to become abnormal structures, which may in turn lead to inappropriate chemical reactions. Thus, when enzyme molecules are damaged by interaction with ionizing particles, essential biochemical processes may not occur in the cell at the appropriate time. For example, if an enzyme is inactivated, it will not be available to facilitate a particular biochemical reaction. Should this occur during the synthesis of a particular protein, the protein will not be manufactured, and if this protein was intended to perform a specific function, its nonexistence will hinder or prevent that function. In the event that other cell operations depend on the suppressed function, these operations sustain some type of damage as well, and so a biologic chain reaction essentially occurs.

Radiolysis of Water

Ionization of Water Molecules

X-ray photons may interact with and ionize water molecules contained within the human body. Such an interaction between an x-ray photon and a water molecule creates an ion pair consisting of a water molecule with a positive charge (HOH^+) and an electron (e^-). After the original ionization of the water molecule, several reactions can occur. One is that the positively charged water molecule (HOH^+) may recombine with the electron (e^-) to re-form a stable water molecule ($HOH^+ + e^- = H_2O$). If this happens, no damage occurs. Alternatively, the electron (the negative ion) may join with another water molecule, producing a negative water ion ($H_2O + e^- = HOH^-$).

Production of Free Radicals

The positive water molecule (HOH^+) and the negative water molecule (HOH^-) are basically unstable. Hence they will break apart into smaller molecules. HOH^+ becomes a hydrogen ion (H^+) and a hydroxyl radical (OH^*), whereas HOH^- becomes a hydroxyl ion (OH^-) and a hydrogen radical (H^*). The asterisk symbolizes a free radical. A free radical is a configuration of one or more atoms having an unpaired electron but no net electrical charge. This object is highly reactive because the unpaired electron will pair up with another electron even if it has to break a chemical bond to do this. Hence, the interaction of radiation with water results in the formation of an ion pair, H^+ and OH^- (hydrogen ion and hydroxyl ion), and two free radicals, H^* and OH^* (a hydrogen radical and a hydroxyl radical) (Fig. 5-4).

Production of Undesirable Chemical Reactions and Biologic Damage

Because the hydrogen and hydroxyl ions usually recombine to form a normal water molecule, the existence of these ions as free agents within the human body is insignificant in terms of biologic damage. The presence of hydrogen and hydroxyl free radicals, however, is not insignificant. As molecules containing an unpaired electron in their outer shell, they are chemically unstable and very reactive. They can produce undesirable chemical reactions and cause biologic damage by transferring their excess energy to

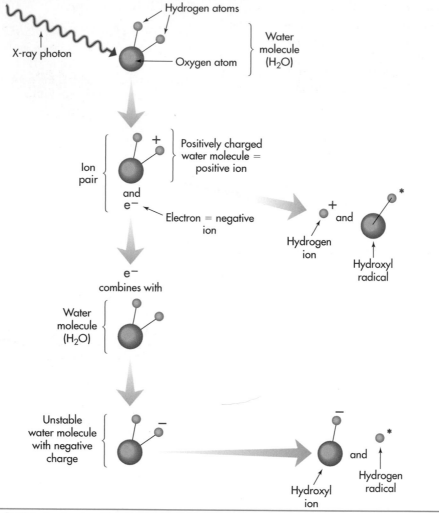

FIG. 5-4. Radiolysis of water. The final result of the interaction of radiation with water is the formation of an ion pair (H^+ and OH^-) and two free radicals (H^* and OH^*).

other molecules, thereby either breaking these molecules' chemical bonds or at the very least causing point lesions (i.e., altered areas caused by the breaking of a single chemical bond) in the molecule. Approximately two thirds of all radiation-induced damage is believed to be ultimately caused by the hydroxyl free radical (OH^*). In addition, because free radicals have excess energy and can travel through the cell, they are capable of destructively interacting with other molecules located at some distance from their place of origin.

Production of Cell-Damaging Substances

Hydrogen and hydroxyl radicals are not the only destructive substances that may be produced during the radiolysis of water. A hydroxyl radical (OH^*) may bond with another hydroxyl radical (OH^*) and form hydrogen peroxide ($OH^* + OH^* = H_2O_2$), a substance that is poisonous to the cell. Also, a hydroperoxyl radical (HO_2*) is formed when a hydrogen free radical ($H*$) combines with molecular oxygen (O_2). This radical and hydrogen peroxide are believed to be among the primary substances that produce biologic damage directly after the interaction of radiation with water.

Organic Free Radical Formation

Absorption of radiation can cause a normal organic molecule (for simplicity, let us call it RH, in which "H" stands for hydrogen and "R" can be any organic molecule) to form the free radicals: $R*$ (an organic neutral free radical) and $H*$. Without oxygen or a force to attract an electron, these radicals will usually react with one another to re-form the original organic molecule (RH). When oxygen is present, however, $R*$ and $H*$ may react with the oxygen to form the radicals RO_2* and HO_2*. Hence the organic molecule (RH) is destroyed and moreover the radicals RO_2* and HO_2* can react with other organic molecules to cause biologic damage. Thus, a small-scale chain reaction of destructive events occurs that results from radiation depositing energy within tissue in the presence of oxygen.

Indirect Action

When free radicals previously produced by the interaction of radiation with water molecules act on a molecule such as DNA, the damaging action of ionizing radiation on the vital biologic macromolecule is indirect in the sense that the radiation is not the immediate cause of injury to the macromolecule. It is the by-products of the radiation, the free radicals, that are the immediate cause of this damage. Because the human body is 80% water and less than 1% DNA, essentially all other effects of irradiation in living cells result from indirect action.[2]

In summary, the process of indirect action (Fig. 5-5) involves the breakdown of a water molecule into smaller molecules, producing both ions and free radicals in the process. As we have seen, the free radicals produced can recombine to form hydrogen peroxide, a cellular poison, and a hydroperoxyl radical, another toxic substance. Both of these agents are highly

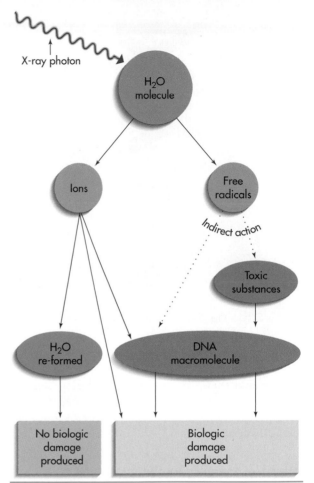

FIG. 5-5. Indirect action of ionizing radiation on biologic molecules. X-ray photons interact directly with a water (H_2O) molecule. The H_2O molecule breaks down into ions and free radicals. The ions can recombine to form a water molecule, thereby creating no biologic damage. The free radicals can migrate to another molecule, such as a DNA molecule located at some distance from the site of the initial ionization, and destructively interact with it by ionizing it or rupturing some chemical bonds. This creates molecular or point lesions in the DNA macromolecule. Free radicals can spread biologic damage by combining with other molecules to form toxic substances that also can migrate to distant DNA molecules and destructively interact.

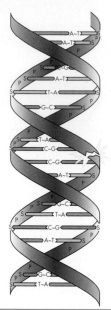

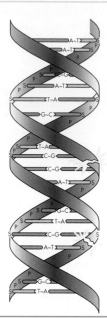

FIG. 5-6. Single-strand break in the ladderlike DNA molecular structure.

FIG. 5-7. A widely spaced double-strand break in the ladder-like DNA molecular structure.

reactive and therefore capable of producing biologic damage. By themselves, free radicals may transfer excess energy to other molecules, thereby breaking their chemical bonds.

Effects of Ionizing Radiation on DNA

Single-Strand Break

If ionizing radiation interacts with a DNA macromolecule, the energy transferred can rupture one of its chemical bonds, possibly severing one of the sugar-phosphate chain side rails or strands of the ladderlike molecular structure (single-strand break) (Fig. 5-6). This type of injury to DNA is called a **point mutation.** Gene mutations may result from a single alteration along the sequence of nitrogenous bases. Point mutations commonly occur with low-LET radiations. Repair enzymes, however, are capable of reversing this damage.

Double-Strand Break

Further exposure of the affected DNA macromolecule to ionizing radiation may result in additional breaks in the sugar-phosphate molecular chain(s). These

breaks might also be repaired, but double-strand breaks (one or more breaks in each of the two sugar-phosphate chains) (Fig. 5-7) are not repaired as easily as single-strand breaks. If repair does not take place, further separation may occur in the DNA chains, threatening the life of the cell. Double-strand breaks occur more commonly with densely ionizing (high-LET) radiations and often are associated with the loss or gain of one or more nitrogenous bases. When high-LET radiation interacts with DNA molecules, the ionization interactions may be so closely spaced that, by chance, both strands of the DNA chain are broken. If both strands are broken at the same nitrogenous base "rung," the result is the same as if both side rails of the ladder were cut at the same step or rung—the ladder would be cut into two pieces. If the DNA is cut into two pieces, the chromosome, which is composed of a long chain of twisted strands of DNA ladders, is itself broken. Thus some types of chromosomal damage that are particularly associated with high-LET radiation are related to double-strand breaks of DNA. Because the chance of repairing this damage is much slighter, the possibility of inducing a lethal alteration

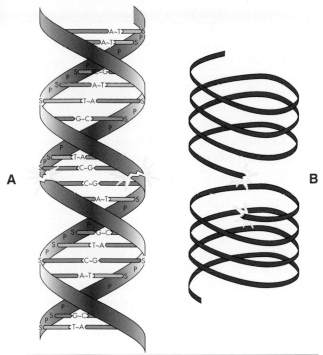

A

B

FIG. 5-8. Double-strand break in same rung of the DNA ladderlike molecular structure **(A)** causes complete chromosome breakage, resulting in a cleaved or broken chromosome **(B)**.

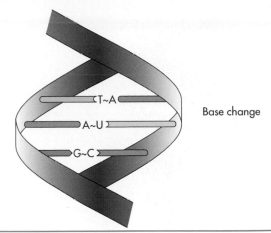

Base change

FIG. 5-9. Alteration of the nitrogen base sequence on the DNA chain caused by the interaction of high-energy radiation directly on a DNA molecule.

of nitrogenous bases within the genetic sequence is far greater.

Double-Strand Break in Same Rung of DNA

When two interactions (hits), one on each of the two sugar-phosphate chains, occur within the same rung of the DNA ladderlike configuration (Fig. 5-8, A), the result is a cleaved or broken chromosome (Fig. 5-8, B), with each new portion containing an unequal amount of genetic material. If this damaged chromosome divides, each new daughter cell will receive an incorrect amount of genetic material. This will culminate in the death or impaired functioning of the new daughter cell.

Mutation

In general, the interaction of high-energy radiation with a DNA molecule causes either a loss of or change in a nitrogenous base on the DNA chain. The direct consequence of this damage is an alteration of the base sequence (Fig. 5-9). Because the genetic information to be passed on to future generations is contained in the strict sequence of these bases, the loss or change of a base in the DNA chain is a **mutation.** It may not be reversible and may cause acute consequences for the cell but, more important, if the cell remains viable, incorrect genetic information will be transferred to one of the two daughter cells when the cell divides.

Covalent Cross-Links

Covalent cross-links are chemical unions created between atoms by the single sharing of one or more pairs of electrons. Covalent cross-links involving DNA are another effect initiated by high-energy radiation. At low energies, however, covalent cross-links are probably caused by the process of indirect action. Following irradiation, some molecules can produce small, spurlike molecules that become very interactive ("sticky") when exposed to radiation. This can cause these molecules to attach to other macromolecules or to other segments of the same macromolecule chain. Cross-linking can occur in many different patterns. For example, a cross-link can form between two places on the same DNA strand. This joining is termed an *intrastrand cross-link.* Cross-linking may also occur between complementary DNA strands (Fig. 5-10) or between entirely different DNA molecules. These

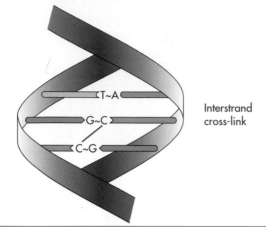

Interstrand cross-link

FIG. 5-10. Interstrand covalent cross-link produced by high-energy radiation interacting directly on a DNA molecule.

joinings are termed *interstrand cross-links*. Finally, DNA molecules also may become covalently linked to a protein molecule.[3] All these linkages are potentially fatal to the cell if they are not properly repaired.

Effects of Ionizing Radiation on Chromosomes

Large-scale structural changes in a chromosome brought about by ionizing radiation may be as grave for the cell as are radiation-induced changes in DNA. When changes occur in the DNA molecule, the chromosome exhibits the alteration. Because DNA modifications are discrete, they do not inevitably result in observable structural chromosome alterations.

Radiation-Induced Chromosome Breaks

After irradiation and during cell division, some radiation-induced chromosome breaks may be viewed microscopically. These alterations manifest themselves during the metaphase and anaphase of the cell division cycle, when the length of the chromosomes is visible. Because the events that have happened before these phases of cell division are not visible, they can only be assumed to have occurred. What can be seen, however, is the effect of these events—the gross or visible alterations in the structure of the chromosome. Both somatic cells and reproductive cells are subject to chromosome breaks induced by radiation.

Chromosomal Fragments

After chromosome breakage, two or more chromosomal fragments are produced. Each of these fragments has a fractured extremity. These broken ends appear sticky and have the ability to adhere to another such sticky end. The broken fragments may rejoin in their original configuration, fail to rejoin and create an aberration (lesion or anomaly), or rejoin other broken ends and create new chromosomes that may not look structurally altered compared with the chromosome before irradiation.

Chromosome Anomalies

Two types of chromosome anomalies have been observed at metaphase. They are called (1) *chromosome aberrations* and (2) *chromatid aberrations*. Chromosome aberrations result when irradiation occurs early in interphase, before DNA synthesis takes place. In this situation, the break caused by ionizing radiation is in a single strand of chromatin; during the DNA synthesis that follows, the resultant break is replicated when this strand of chromatin lays down an identical strand adjacent to itself if repair is not complete before the start of DNA synthesis. This leads to a chromosome aberration in which both chromatids exhibit the break. This break is visible at the next mitosis. Each daughter cell generated will have inherited a damaged chromatid as a consequence of a failure in the repair mechanism. Chromatid aberrations, on the other hand, result when irradiation of individual chromatids occurs later in interphase, after DNA synthesis has taken place. In this situation, only one chromatid of a pair might suffer a radiation-induced break. Therefore only one daughter cell is affected.

Structural Changes in Biologic Tissue Caused by Ionizing Radiation

Ionizing radiation interacts randomly with matter. Because of this phenomenon, exposure to radiation produces a variety of structural changes in biologic tissue. Some of these changes are as follows:
- A single-strand break in one chromosome
- A single-strand break in one chromatid
- A single-strand break in separate chromosomes
- A strand break in separate chromatids
- More than one break in the same chromosome

- More than one break in the same chromatid
- Chromosome stickiness, or clumping together

Consequences to the Cell from Structural Changes in Biologic Tissue

These structural changes may result in one of the following consequences to the cell:

1. Restitution, whereby the breaks rejoin in their original configuration with no visible damage (Fig. 5-11). In this case no damage to the cell occurs because the chromosome has been restored to the condition it was in before irradiation. The process of healing by restitution is believed to be the way in which 95% of single-chromosome breaks mend.[3]
2. Deletion, whereby a part of the chromosome or chromatid is lost at the next cell division, creating an aberration known as an acentric fragment (Fig. 5-12).
3. Broken-end rearrangement, whereby a grossly misshapen chromosome may be produced. Ring chromosomes, dicentric chromosomes, and anaphase bridges are examples of such distorted chromosomes (Fig. 5-13).
4. Broken-end rearrangement without visible damage to the chromosomes, whereby the chromosome's genetic material has been rearranged even though the chromosome appears normal. Translocations are an example of such rearrangements (Fig. 5-14). Changes such as these inevitably result in mutation because the positions of the genes on the chromosomes have been rearranged, thus altering the heritable characteristics of the cell.

Target Theory

Amid the many different types of molecules that lie within the cell, a master, or key, molecule that maintains normal cell function also is believed to be present (Fig. 5-15). This master molecule is necessary for the survival of the cell. Because this molecule is unique in any given cell, no similar molecules in the cell are available to replace it; if the master molecule is inactivated by exposure to radiation, the cell will die (Fig. 5-16). Experimental data strongly support this concept and indicate that DNA is the irreplaceable master, or key, molecule that serves as the vital target. Destruction of some of the molecules that are plentiful in the cell does not result in cell death. The reason for this is simply that cells have an abundance of similar molecules to take over and perform necessary functions for them in the event of their demise. If only a few non-DNA cell molecules are destroyed by radiation

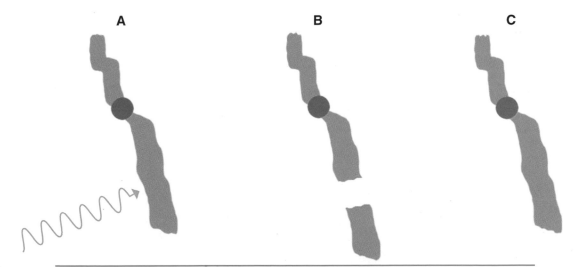

A   **B**   **C**

FIG. 5-11. The process of restitution, whereby the breaks rejoin in the original configuration with no visible damage. **A,** Chromosome break occurs because of a photon interaction. **B,** Fragment is fully separated from the rest of the chromosome. **C,** Broken fragment has reattached in its original location through the action of repair enzymes.

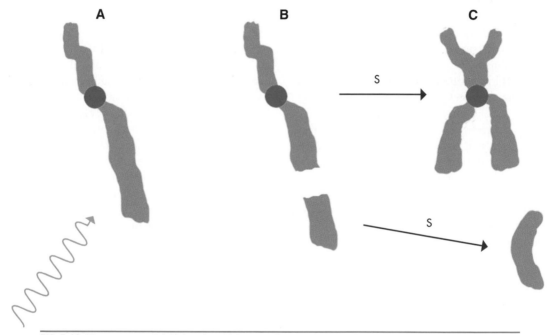

FIG. 5-12. The process of deletion, in which part of a chromosome is lost at the next cell division, creating an acentric fragment. **A,** Chromosome break results from a photon interaction. **B,** Fragment is fully separated from the rest of the chromosome. **C,** After the next DNA synthesis phase of the cell cycle (labeled *S*), the remainder of the chromosome has been replicated normally but with fragments missing from the two arms of the chromosome. The replicated fragment is acentric, a section of genetic material without a centromere.

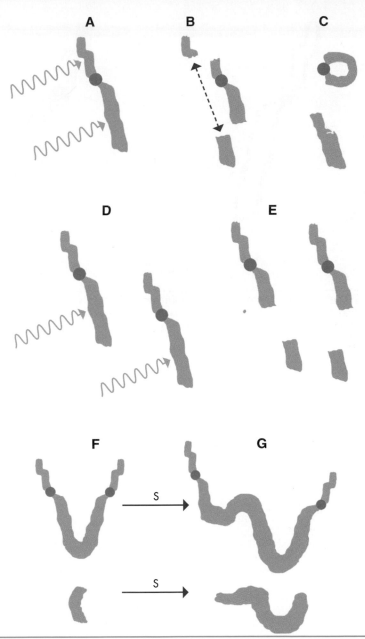

FIG. 5-13. The process of broken-end rearrangement may result in grossly misshapen chromosomes. **A,** Two chromosome breaks occur in a single chromosome as a result of the interactions of two photons. **B,** The fragments from opposite ends unite before the DNA synthesis phase. **C,** The ends of the chromosome that are still attached to the centromere also unite, forming a "ring" chromosome. **D,** Chromosome breaks occur in two different chromosomes. **E,** The fragments are fully separated from the rest of their respective chromosomes. **F,** The ends of the chromosomes and the ends of the fragments have joined before DNA synthesis, forming a dicentric (two centromeres) and an acentric (no centromere) fragment. **G,** After DNA synthesis (labeled *S*), the chromosome is elongated but cannot split in two. The two centromeres are "bridged." This type of chromosomal damage leads to reproductive death of the cell (i.e., it cannot replicate or divide into two cells).

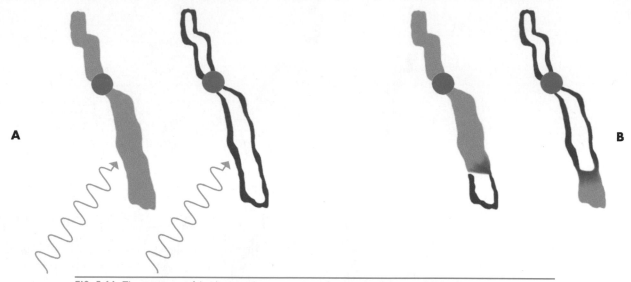

FIG. 5-14. The process of broken-end rearrangement may result in no visible damage to the chromosome, although the chromosome's genetic material has been rearranged—a result that will drastically alter its function within the cell, probably leading to cell death or failure to replicate.

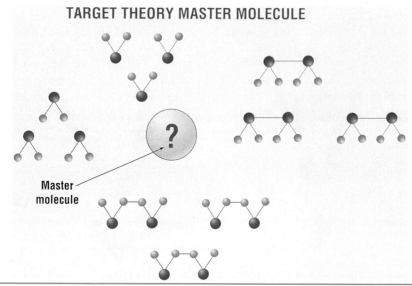

FIG. 5-15. A master, or key, molecule that maintains normal cell function is believed to be present in every cell. This molecule is vital to the survival of the cell and is presumed to be DNA. (From *Mosby's radiographic instructional series: radiobiology and radiation protection,* St. Louis, 1999, Mosby.)

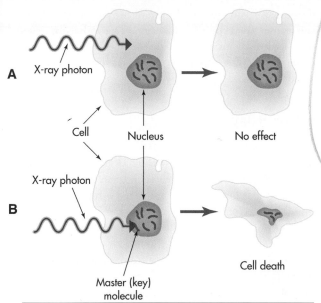

A, X-ray photon — Cell — Nucleus — No effect

B, X-ray photon — Master (key) molecule — Cell death

FIG. 5-16. The target theory holds that the cell will die after exposure to ionizing radiation only if the master, or key, molecule (DNA) is inactivated in the process. **A,** X-ray photon passes through the cell without interacting with the master molecule, which is located in the cell nucleus; no measurable effect results. **B,** X-ray photon enters the nucleus and interacts with and inactivates the master molecule; the cell dies as a result.

exposure, the cell will probably not show any evidence of injury after irradiation.

In its passage through the molecular structure of living systems, radiation does not seek out master molecules in cells to destroy them; it interacts with these key molecules only by chance. The **target theory** may be used to explain cell death and nonfatal cell abnormalities caused by exposure to radiation.

Interactions between ionizing radiation and molecular targets such as DNA occur through both direct and indirect action. However, discerning which of the two types of effects or actions has been at work in any given case of cell death is virtually impossible.

CELLULAR EFFECTS OF IRRADIATION

Ionizing radiation can adversely affect the cell. Damage to the cell's nucleus reveals itself in one of the following ways:

1. Instant death
2. Reproductive death
3. Apoptosis, or programmed cell death (interphase death)
4. Mitotic, or genetic, death
5. Mitotic delay
6. Interference of function
7. Chromosome breakage

Instant Death

Instant death of large numbers of cells occurs when a volume is irradiated with an x-ray or gamma-ray dose of about 1000 Gy (100,000 rads) in a period of seconds or a few minutes. This large influx of energy causes gross disruption of cellular form and structure and severe changes in chemical machinery. As a result of receiving such a massive dose of ionizing radiation, a cell's DNA macromolecule breaks up and cellular proteins coagulate. Radiation doses high enough to cause this type of damage are vastly greater than those used for diagnostic examinations or even therapeutic treatments.

Reproductive Death

Reproductive death generally results from exposure of cells to doses of ionizing radiation in the range of 1 to 10 Gy (100 to 1000 rads). Although the cell does not die when reproductive death occurs, it permanently loses its ability to procreate. Even though the cell has lost its reproductive capacity, it continues to metabolize and synthesize nucleic acids and proteins. The termination of cells' reproductive abilities does, however, prevent the transmission of damage to future generations of cells.

Apoptosis

A nonmitotic, or nondivision, form of cell death that occurs when cells die without attempting division during the interphase portion of the cell life cycle is termed **apoptosis,** or programmed cell death. This was formerly called *interphase death*. Apoptosis occurs spontaneously in both normal tissue and in tumors. It can occur in human beings and other vertebrate animals and amphibians—in the embryo and in the adult. An example of this process is the sequence of events during embryonic development whereby tadpoles lose their tails.

Programmed Cell Death for Development and Maintenance of Organisms

Certain types of *programmed cell death* are integral to the development and maintenance of organisms. Many types of cells are destined to die for the good of the organism. For example, human beings lose webbing between their digits during embryonic development, and all through life, human skin cells die and form the protective outer coating we usually refer to as *skin*. In apoptosis, the cell shrinks and produces tiny membrane-enclosed structures called *blebs*. The cell nucleus breaks up and then the cell itself breaks up, and its fragments are usually ingested by other neighboring cells.

Apoptosis Research

Researchers believe that apoptosis may be instigated by radiation under some circumstances. The mechanisms of apoptosis and its relationship to radiosensitivity are areas of active research in radiobiology as of this writing. A new type of radiation therapy may involve activation of the genes that regulate apoptosis so that the occurrence of apoptosis becomes much more likely after irradiation in a tumor.

Radiosensitivity

Radiosensitivity of the individual cell governs the dose required to cause apoptosis; the more radiosensitive the cell, the smaller the dose required to cause apoptotic death during interphase. A few hundred centigray (cGy [rads]) can kill very sensitive cells such as lymphocytes or spermatogonia. Programmed cell death of less radiosensitive cells such as those in bone may require radiation doses of several thousand cGy (rads).

Mitotic Death

Ionizing radiation can adversely affect cell division. It may retard the mitotic process or permanently inhibit it; cell death follows permanent inhibition. *Mitotic, or genetic, death* occurs when a cell dies after one or more

divisions. Even relatively small doses of radiation can cause this type of cell death. The radiation dose required to produce mitotic death is less than the dose needed to produce apoptosis in slowly dividing cells or nondividing cells.

Mitotic Delay

Exposing a cell to as little as 0.01 Gy (1 rad) of ionizing radiation just before it begins dividing can cause *mitotic delay*, the failure of the cell to start dividing on time. After this delay, the cell may resume its normal mitotic function. The underlying cause of this phenomenon is not known. Possible reasons for the delay may be (1) irradiation causing alteration of a chemical involved in mitosis, (2) proteins required for cell division not being synthesized, and (3) a change in the rate of DNA synthesis after irradiation.

Interference of Function

Permanent or temporary interference of cellular function independent of the cell's ability to divide can be brought about by exposure to ionizing radiation. If repair enzymes are able to fix the damage, the cell can recover and continue to function.

Chromosome Breakage

Chromosome breakage is a potential outcome when ionizing radiation interacts with a DNA macromolecule. These breaks may occur in one or both strands (sugar-phosphate chains) of the DNA ladderlike structure and were discussed previously (see Direct Action).

If cells are irradiated during mitosis and chromosome breakage occurs, permanent chromosome abnormalities will be evident in future mitotic cycles. Because chromosome breakage results in a loss of genetic material, this may lead to genetic mutations in succeeding generations.

SURVIVAL CURVES FOR MAMMALIAN CELLS

Cells vary in their radiosensitivity. This fact is particularly important in determining the type of cancer

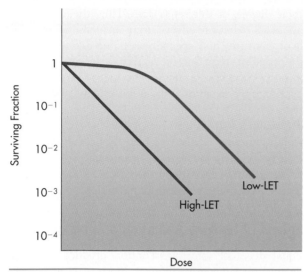

FIG. 5-17. Cell survival curves for the same cell line irradiated with both low- and high-LET radiation. With low-LET radiation, a "shoulder" to the curve at lower doses indicates the cell's ability to repair some damage at low doses. High-LET radiation typically has no shoulder, indicating that little or no repair takes place.

cells that will respond to radiation therapy. A classic method of displaying the sensitivity of a particular type of cell to radiation is the **cell survival curve**.[4] A cell survival curve is constructed from data obtained by a series of experiments. First, the cells are made to grow "in culture," meaning in a laboratory environment such as a Petri dish. Then the cells are exposed to a specified dose of radiation. After radiation exposure, the ability of the cells to divide, or form new "colonies" of cells, is measured. The fraction of cells that are able to form new colonies through cell division is then reported as the fraction of cells that have survived irradiation. The process is repeated for a range of radiation doses, and the results are graphed with the logarithm of the surviving fraction on the vertical axis and the dose on the horizontal axis.

Fig. 5-17 shows two cell survival curves, one for high-LET radiation and one for low-LET radiation. The curve for low-LET radiation shows very little change in survival at low doses, followed by a linear portion in which survival decreases in regular proportions at higher doses. This indicates that at low doses the cell is able to find and repair some of the damage.

At higher doses the repair mechanism is overwhelmed. For the high-LET curve, no survival shoulder exists. If damage occurs, it is usually so extensive that it is irreparable.

CELL RADIOSENSITIVITY

Cell Maturity and Specialization

The human body is composed of different types of cells and tissues, which vary in their degree of radiosensitivity. Immature cells are nonspecialized (undifferentiated) and undergo rapid cell division, whereas more mature cells are specialized in their function (highly differentiated) and divide at a slower rate or else do not divide. These factors affect the cells' degree of radiosensitivity. Examples of radiosensitive and radioinsensitive cells are listed in Box 5-4. Because combinations of both immature and mature cells in various ratios form the different body tissues and organs, radiosensitivity varies from one tissue and organ to another.

Amount of Radiation Energy Transferred to Biologic Tissue

When ionizing radiation interacts with cell atoms and molecules, the amount of radiation energy transferred (absorbed in the tissue) plays a major role in determining the amount of biologic response. As LET increases (i.e., as the radiation transfers more energy per unit length of track), the ability of the radiation to cause biologic effects also generally increases until it reaches a maximal value. Hence LET affects cell radiosensitivity.

BOX 5-4	
Examples of Radiosensitive and Radioinsensitive Cells	
Radiosensitive Cells	**Radioinsensitive Cells**
Basal cells of the skin	Brain cells
Intestinal crypt cells	Muscle cells
Reproductive (germ) cells	Nerve cells

Oxygen Enhancement Effects

As addressed earlier in this chapter, oxygen enhances the effects of ionizing radiation on biologic tissue by increasing tissue radiosensitivity. If oxygen is present when a tissue is irradiated, more free radicals (which possess the ability to attack and damage organic molecules) are formed in the tissue; this increases the indirect damage potential of the radiation.

During diagnostic radiologic procedures, fully oxygenated human tissues are exposed to x-radiation. However, diagnostic radiologic and nuclear medicine procedures employ low doses of radiation (x-rays and/or gamma rays) that are also low-LET. Consequently, very few cells are killed by the radiations used in these procedures.

In radiotherapy, the presence of oxygen plays a significant role in radiosensitivity. When radiation is used to treat certain types of cancerous tumors, high-pressure (hyperbaric) oxygen has sometimes been used in conjunction with it to increase tumor radiosensitivity. Cancerous tumors often contain hypoxic cells, which lack an adequate amount of oxygen, and normally aerated cells. The poorly oxygenated cells severely inhibit the indirect mechanism of radiation interaction with cells and therefore are radioresistant (particularly to low-LET radiations); hence, hypoxic cells are more difficult to destroy than normally oxygenated cells. However, when oxygen tensions in capillaries are increased by hyperbaric oxygenation, hypoxic cells may reoxygenate and become sensitive to radiation; consequently, the chances of their being destroyed by therapeutic radiation increase. Radiosensitization also may be accomplished with chemical-enhancing agents such as misonidazole.[1]

Law of Bergonié and Tribondeau

In 1906, two French scientists, J. Bergonié and L. Tribondeau, observed the effects of ionizing radiation on testicular germ cells of rabbits they had exposed to x-rays. They established that radiosensitivity was a function of the metabolic state of the cell receiving the exposure. Their findings eventually became known as the **law of Bergonié and Tribondeau.** It states that the radiosensitivity of cells is directly proportional to their reproductive activity and inversely proportional to their degree of differentiation. Thus the most pronounced radiation effects occur in cells having the least maturity and specialization, or differentiation; the greatest reproductive activity; and the longest mitotic phases.[5] Although the law was originally applied only to germ cells, it is actually true for all types of cells in the human body. Consequently, within the realm of diagnostic radiology, the embryo-fetus, which contains a large number of immature, nonspecialized cells, is much more susceptible to radiation damage than is the child or the adult. All imaging professionals should be ever mindful of this.

Effects of Ionizing Radiation on Human Cells

Equal doses of ionizing radiation produce different degrees of damage in different kinds of human cells because of differences in cell radiosensitivity. The more mature and specialized in performing functions a cell is, the less sensitive it is to radiation. In the following sections the radiation response of some of the most important cell groups is examined in detail.

Blood Cells

Hematologic Depression Ionizing radiation adversely affects blood cells by depressing the number of cells in the peripheral circulation. A whole-body dose of 0.25 Gy (25 rads) delivered within a few days produces a measurable hematologic depression. This dose by far exceeds normal doses sustained by the working population of the radiation industry. Therefore, the use of blood tests for purposes of dosimetry is not valid.

Depletion of Immature Blood Cells Most blood cells are manufactured in bone marrow. Radiation causes a decrease in the number of immature blood cells (stem, or precursor) produced in bone marrow and hence a reduction, ultimately, of the number of mature blood cells in the bloodstream. The higher the radiation dose received by the bone marrow, the greater the severity of the resulting cell depletion.

Repopulation After a Period of Recovery If the bone marrow cells have not been destroyed by exposure to ionizing radiation, they can repopulate after a period of recovery. The time necessary for recovery depends on the magnitude of the radiation dose received. If a relatively low dose (below 1 Gy, or 100 rads) of radiation is received, bone marrow repopulation occurs within weeks after irradiation. Moderate (1 to 10 Gy, or 100 to 1000 rads) to high (10 or more Gy, or 1000 or more rads) doses, which severely deplete the number of bone marrow cells, require a longer recovery period. Very high doses of radiation can cause a permanent decrease in the number of stem cells.

Effects on Stem Cells of the Hematopoietic System Radiation affects primarily the stem cells of the hematopoietic (blood-forming) system. Erythrocytes (precursors of red blood cells) are among the most sensitive of human tissues. As with all cells that transform from an immature, undifferentiated state to a mature, functional state, the mature red blood cells are much less radiosensitive. Because the population of circulating red blood cells is high and their life span is long, depletion of red cells is not usually the cause of death in high-dose (i.e., several Gy delivered to the whole body) irradiation. Death, if it occurs, is more typically caused by infection that cannot be overcome by the immune system because of the destruction of myeloblasts (precursors of granulocytes, a type of white blood cell) and internal hemorrhage resulting from destruction of megakaryoblasts (precursor of platelets).

Whole-Body Doses in Excess of 5 Gy (500 rads) Human beings who receive whole-body doses in excess of 5 Gy (500 rads) may die within 30 to 60 days because of effects related to initial depletion of the stem cells of the hematopoietic system. The use of antibiotics or isolation from pathogens in the environment (e.g., placing the patient in a sterile environment, feeding only sterilized food) has been shown to mitigate these effects in animals and human beings. Human beings, however, recover more slowly than do laboratory animals. Thus the lethal dose in animals is usually specified as LD 50/30 (dose that produces death in 50% of the subjects within 30 days). The lethal dose in human beings is usually given as LD 50/60 since a human's recovery is slower than that of the laboratory animals and death may still occur at a later time following a substantial whole-body exposure. Whether survival lasts for 30 days or 60 days, the lethal dose for human beings is generally estimated to be 3.0 to 4.0 Gy (300 to 400 rads) without treatment

TABLE 5-1

LD 50/30 Values for Various Species

Species	LD 50/30	
	Gy	Rads
Human beings	3.0-4.0*	300-400*
Monkey	4.0-4.75	400-475
Dog	3.0	300
Hamster	7.0	700
Rabbit	7.25	725
Rat	9.0	900
Turtle	15.0	1500
Newt	30.0	3000

*Depending on the source of the radiation exposure, LD 50/30 varies. LD 50 may be higher if medical intervention is available. For humans, LD 50/60 may be more realistic because humans are more likely to survive longer than 30 days following an acute whole-body exposure, especially if medical treatment is provided.

and higher if medical intervention is available. Table 5-1 presents an overview of LD 50/30 for various species. Additional information pertaining to the measurement of acute radiation lethality is presented in Chapter 6.

Effects of Ionizing Radiation on Lymphocytes White blood cells are collectively called leukocytes. Lymphocytes *are* a very important subgroup of white blood cells. These cells defend the body against foreign antigens by producing antibodies to combat disease. Lymphocytes live only for about 24 hours, having the shortest life span of all the blood cells. Lymphocytes manufactured in bone marrow are the most radiosensitive blood cells in the human body. A radiation dose as low as 0.25 Gy (25 rads) is sufficient to depress the number of cells present in the circulating blood. When significant numbers of lymphocytes are damaged by radiation exposure, the body loses its natural ability to combat infection and becomes more susceptible to bacteria and viral antigens.

The normal white blood cell count for an adult ranges from 5000 to 10,000/mm^3 of blood. The number of lymphocytes present in circulating blood decreases when low doses of radiation (0.25 Gy or less, or 25 rads or less) are received. At this dose level, complete blood cell recovery occurs shortly after irradiation. However, when a higher dose of whole-body radiation (0.5 to 1 Gy, or 50 to 100 rads) is received, the lymphocyte count decreases to zero within a few days. Full recovery generally requires a period of several months after the exposure.

Effects of Ionizing Radiation on Neutrophils

Neutrophils, another kind of white blood cell, also play an important role in fighting infection. If radiation exposure causes a decrease in the number of these cells, a person's susceptibility to infection increases. A dose of 0.5 Gy (50 rads) of ionizing radiation can cause a reduction in the number of neutrophils present in the circulating blood. When they receive moderate doses of radiation, however, these cells decrease in number to the lowest level possible within a few weeks of irradiation. A few months after the exposure, the number of neutrophils present in the blood returns to its original value.

Effects of Ionizing Radiation on Granulocytes

Granulocytes are a scavenger type of white blood cell that fight bacteria. They remain in the circulating blood for only a few days. These cells respond to irradiation by suddenly increasing in number. After this sudden increase, the granulocytes decrease in number, rapidly at first and then more slowly. Depending on the dose of radiation received, these cells may fully repopulate within about 2 months after their irradiation.

Effects of Ionizing Radiation on Thrombocytes (Platelets)

Thrombocytes, or platelets, initiate blood clotting and prevent hemorrhage. They have a life span of about 30 days. The normal platelet count in the human adult ranges from 150,000 to 350,000/mm³ of blood. A dose of radiation greater than 0.5 Gy (50 rads) lessens the number of platelets in the circulating blood, but when exposed in the range of 1 to 10 Gy (100 to 1000 rads), these cells only begin to regain their original numbers approximately 2 months after being irradiated.

Radiation Exposure During Diagnostic Radiologic Procedures

Neither the blood nor the blood-forming organs of patients should suffer appreciable damage from radiation exposure received during diagnostic radiologic procedures. However, numerous studies indicate chromosome aberrations in circulating lymphocytes that received radiation doses within the diagnostic radiology range. Prime candidates for such aberrations are those in whom high-level fluoroscopy was employed and those in whom very long fluoroscopic exposure times occurred (e.g., cardiac catheterization).

Monitoring of Patients Undergoing Radiation Therapy Treatment

A therapeutic dose of ionizing radiation causes a decrease in the blood count. Patients who are undergoing radiation therapy treatment are monitored frequently (in the form of weekly or biweekly blood counts) to determine whether their platelet counts are adequate.

Occupational Radiation Exposure Monitoring

As previously discussed, a periodic blood count is not recommended as a method for monitoring occupational radiation exposure because biologic damage has already been sustained when an irregularity is seen in the blood count. Also, a blood count is a relatively insensitive test that is unable to indicate exposures of less than 10 cGy (10 rads). Traditional film badge dosimetry, and state-of-the-art, optically stimulated luminescence (OSL) dosimetry (see Chapter 10) detect exposures in the millirem range and therefore may be used to discover potentially hazardous working conditions before actual hazards appear.

Epithelial Tissue

Epithelial tissue lines and covers body tissue. The cells of these tissues lie close together, with few or no substances between them. Epithelial tissue contains no blood vessels, and it regenerates through the process of mitosis. These cells are found in the lining of the intestines, the mucous lining of the respiratory tract, the pulmonary alveoli, and the lining of blood and lymphatic vessels. Because the body constantly regenerates epithelial tissue, the cells that compose this tissue are highly radiosensitive.

Muscle Tissue

Muscle tissue contains fibers that affect movement of an organ or part of the body. Because muscle tissue cells are highly specialized and do not divide, they are relatively insensitive to radiation.

Nervous Tissue

Nervous tissue (conductive tissue) is found in the brain and spinal cord. A nerve cell (neuron) (Fig. 5-18) consists of a cell body and two kinds of very fine stringlike tissue segments that extend outward called

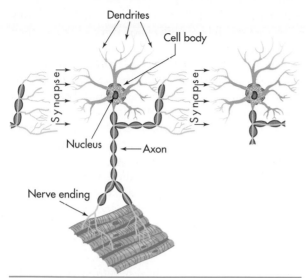

FIG. 5-18. A nerve cell (neuron). Nerve cells relay messages to and from the brain. A message enters a nerve cell through its dendrites, passes through the cell body, and exits the cell through the axon, which transmits the message across a synapse, the communication area leading to the next nerve cell in the chain.

processes: namely, *dendrites* (tentacle-like extensions from the cell body that carry impulses toward the cell) and the *axon* (a long single tentacle from the cell body that carries impulses away from it). Nerve cells relay messages to and from the brain. A message enters the nerve cell through the dendrites. It passes through the cell body and exits the cell through the axon, which transmits the message across a synapse, the communicating area leading to the next nerve cell in the chain.

Nerve Tissue in the Human Adult In the adult, nerve cells are highly specialized. They perform specific functions for the body and, similar to muscle cells, do not divide. Nerve cells contain a nucleus. If the nucleus of one of these cells is destroyed, the cell dies and is never restored. If the cell nucleus has been damaged but not destroyed by exposure to radiation, the damaged nerve cell may still be able to function but in a partially impaired fashion. Radiation also can cause temporary or permanent damage to a nerve's processes (dendrites and axon). When this occurs, communication with and control of some areas of the body may be disrupted. Whole-body exposure to very

high doses of radiation causes severe damage to the central nervous system. A single exposure in excess of 50 Gy (5000 rads) of ionizing radiation may lead to death within a few hours or days.

Nerve Tissue in the Embryo-Fetus Developing nerve cells in the embryo-fetus are more radiosensitive than the mature nerve cells of the adult. Irradiation of the embryo may lead to central nervous system anomalies, microcephaly (small head circumference), and mental retardation. The Japanese atomic bomb survivors provide strong evidence of a "window of maximal sensitivity" extending from 8 to 15 weeks after gestation. This time span covers the end of the period of *neuron organogenesis*, a period of development and change of the nerve cells, and extends into the beginning of the fetal period. A lower level of risk remains until week 25, at which time the risk is not found to be significantly different from that for young adults. During the window of maximal sensitivity, a 0.1-Sv (10-rem) fetal equivalent dose is associated with as much as a 4% risk of mental retardation. This level of risk is considered significant compared with risks during a normal pregnancy. Therefore, special consideration is given to the irradiation of the abdomen or pelvis of a pregnant patient, particularly during the period of greatest sensitivity. However, the fetal equivalent dose associated with routine abdominal fluoroscopy is generally less than 0.05 Sv (5 rem). Thus, if the referring physician and radiologist believe that the diagnostic imaging procedure is vital to the medical management of the mother or offspring, the risk associated with radiation exposure may be justified.

Reproductive Cells

Spermatogonia Human reproductive cells (germ cells) are relatively radiosensitive, although the exact responses of male and female germ cells to ionizing radiation differ because their processes of development from immature to mature status differ. The male testes contain both mature and immature spermatogonia. Because the mature spermatogonia are specialized and do not divide, they are relatively insensitive to ionizing radiation. The immature spermatogonia, however, are unspecialized and divide rapidly, and therefore these germ cells are extremely radiosensitive. A radiation dose of 2 Gy (200 rads) may cause temporary sterility for as long as 12 months, and a dose of 5 or 6 Gy (500 to 600 rads) may cause permanent sterility. Even small doses of ionizing radiation (doses as low as 0.1 Gy [10 rads]) may depress the male sperm population. Male reproductive cells that have been exposed to a radiation dose of 0.1 Gy (10 rads) or more may cause genetic mutations in future generations. To prevent mutations from being passed on to offspring, males receiving this level of testicular radiation dose should refrain from unprotected sex for a few months after such an exposure. By that time, cells that were irradiated during their most sensitive stages will have matured and disappeared. It is highly unlikely that germ cells of patients undergoing diagnostic radiologic procedures would ever receive doses of 0.1 Gy (10 rads), and radiographers working under normal occupational conditions would never receive a gonadal dose of this level.

Ova The ova, the mature female germ cells, do not divide constantly. After puberty, one of the two ovaries expels a mature ovum about every 28 to 36 days (the exact number of days varies among women). During the reproductive life of a woman (from approximately age 12 to 50), 400 to 500 mature ova are produced. Radiosensitivity of ova varies considerably throughout the lifetime of the germ cell. Immature ova are very radiosensitive, whereas more mature ova have little radiosensitivity. After irradiation, a mature ovum can still unite with a male germ cell during conception. However, these irradiated cells may contain damaged chromosomes. If fertilization of an ovum with damaged chromosomes occurs, genetic damage may be passed on to the offspring. If the offspring receives damaged chromosomes, the child might be born with congenital abnormalities. In general, whenever chromosomes in male or female germ cells are damaged by exposure to ionizing radiation, it is possible for mutations to be passed on to succeeding generations. Even low doses received from diagnostic imaging procedures could cause chromosomal damage. For this reason, the reproductive organs should be shielded whenever possible.

Exposure to ionizing radiation also may cause female sterility. The dose necessary to produce this consequence depends partly on the age of the subject. Sterility occurs when radiation exposure destroys new and/or mature ova. The ovaries of the female fetus and a young child are very radiosensitive because they contain a large number of stem cells (oogonia) and immature cells (oocytes). As the female child matures from birth to puberty, the number of immature cells (oocytes) decreases. Hence the ovaries become less radiosensitive. This decrease continues up to the age of 30 years, with women between the ages of 20 and 30 exhibiting the lowest level in sensitivity. After a woman reaches age 30, the overall sensitivity of the ovaries increases constantly until menopause because the new ova being destroyed are not replenished.[6-8] Because the ovaries of a younger woman are less sensitive than the ovaries of an older woman, a higher dose of radiation is required to cause sterility in the younger woman.

Temporary sterility usually results from a single radiation dose of 2 Gy (200 rads) to the ovaries. If the radiation dose is fractionated (i.e., given as a combination of smaller doses with time between doses, which permits the cells to repair some of the damage) over a period of several weeks, doses as high as 20 Gy (2000 rads) may be tolerated.[9,10] A single dose of 5 Gy (500 rads) generally causes permanent sterility in mature women. Even small doses of ionizing radiation (doses as low as 0.1 Gy [10 rads]) may cause menstrual irregularities such as delay or suppression of menstruation. Although some evidence suggests that immature ova are capable of repairing radiation damage, women who have received 0.1 Gy (10 rads) or more are sometimes advised to postpone attempting conception for 30 days or more to allow the damaged immature ova to be expelled. Because all the ova a woman will ever possess are present from birth until the time they are fertilized or expelled, the best solution is to avoid substantial exposures in the first place.

SUMMARY

➤ Linear energy transfer (LET)
  - LET is the average energy deposited per unit length of track by ionizing radiation as it passes through and interacts with a medium along its path.
  - It is described in units of keV per micron (1 micron [μm] = 10^{-6} m).

- Low-LET radiation (x-rays and gamma rays) mainly causes indirect damage to biologic tissues, which usually can be reversed by repair enzymes.
- High-LET radiation (alpha particles, ions of heavy nuclei, and low-energy neutrons) can cause irreparable damage to DNA because multiple-strand breaks in DNA that cannot be undone by repair enzymes may result.

➤ Relative biologic effectiveness (RBE).
- RBE for the type of radiation being used is the ratio of the dose of a reference radiation (conventionally 250-kVp x-rays) to the dose that is necessary to produce the same biologic reaction in a given experiment; the reaction is produced by a dose of test radiation delivered under the same conditions.
- As the LET of radiation increases, so do biologic effects; RBE quantitatively describes this relative effect.
- RBE describes the relative capabilities of radiation with differing LETs to produce a particular biologic reaction.

➤ Oxygen enhancement ratio (OER)
- OER is a comparative measure used to obtain the amount of cellular injury for a species of ionizing radiation.

➤ Radiation-induced damage is observed on the molecular, cellular, and organic levels.

➤ Radiation action on the cell is either direct or indirect, depending on site of interaction.
- Action is direct when biologic damage occurs as a result of the ionization of atoms on DNA, causing them to become inactive or functionally altered.
- Action is indirect when effects are produced by reactive free radicals created by the interaction of radiation with water molecules; these unstable, highly reactive free radicals can cause substantial disruption to DNA molecules, which results in cell death.
- High-LET radiation is more likely to cause biologic damage through direct action than is low-LET.
- Most x-ray damage to macromolecules is the result of indirect action.

- Point mutations commonly occur with low-LET radiation and are reversible through the action of repair enzymes.
- Double-strand breaks of DNA are associated with high-LET radiation, and repair of this type of damage is not likely to occur.
- Target theory states that when cell DNA is directly or indirectly inactivated by exposure to radiation the cell will die.
- When a cell nucleus is significantly damaged by exposure to ionizing radiation, the cell can die or experience reproductive death, apoptosis, mitotic death, mitotic delay, interference of function, or chromosome breakage.

➤ Cell survival curve is used to display the radiosensitivity of a particular type of cell, which helps determine the types of cancer cells that will respond to radiation therapy.

➤ The law of Bergonié and Tribondeau states that the most pronounced radiation effects occur in cells having the least maturity and specialization, the greatest reproductive activity, and the longest mitotic phases.
- The embryo-fetus is very susceptible to radiation damage, which can cause CNS anomalies, microcephaly, and mental retardation.
- Lymphocytes are the most radiosensitive blood cells, and when they are damaged the body loses its natural ability to combat infection and becomes more susceptible to bacterial and viral antigens.
- Human germ cells are relatively radiosensitive; temporary sterilization occurs at 2 Gy (200 rads); permanent sterilization occurs at 5 to 6 Gy (500 to 600 rads).

References

1. Hall EJ: *Radiobiology for the radiologist,* ed 5, Philadelphia, 2000, Lippincott Williams & Wilkins.
2. Bushong SC: *Radiologic science for technologists: physics, biology and protection,* ed 8, St. Louis, 2004, Mosby.
3. Travis EL: *Primer of medical radiobiology,* ed 2, Chicago, 1989, Year Book Medical Publishers.
4. Puck TT, Marcus PI: Action of x-rays on mammalian cells, *J Exp Med* 103:653, 1956.

5. Bergonié J, Tribondeau L: De quelques resultants de la radiotherapie et assai de fixation d'une technique rationelle, *CR Acad Sci* (Paris) 143:983, 1906.

6. United Nations Scientific Committee on the Effects of Atomic Radiation (UNSCEAR): *Ionizing radiation sources and biologic effects. Report E.82.IX.8*, New York, 1992, United Nations.

7. International Commission on Radiological Protection (ICRP): *Non-stochastic effects of ionizing radiation, ICRP Publication 41*, Oxford, 1984, Pergamon.

8. Upton AR: Cancer induction and non-stochastic effects, *Br J Radiol* 60:1-16, 1987.

9. Lushbaugh CC, Ricks RC: Some cytokinetic and histopathologic consideration of irradiated male and female gonadal tissue. In Vath JM, editor: *Frontiers of radiation therapy and oncology*, vol 6, Basel, 1972, Karger, pp 228-248.

10. Lushbaugh CC, Casarett: The effects of gonadal irradiation in clinical radiation therapy: a review, *Cancer* 37:1111-1120, 1976.

GENERAL DISCUSSION QUESTIONS

1. Why is it necessary for persons who administer radiation to humans for medical purposes to have a basic understanding of cell structure, composition, and function as well as adverse effects on these of ionizing radiation?

2. What will an ionized atom of biologic tissue not be able to do?

3. Why is LET an important factor in assessing potential tissue and organ damage from exposure to ionizing radiation?

4. Why are high-LET radiations more destructive to biologic matter than are low-LET radiations?

5. Why is the concept of relative biologic effectiveness (RBE) not practical for specifying radiation protection dose levels in humans?

6. Why does the presence of oxygen in biologic tissue make the damage produced in that tissue by free radicals permanent?

7. What consequences can occur if ionizing radiation damages germ (reproductive) cells?

8. How can ionizing radiation interact with a DNA macromolecule and create a point mutation?

9. Why is the embryo-fetus more susceptible to radiation damage than either the child or the adult?

10. Why is LD 50/60 a more accurate way to assess lethal dose for humans in comparison to LD 50/30?

REVIEW QUESTIONS

1. **For radiation protection, high-LET radiation is of *greatest* concern when a radionuclide has been implanted, ingested, injected, or inhaled because:**
   A. Only single-strand breaks in DNA are possible
   B. The potential exists for repairable damage of single-strand breaks in DNA
   C. The potential exists for irreparable damage because multiple-strand breaks in DNA are possible
   D. The potential exists for repairable damage in DNA resulting from multiple-strand breaks

2. **Free radicals behave as an extremely reactive single entity as a result of the presence of:**
   A. Paired electrons
   B. Unpaired electrons
   C. Paired neutrons and protons
   D. Unpaired neutrons and protons

3. **Which of the following are classified as high-LET radiations?**
   1. **Alpha particles**
   2. **Gamma rays**
   3. **X-rays**
   A. 1 only
   B. 2 only
   C. 3 only
   D. 1, 2, and 3

4. **A biologic reaction is produced by 3 Gy of a test radiation. It takes 12 Gy of 250-kVp x-radiation to produce the same biologic reaction. What is the relative biologic effectiveness (RBE) of the test radiation?**
   A. 2.5
   B. 3
   C. 4
   D. 8

5. **Which action of ionizing radiation is *most* harmful to the human body?**
   A. Direct action
   B. Indirect action
   C. Epidemiologic action
   D. Mitotic action

6. **Which molecules in the human body are most commonly directly acted on by ionizing radiation to produce molecular damage through an indirect action?**
   A. Protein
   B. Carbohydrate
   C. Fat
   D. Water

7. **When does ionizing radiation cause complete chromosome breakage?**
   A. When a single strand of the sugar-phosphate chain sustains a direct hit
   B. When two direct hits occur in the same rung of the DNA macromolecule
   C. When two direct hits occur in different rungs of the DNA macromolecule
   D. When two direct hits are sustained at opposite ends of the DNA macromolecule

8. **When significant numbers of lymphocytes are damaged by exposure from ionizing radiation, the body:**
   1. **Loses its natural ability to combat infection**
   2. **Becomes more susceptible to bacteria**
   3. **Becomes more susceptible to viral antigens**
   A. 1 and 2 only
   B. 1 and 3 only
   C. 2 and 3 only
   D. 1, 2, and 3

9. **With respect to the law of Bergonié and Tribondeau, which of the following would *best* complete this statement? "The most pronounced radiation effects occur in cells having the _____."**
   A. Least reproductive activity, shortest mitotic phases, and most maturity
   B. Greatest reproductive activity, shortest mitotic phases, and most maturity
   C. Greatest reproductive activity, longest mitotic phases, and least maturity
   D. Least reproductive activity, shortest mitotic phases, and least maturity

10. **What do basal cells of the skin, intestinal crypt cells, and reproductive cells have in common?**
   A. All cells are hypoxic
   B. All cells are premalignant
   C. All cells are radioinsensitive
   D. All cells are radiosensitive

6 Radiation Effects on Organ Systems

KEY TERMS

absolute risk
acute radiation syndrome (ARS)
biologic dosimetry
carcinogenesis
cataractogenesis
doubling dose
early nonstochastic somatic effects
embryologic effects (birth defects)
genetic effects
late nonstochastic (deterministic) somatic effects

late somatic effects
late stochastic (probabilistic) somatic effects
latent period
linear, nonthreshold curve
linear-quadratic, nonthreshold curve
manifest illness
nonstochastic (deterministic) somatic effects
nonthreshold

prodromal, or initial, stage
radiation dose-response relationship
recovery
relative risk
sigmoid, or "s-shaped" (nonlinear) threshold curve
somatic effects
stochastic (probabilistic) somatic effects
threshold

OBJECTIVES

After completing this chapter, the reader will be able to perform the following:

- Explain the purpose of a radiation dose-response curve.
- Draw diagrams demonstrating the various dose-response relationships.
- Explain why regulatory agencies continue to use the linear dose-response model for establishing radiation protection standards.
- Differentiate between threshold and nonthreshold relationships.
- List four factors on which the amount of somatic and genetic biologic damage resulting from radiation exposure depend.
- List and describe the various early nonstochastic somatic effects, late nonstochastic somatic effects, and late stochastic somatic effects of ionizing radiation on living systems.
- Describe acute radiation syndrome and list 3 separate dose-related syndromes that occur as part of this total body syndrome.
- Identify and describe the 4 major response stages of acute radiation syndrome.
- Recall the LD 50/30 for human adults, explain its significance, and explain why LD 50/60 is more accurate for humans as a measure of lethality.
- Describe the concept of risk for radiation-induced malignancies and explain the models that are used to give risk estimates.
- Identify ionizing radiation–exposed human populations or groups that prove radiation induces cancer.
- Explain how spontaneous mutations occur and discuss the concept of radiation-induced genetic effects; also explain how ionizing radiation causes these effects and how they can be passed on to future generations.
- Differentiate between dominant and recessive gene mutations.
- Explain the doubling dose concept and give an example of how the number of mutations increases as dose increases.

R adiation-induced damage at the cellular level may lead to measurable somatic and genetic damage in the living organism as a whole. Some examples of measurable biologic damage are cataracts, leukemia, and genetic mutations. This chapter focuses on organic damage resulting from ionizing radiation exposure.

RADIATION DOSE–RESPONSE RELATIONSHIP

Dose-Response Curves

Radiobiologists engaged in research have a common goal to establish relationships between radiation and dose-response. The information obtained can be used to predict the risk of malignancy in human populations that have been exposed to low levels of ionizing radiation. The **radiation dose-response relationship** is demonstrated graphically through a *curve* that maps the observed effects of radiation exposure in relation to the dose of radiation received. As the dose escalates, so do most effects. In such a dose-response curve the variables, or numbers, are plotted along the axes of the graph to demonstrate the relationship between the dose received (horizontal axis) and the biologic effects observed (vertical axis). The curve is either linear (straight line) or nonlinear (curved to some degree) and depicts either a threshold dose or a nonthreshold dose (Fig. 6-1, A and B).

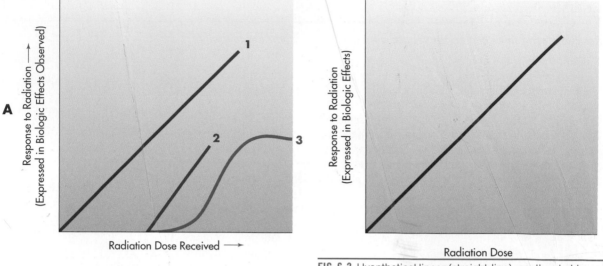

A

B

(Threshold)

FIG. 6-1. **A,** *1* represents a hypothetical linear (straight-line), nonthreshold curve of radiation dose-response relationship. *2* represents a hypothetical linear (straight-line), threshold curve of radiation dose-response relationship. *3* represents a hypothetical nonlinear, threshold curve of radiation dose-response relationship. **B,** Hypothetical sigmoid (S-shaped, hence nonlinear) threshold curve of radiation dose-response relationship generally employed in radiation therapy to demonstrate high-dose cellular response.

FIG. 6-2. Hyopthetical linear (straight-line), nonthreshold curve of radiation dose-response relationship. The straight-line curve passing through the origin in this graph indicates both that the response to radiation (in terms of biologic effects) is directly proportional to the dose of radiation and that no known level of radiation dose exists below which the chance of sustaining biologic damage is zero. In contrast to a cell-survival curve, both the vertical and horizontal axes of a dose-response curve are ordinary linear scales.

Threshold and Nonthreshold Relationships

The term **threshold** may be defined as a point at which a response or reaction to an increasing stimulation first occurs. With reference to ionizing radiation, this means that below a certain radiation level or dose, no biologic effects are observed. Biologic effects are observed only when the threshold level or dose is reached. A **nonthreshold** relationship means that any radiation dose will produce a biologic effect. No radiation dose is believed to be absolutely "safe." Therefore, if ionizing radiation functions as the stimulus and the biologic effect it produces is the response, and if a nonthreshold relationship exists between radiation dose and a biologic response (Fig. 6-2), some biologic effects will be caused in living organisms by even the smallest dose of ionizing radiation.

Risk Models Used to Predict Cancer Risk and Genetic Damage in Human Populations

In a 1980 report the Committee on the Biological Effects of Ionizing Radiation (BEIR), under the auspices of the National Academy of Sciences, revealed that the majority of stochastic somatic effects (e.g., cancer) and genetic effects at low-dose levels from low-LET radiations, such as those employed in diagnostic radiology, appear to follow a linear-quadratic non-threshold curve. New risk models and updated dosimetry techniques have provided a better follow-up study of Hiroshima and Nagasaki atomic bomb survivors. In 1990 the BEIR Committee's revised risk estimates indicated that the risk of radiation exposure was about three to four times greater than previously projected. Currently the committee recommends the use of the **linear, nonthreshold curve** of radiation dose-response for most types of cancer. The linear, nonthreshold curve implies that the biologic response to ionizing radiation is directly proportional to the dose (see Fig. 6-2).

Risk Models Used to Predict Leukemia, Breast Cancer, and Heritable Damage

As previously stated, no radiation exposure level is assumed to be "absolutely" safe. Currently, some experts theorize that all radiation exposure levels possess the potential to cause biologic damage and radiographers must employ thoughtful radiation safety measures whenever humans are exposed to radiation during diagnostic imaging procedures. The **linear-quadratic, nonthreshold curve** (Fig. 6-3) estimates the risk associated with low-level radiation. As previously stated, the BEIR Committee believes it is a more accurate reflection of stochastic somatic and genetic effects at low-dose levels from low-LET radiations. Leukemia, breast cancer, and heritable damage are presumed to follow this curve. For leukemia, the linear-quadratic, nonthreshold curve is supported by an analysis of the leukemia occurrences in Nagasaki and Hiroshima using a recent reevaluation of the radiation dose distribution in these two cities.[1,2]

Rationale for Risk Model Selection

The continued use of the linear dose-response model for radiation protection standards has the potential to

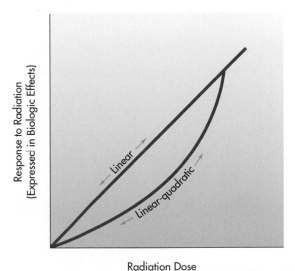

FIG. 6-3. Hypothetical linear-quadratic, nonthreshold dose-response relationship. The curve estimates the risk associated with low-dose levels from low-LET radiations.

exaggerate the seriousness of radiation effects at lower-dose levels from low-LET radiations. However, it accurately reflects the effects of high-LET radiations (neutrons and alpha rays) at higher doses. In establishing radiation protection standards, the regulatory agencies have chosen to be conservative—that is, to use a model that might overestimate risk but is not expected to underestimate risk.

Risk Model Used to Predict High-Dose Cellular Response

Nonstochastic effects of significant radiation exposure such as skin erythema and hematologic depression may be demonstrated graphically through the use of a linear, threshold curve of radiation dose-response (Fig. 6-4). Here, a biologic response does not occur below a specific dose level. Laboratory experiments on animals and data from human populations observed after acute high doses of radiation provided the foundation for this curve. The **sigmoid or "S-shaped" (nonlinear), threshold curve** of radiation dose–response relationship (see Fig. 6-1, B) is generally employed in radiation therapy to demonstrate high-dose cellular response. This curve indicates the existence of a threshold, a minimal dose of ionizing radiation below which

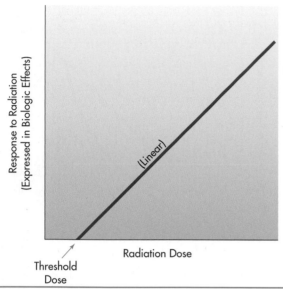

FIG. 6-4. Hypothetical linear, threshold curve of radiation dose-response. This depicts those cases for which a biologic response does not occur below a specific radiation dose.

observable effects will not occur. Different effects require different minimal doses. The tail of the curve indicates that limited recovery occurs at low radiation doses. At the highest radiation doses, the curve gradually levels off and then veers downward because the affected living specimen or tissue dies before the observable effect appears.

SOMATIC AND GENETIC DAMAGE FACTORS

The amount of somatic and genetic biologic damage a human being suffers as a result of radiation exposure depends on several factors (Box 6-1). Ionizing radiation produces the greatest amount of biologic damage in the human body when a large dose of densely ionizing (high-LET) radiation is delivered to a large or radiosensitive area of the body.

SOMATIC EFFECTS

When living organisms (such as human beings) that have been exposed to radiation suffer biologic damage, the effects of this exposure are classified as **somatic**

BOX 6-1
Somatic and Genetic Damage Factors

1. The quantity of ionizing radiation to which the subject is exposed
2. The ability of the ionizing radiation to cause ionization of human tissue
3. The amount of body area exposed
4. The specific body parts exposed

---

effects. Depending on the length of time from the moment of irradiation to the first appearance of symptoms of radiation damage, the effects are classified as either *early or late somatic effects.* If these effects are cell-killing and directly related to the dose received, they are termed **nonstochastic (deterministic) somatic effects** (see Chapter 7 for additional information). Late effects of ionizing radiation that are mutational or randomly occurring biologic somatic changes, independent of dose, are termed **stochastic (probabilistic) somatic effects** (see Chapter 7 for additional information).

Early Nonstochastic (Deterministic) Somatic Effects

Early nonstochastic (deterministic) somatic effects are those that appear within minutes, hours, days, or weeks of the time of radiation exposure. A substantial dose of ionizing radiation is required to produce biologic effects so soon after irradiation. The severity of these effects is dose-related. With the exception of certain lengthy high-dose-rate fluoroscopic procedures, diagnostic radiologic examinations do not usually impose radiation doses sufficient to cause early deterministic effects. Therefore, they are of little concern in diagnostic imaging. High-dose effects include nausea, fatigue, erythema (diffuse redness over an area of skin after irradiation) (Fig. 6-5), epilation (loss of hair), blood disorders, intestinal disorders, fever, dry and moist desquamation (shedding of the outer layer of skin) (Fig. 6-6), depressed sperm count in the male, temporary or permanent sterility in the male and female, and injury to the central nervous system (at extremely high radiation doses). The various types of organic damage may be related to the

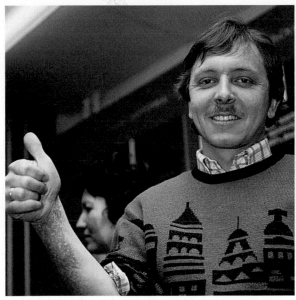

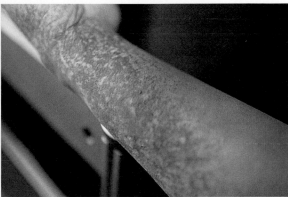

FIG. 6-5. Radiation burn or erythema on the arm of a former worker who was present at the Chernobyl nuclear power plant during the 1986 radiation accident. (Courtesy Ken Graham Photography.)

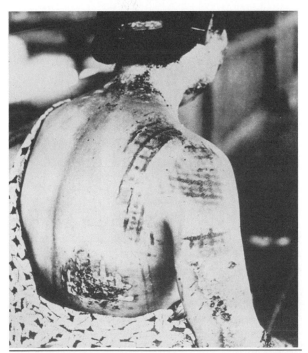

FIG. 6-6. Dry and moist desquamation. The back of this female Japanese atomic bomb survivor demonstrates the pattern of the kimono she was wearing at the time of the bombing. Radiation burns resulting in the shedding of the outer layer of skin are visible. (From PhotoAssist, Inc.)

cellular effects discussed previously in Chapter 5. For example, intestinal disorders are caused by damage to the sensitive epithelial tissue lining the intestines (Fig. 6-7). When the whole body is exposed to a dose of 6 Gy (600 rads) of ionizing radiation, many of these manifestations of organic damage occur in succession. These early somatic effects are called **acute radiation syndrome (ARS).**

Acute Radiation Syndrome (ARS)

ARS, or radiation sickness, occurs in humans after whole-body reception of large doses of ionizing radiation delivered over a short period of time. Data from epidemiologic studies of human populations exposed to doses of ionizing radiation sufficient to cause this syndrome have been obtained from atomic bomb survivors of Hiroshima and Nagasaki, the Marshall Islanders who were inadvertently subjected to high levels of fallout during an atomic bomb test in 1954, nuclear radiation accident victims such as those injured in the 1986 Chernobyl disaster, and radiation therapy patients.

ARS Symptoms *Syndrome* is the medical term that means a collection of symptoms. ARS is a collection of symptoms associated with high-level radiation exposure. Three separate dose-related syndromes occur

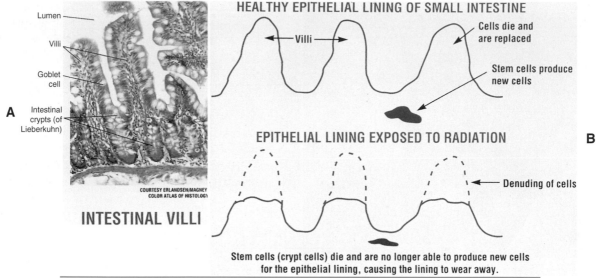

FIG. 6-7. **A,** Intestinal villi. **B,** The top drawing depicts the healthy lining of the small intestine. The bottom drawing shows the epithelial lining of the small intestine after it is exposed to radiation. Stem cells (crypt cells) die and are no longer able to produce new cells for the epithelial lining, causing the lining to wear away. (From *Mosby's radiographic instructional series radiobiology and radiation protection,* St. Louis, 1999, Mosby.)

as part of the total-body syndrome: hematopoietic syndrome, gastrointestinal syndrome, and cerebrovascular syndrome.

Major Response Stages of ARS ARS presents in four major response stages: prodromal, latent period, manifest illness, and recovery or death (Fig. 6-8). The **prodromal, or initial, stage,** also called the *prodromal syndrome,* occurs within hours after a whole-body absorbed dose of 1 Gy (100 rads) or more (Fig. 6-9). Nausea, vomiting, diarrhea, fatigue, and leukopenia (an abnormal decrease in white blood corpuscles, usually below 5000/mm^3) characterize this initial stage. The severity of these symptoms is dose-related; the higher the dose, the more severe the symptoms. The length of time involved for this stage to run its course may be hours or a few days. After the prodromal stage, a **latent period** of about 1 week occurs, during which no visible symptoms occur. Actually, it is during this period that either recovery or lethal effects begin. Toward the end of the first week, the next stage commences. This stage is called **manifest illness** because it is the period when symptoms that affect the hematopoietic, gastrointestinal, and

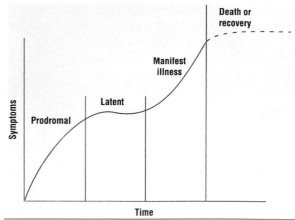

FIG. 6-8. The graph depicts the stages of acute radiation syndrome following a whole-body reception of large doses of ionizing radiation delivered over a short period of time. The length of time involved for the syndrome to run its course and the final outcome of the syndrome depend on the dose received. (From *Mosby's radiographic instructional series: radiobiology and radiation protection,* St. Louis, 1999, Mosby.)

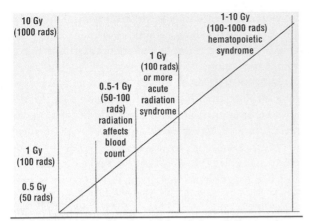

FIG. 6-9. The prodromal stage of the acute radiation syndrome occurs within hours after a whole-body absorbed dose of 1 Gy (100 rads) or more is received. Doses ranging from 1 to 10 Gy (100 to 1000 rads) are responsible for causing the hematopoietic form of the acute radiation syndrome. (From *Mosby's radiographic instructional series: radiobiology and radiation protection,* St. Louis, 1999, Mosby.)

cerebrovascular systems become visible. Some of these symptoms are apathy, confusion, a decrease in the number of red and white blood cells and platelets in the circulating blood, fluid loss, dehydration, epilation, exhaustion, vomiting, severe diarrhea, fever, headaches, infection, hemorrhage, and cardiovascular collapse. In severe high-dose cases, emaciated human beings eventually die.

If after a whole-body sublethal dose such as 2 to 3 Gy (200 to 300 rads), exposed persons pass through the first three stages but show less severe symptoms than those seen after super-lethal doses of 6 to 10 Gy (600 to 1000 rads), **recovery** may occur in about 3 months. However, those who recover may show some signs of radiation damage and experience late effects.

ARS as a Consequence of the Chernobyl Nuclear Power Plant Accident

The massive explosion that blew apart a reactor (Unit #4) at the nuclear power station in Chernobyl, Russia (see Fig. 1-12, A-C) on April 26, 1986 provides a recent example of humans suffering from ARS. During the explosion, several tons of burning graphite, uranium dioxide fuel, and other contaminants such as cesium-137, iodine-131, and plutonium-239 were ejected vertically into the atmosphere in a 3-mile-high radioactive plume of intense heat. Of 444 people working at the power plant at the time of the explosion, 2 died instantly and 29 died within 3 months of the accident as a consequence of thermal trauma (burns) and severe injuries from doses of whole-body ionizing radiation of approximately 6 Gy (600 rads) or more.[3-5]

Without effective physical monitoring devices, biologic criteria such as the occurrence of nausea and vomiting played an important role in the identification of radiation casualties during the first 2 days after the nuclear disaster. ARS caused the hospitalization of at least 203 people.[5,6] A determination of the lapse of time from the incidental exposure of the victims to the onset of nausea and/or regurgitation completed the biologic criteria. Dose assessment was determined from **biologic dosimetry.** This included serial measurements of levels of lymphocytes and granulocytes in the blood and a quantitative analysis of dicentric chromosomes (chromosomes having two centromeres) in blood and hematopoietic cells coming from bone marrow. The data were compared with doses and effects from earlier radiation mishaps.[4,5]

ARS as a Consequence of the Atomic Bombing of Hiroshima and Nagasaki

The Japanese atomic bomb survivors of Hiroshima and Nagasaki are examples of a human population afflicted with ARS as a consequence of war. Follow-up studies of the survivors who did not die of ARS have demonstrated late deterministic and stochastic effects of ionizing radiation. The atomic bombing of Japan and the nuclear accident at Chernobyl have made the medical community recognize the need for a thorough understanding of ARS and appropriate medical support of persons afflicted.

Forms of ARS

Hematopoietic syndrome, gastrointestinal syndrome, and cerebrovascular syndrome are forms of acute radiation syndrome.

Hematopoietic syndrome

The hematopoietic form of ARS, or "bone marrow syndrome," occurs when human beings receive whole-body doses of ionizing radiation ranging from 1 to 10 Gy (100 to 1000 rads) (see Fig. 6-9). The hematopoietic system manufactures the corpuscular elements of the blood and is the most radiosensitive vital organ system in humans. Radiation exposure causes the number of red cells, white cells, and platelets in the circulating blood to decrease. Dose levels that cause this syndrome also may damage cells in other organ systems, causing the affected organ or organ system to fail. For example, radiation doses ranging from 1 to 10 Gy (100 to 1000 rads) produce a decrease in the number of bone marrow stem cells. When the cells of the lymphatic system are damaged, the body loses some of its ability to combat infection. Because the number of platelets also decreases with loss of bone marrow function, the body loses a corresponding amount of its blood-clotting ability. This makes the body more susceptible to hemorrhage.

For persons affected with hematopoietic syndrome, survival time shortens as the radiation dose increases. Because additional bone marrow cells are destroyed as the radiation dose escalates, the body becomes more susceptible to infection (mostly from its own intestinal bacteria) and more prone to hemorrhage. When death occurs, it is a consequence of bone marrow destruction.

Death may occur 6 to 8 weeks after irradiation in some sensitive human subjects who receive a whole-body dose exceeding 2 Gy (200 rads). As the whole-body dose increases from 2 to 10 Gy (200 to 1000 rads), irradiated individuals die sooner. If the radiation exposure is not lethal, perhaps in the range of 1 to 2 Gy (100 to 200 rads), bone marrow cells will eventually repopulate to a level adequate to support life in most individuals. Many of these people recover 3 weeks to 6 months after irradiation. The actual dose of radiation received and the irradiated person's general state of health at the time of irradiation determine the possibility of recovery. When death occurs in exposed individuals, it results from bone marrow destruction. The severe reduction of blood cells causes anemia and permits exposed individuals to become susceptible to infection. This results in death of those individuals.

Survival probability of patients with hematopoietic syndrome is enhanced by intense supportive care and special hematologic procedures. As an illustration, victims who received doses in excess of 5 Gy (500 rads), like those of the nuclear power station accident in Chernobyl, benefited from bone marrow transplants from appropriate histocompatible donors. During the operation, hematopoietic stem cells are transplanted to facilitate bone marrow recovery. This operation, however, is not an absolute cure for patients suffering from hematopoietic syndrome because many individuals undergoing bone marrow transplant die of burns or other radiation-induced damage they sustained before the transplanted stem cells have had a chance to support recovery.

Gastrointestinal syndrome In human beings the gastrointestinal form of ARS appears at a threshold dose of approximately 6 Gy (600 rads) and peaks after a dose of 10 Gy (1000 rads). Without medical support to sustain life, exposed persons receiving doses of 6 to 10 Gy (600 to 1000 rads) may die 3 to 10 days after being exposed. Even if medical support is provided, the exposed person will live only a few days longer. Survival time does not change with dose in this syndrome.

A few hours after the dose required to cause the gastrointestinal syndrome has been received, the prodromal stage occurs. Severe nausea, vomiting, and diarrhea persist for as long as 24 hours. This is followed by a latent period, which lasts as long as 5 days. During this time the symptoms disappear. The manifest illness stage follows this period of false calm. Again, the human subject experiences severe nausea, vomiting, and diarrhea. Other symptoms that may occur include fever (as in hematopoietic syndrome), fatigue, loss of appetite, lethargy, anemia, leukopenia (decrease in the number of white blood cells), hemorrhage (gastrointestinal tract bleeding occurs because the body loses its blood-clotting ability), infection, electrolyte imbalance, and emaciation. Death occurs primarily because of catastrophic damage to the epithelial cells that line the gastrointestinal tract. Such severe damage to these cells results in the death of the exposed person within 3 to 5 days of irradiation, as a result of infection, fluid loss, or electrolytic imbalance. Death from gastrointestinal syndrome is not exclusively from damage to the bowel but also can be induced from damage to the bone marrow. The latter is usually sufficient to cause death in hematopoietic syndrome.

The small intestine is the most severely affected part of the gastrointestinal tract. Because epithelial cells function as an essential biologic barrier, their breakdown leaves the body vulnerable to infection (mostly from its own intestinal bacteria), dehydration, and severe diarrhea. Some epithelial cells regenerate before death occurs. However, because of the large number of epithelial cells damaged by the radiation, death may occur before cell regeneration is accomplished. The workers and firefighters at Chernobyl are examples of humans who died as a result of gastrointestinal syndrome.

Cerebrovascular syndrome The cerebrovascular form of the ARS results when the central nervous system and cardiovascular system receive doses of 50 Gy (5000 rads) or more of ionizing radiation. A dose of this magnitude can cause death within a few hours to 2 or 3 days after exposure. After irradiation the prodromal stage begins. Symptoms include excessive nervousness, confusion, severe nausea, vomiting, diarrhea, loss of vision, a burning sensation of the skin, and loss of consciousness. A latent period lasting up to 12 hours follows. During this time, symptoms lessen or disappear. After the latent period the manifest illness stage occurs. During this period the prodromal syndrome recurs with increased severity, and other symptoms appear, including disorientation and shock, periods of agitation alternating with stupor, ataxia (confusion and lack of muscular coordination), edema in the cranial vault, loss of equilibrium, fatigue, lethargy, convulsive seizures, electrolytic imbalance, meningitis, prostration, respiratory distress, vasculitis, and coma. Damaged blood vessels and permeable capillaries permit fluid to leak into the brain, causing an increase in fluid content. This creates an increase in intracranial pressure, which causes more tissue damage. The final result of this damage is failure of the central nervous and cardiovascular systems, which causes death in a matter of minutes. Because the gastrointestinal and hematopoietic systems are more radiosensitive than the central nervous system, they also are severely damaged and fail to function after a dose of this magnitude. However, because death occurs quickly, the consequences of the failure of these two systems are not demonstrated.

An overview of acute radiation lethality is presented in Table 6-1. The radiation dose required to cause a particular syndrome and the average survival time are the most important measures used to quantify human radiation lethality. The progression of each syndrome, the length of time required for the consequential chain of events to occur, and the final outcome depend on the effective dose received.

Lethal Dose (LD)

LD 50/30 The term *LD 50/30* signifies the whole-body dose of radiation that can be lethal to 50% of the

---

TABLE 6-1

Overview of Acute Radiation Lethality

Stage	Dose—Gy (Rads)	Average Survival Time	Symptoms
Prodromal	1 (100)	—	Nausea, vomiting, diarrhea, fatigue, leukopenia
Latent	1-100 (100-10,000)	—	None
Hematopoietic	1-10 (100-1000)	6 to 8 wk (doses over 2 Gy)	Nausea; vomiting; diarrhea; decrease in number of red blood cells, white blood cells, and platelets in the circulating blood; hemorrhage; infection
Gastrointestinal	6-10 (600-1000)	3-10 days	Severe nausea, vomiting, diarrhea, fever, fatigue, loss of appetite, lethargy, anemia, leukopenia, hemorrhage, infection, electrolytic imbalance, and emaciation
Cerebrovascular	5 and above (5000 and above)	Several hours to 2 or 3 days	Same as hematopoietic and gastrointestinal, plus excessive nervousness, confusion, lack of coordination, loss of vision, a burning sensation of the skin, loss of consciousness, disorientation, shock, periods of agitation alternating with stupor, edema, loss of equilibrium, meningitis, prostration, respiratory distress, vasculitis, coma

exposed population within 30 days. This is a quantitative measurement that is fairly precise when applied to experimental animals. Humans exposed to substantial whole-body doses of ionizing radiation, however, take longer to recover than do laboratory animals. Hence, the LD 50 for humans may require more than 30 days for its full expression. As stated in Chapter 5, the LD 50/30 for adult humans is estimated to be 3.0 to 4.0 Gy (300 to 400 rads) without medical support (Fig. 6-10). For x-rays and gamma rays, this is equal to an equivalent dose of 3.0 to 4.0 Sv (300 to 400 rem). Whole-body doses greater than 6 Gy (600 rads) may cause the death of the entire population in 30 days without medical support. With medical support, human beings have tolerated doses as high as 8.5 Gy (850 rads).[7]

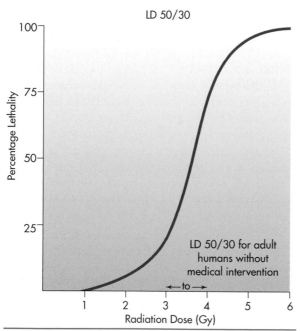

FIG. 6-10. LD 50/30 refers to the whole-body dose of radiation that can be lethal to 50% of the exposed population within 30 days. As can be seen in the graph, no deaths are expected below 1 Gy (100 rads). In this particular graph, which represents human response to radiation exposure, LD 50/30 is reached at 3.5 Gy (350 rads), a dose that falls between 3.0 and 4.0 Gy (300 to 400 rads). This is the point at which half of those exposed to 3.5 Gy (350 rads) of ionizing radiation would die. The graph also demonstrates that at a dose of 6 Gy (600 rads) no one is expected to survive. In reality, survival is possible with extensive medical intervention.

LD 10/30, LD 50/60, and LD 100/60 Other measures of lethality also are quoted, such as *LD 10/30, LD 50/60,* and *LD 100/60.* All these measures refer to the percentage of subjects who survive after a certain number of days. The values reported in the literature vary widely because most lethal dose data represent an estimate of the role played by radiation in fatalities in which other factors (e.g., fire at Chernobyl, physical effects of a large explosion at Hiroshima and Nagasaki, chemical contamination in a few nuclear accidents) were present. Specifications of lethal effects are further complicated by the medical treatment that the patient may receive during the prodromal and latent stages, before many of the symptoms of ARS appear. When medical treatment is given promptly, the patient is supported through initial symptoms, but the question of long-term survival may simply be delayed. Thus survival over a 60-day period may be a more relevant indicator of outcome for humans than survival over a 30-day period. This is the reason that LD 50/60 for humans may be more accurate. Table 6-2 gives estimates of lethal doses, including the treatment that has been given in populations studied. Regardless of treatment, whole-body equivalent doses of greater than 12 Gy (1200 rads) are considered fatal.[8]

Repair and Recovery

Because cells contain a repair mechanism inherent in their biochemistry (repair enzymes), repair and recovery may occur when cells are exposed to sublethal

---

TABLE 6-2

Lethal Dose Values for Healthy Adults Who Receive the Specified Medical Treatment After Exposure to Low-LET Radiation at Dose Rates of More Than 100 mGy/min

Effect	Treatment	Dose (Gy)
LD 50/60	Minimal	3.2-4.5
LD 50/60	Optimal supportive	4.8-5.4
LD 50/60	Autologous bone marrow transplantation	11

From Fry RJM: Acute radiation effects. In Wagner LK et al: *Radiation bioeffects and management: test and syllabus,* Reston, Va, 1991, American College of Radiology.

doses of ionizing radiation. After irradiation, surviving cells begin to repopulate. This permits an organ that has sustained functional damage as a result of radiation exposure to regain some or most of its functional ability. However, the amount of functional damage sustained determines the organ's potential for recovery. In the repair of sublethal damage, oxygenated cells receiving more nutrients have a better prospect for recovery than do hypoxic (poorly oxygenated) cells receiving less nutrients. If both oxygenated and hypoxic cells receive a comparable dose of low-LET radiation, the oxygenated cells are more severely damaged but those that survive repair themselves and recover from the injury. Even though they are less severely damaged, the hypoxic cells do not repair and recover as efficiently.

Research has shown that repeated radiation injuries have a cumulative effect. Hence a percentage (about 10%) of the radiation-induced damage is irreparable, whereas the remaining 90% may be repaired over time. When the processes of repair and repopulation work together, they aid in healing the body from radiation injury and promote recovery.

Late Somatic Effects

Late somatic effects are effects that appear months or years after exposure to ionizing radiation. These effects may result from previous whole- or partial-body acute, high-radiation doses, or they may be the product of individual low doses and chronic low-level doses sustained over several years. Late effects that can be directly related to the dose received and occur months or years after a high-level radiation exposure are classified as **late nonstochastic (deterministic) somatic effects.** Late effects that do not have a threshold, occur in an arbitrary or probabilistic manner, whose severity does not depend on dose, and occur months or years after high-level and possibly after low-level radiation exposure are classified as **late stochastic (probabilistic) somatic effects.** Examples of late nonstochastic and stochastic somatic effects are listed in Box 6-2.

Risk Estimate for Contracting Cancer from Low-Level Radiation Exposure

Low-level doses are a consideration for patients and personnel exposed to ionizing radiation as a result of

---

BOX 6-2

Late Somatic Effects

Late Nonstochastic Somatic Effects
Cataract formation
Fibrosis
Organ atrophy
Loss of parenchymal cells
Reduced fertility
Sterility

Late Stochastic Somatic Effects
Cancer
Embryologic effects (birth defects)

---

diagnostic imaging procedures. The risk estimate for human beings of contracting cancer from low-level radiation exposure is still controversial. No conclusive proof exists that low-level ionizing radiation doses below 0.1 Sv (10 rem) cause a significant increase in the risk of malignancy. The risk, in fact, may be negligible or even nonexistent. Low-level radiation must be defined in broad terms to encompass the various sources of ionizing radiation, such as x-rays and radioactive materials used for diagnostic purposes in the healing arts, employment-related exposures in medicine and industry, and natural background exposure. Such low-level radiation has been defined as "an absorbed dose of [0.1 Sv] 10 rem or less delivered over a short period of time" and as "a larger dose delivered over a long period of time—for instance, [0.5 Sv] 50 rem in 10 years."[9] Numerous laboratory experiments on animals and studies on human populations exposed to high doses of ionizing radiation have been conducted to determine health effects. Using all data available on high radiation exposure, members of the scientific and medical communities have determined that three categories of health effects require study at low-level exposures: cancer induction, damage to the unborn from irradiation in utero, and genetic effects.

Late Stochastic and Nonstochastic Somatic Effects

Cells that survive the initial irradiation and then retain a "memory" of that event are responsible for producing late effects. Such randomly occurring effects are nonthreshold and referred to as *stochastic events*. For these, it is the probability of occurrence rather than the severity that is proportional to dose. This means that the greater the dose received by an individual, the greater the chance that a specific late effect will be seen. However, the severity of the effect does not increase as a consequence of increased dose. Cancer and genetic disorders are examples of stochastic effects that probably do not have a threshold. Theoretically, radiation damage to one or more cells could actually produce a cancer or genetic disorder. When the biologic effects demonstrate the existence of a threshold, a dose below which a person has a negligible chance of sustaining specific biologic damage, and the severity of that biologic damage increases as a consequence of increased absorbed dose, the events are considered nonstochastic. Cataract formation and reproductive cell damage leading to impaired fertility are examples of such late deterministic somatic effects. These effects usually occur at much higher doses that those initiating stochastic effects. It is important for the reader to understand that deterministic effects are not likely to occur from diagnostic imaging procedures. Stochastic and nonstochastic effects are discussed in detail in Chapter 7.

Major Types of Late Somatic Effects

The three major types of late somatic effects are **carcinogenesis, cataractogenesis,** and **embryologic effects (birth defects).** Of these, carcinogenesis and embryologic effects are considered stochastic events, and cataractogenesis is regarded as nonstochastic (deterministic).

Risk Estimates for Cancer

Exposure to ionizing radiation may cause cancer as a late stochastic somatic effect. At high doses, for groups such as the atomic bomb survivors, the risk is measurable in human populations. At low doses, below 0.1 Sv (less than 10 rem), which includes groups such as occupationally exposed individuals and virtually all patients in diagnostic radiology, this risk is not directly measurable in population studies. Either the risk is overshadowed by the natural incidence of cancer in humans, or the risk is zero. Current radiation protection philosophy assumes that risk still exists and may

be determined by extrapolating (scaling down the risk versus dose curve) from high-dose data, where risk has been directly observed, down to the low doses, where it has not been observed. This remains a very controversial concept.

Absolute Risk and Relative Risk Models Risk estimates to predict cancer incidence may be given in terms of absolute risk or relative risk caused by a specific exposure to ionizing radiation (over and above background exposure). Both models predict the number of excess cancers, or cancers that would not have occurred in the population in question without the exposure to ionizing radiation. The **absolute risk** model predicts that a specific number of excess cancers will occur as a result of exposure (Fig. 6-11). The **relative risk** model predicts that the number of excess cancers will increase as the natural incidence of cancer increases with advancing age in a population (Fig. 6-12). It is relative in the sense that it predicts a percentage increase in incidence rather than a specific number of cases. Recent studies of atomic bomb survivors tend to support the relative risk model over the absolute risk model.

Epidemiologic Studies for Determining the Risk of Cancer Epidemiologic studies suggest that although the radiation doses encountered in diagnostic radiology should be considered, the benefit to the patient of the

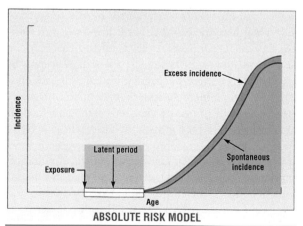

FIG. 6-11. Absolute risk model. This model predicts that a specific number of excess cancers will occur as a result of exposure. (From *Mosby's radiographic instructional series: radiobiology and radiation protection,* St. Louis, 1999, Mosby.)

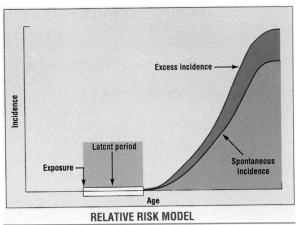

FIG. 6-12. Relative risk model. This model predicts that the number of excess cancers will increase as the natural incidence of cancer increases with advancing age in a population. (From *Mosby's radiographic instructional series: radiobiology and radiation protection,* St. Louis, 1999, Mosby.)

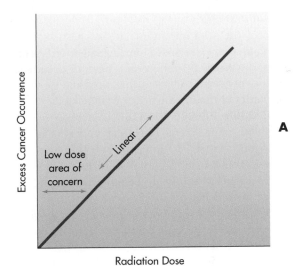

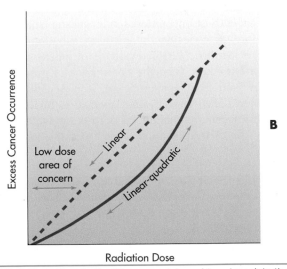

FIG. 6-13. **A,** Hypothetical linear model used to extrapolate the occurrence of cancer from high-dose information to low doses. This model suits current high-dose information satisfactorily but exaggerates the actual risk at low doses and dose rates. **B,** Hypothetical linear-quadratic model used to extrapolate the occurrence of cancer from high-dose information to low doses. This model suits current high-dose information satisfactorily, but risk at low doses may be underestimated.

information gained from an imaging procedure greatly exceeds the minimal theoretical risk to the patient of developing cancer as a stochastic late somatic effect. Even at the relatively high doses encountered by the Japanese atomic bomb survivors, the probability of causation of an excess fatal cancer is surprisingly low—approximately 5% per Sv (100 rem).[10]

Models for Extrapolation of Cancer Risk from High-Dose to Low-Dose Data Researchers commonly use two models for extrapolation of risk from high-dose to low-dose data. These are linear and linear-quadratic models. In the linear model (Fig. 6-13, A), the risk per centigray (rad) is constant; the occurrence of cancer follows a straight-line or dose-proportional progression throughout the entire dose range. Although this model appears to fit the high-dose data, it may substantially overestimate the risk at low doses. The linear-quadratic model (Fig. 6-13, B) includes extra mathematical terms that produce a deviation from straight-line behavior at low doses so that the risk per additional centigray (rad) at low doses is predicted to be less than at high doses. The 1989 BEIR V report supported the linear-quadratic model for leukemia only. For all other cancers the BEIR V Committee recommended adoption of the linear model to fit the available data.[11]

Carcinogenesis

Cancer is the most important late stochastic somatic effect caused by exposure to ionizing radiation. As previously discussed, this effect is a random occurrence that does not seem to have a threshold and for which the severity of the disease is not dose-related.

Radiation-induced Cancer Laboratory experiments with animals and statistical studies of human populations exposed to ionizing radiation (e.g., the Japanese atomic bomb survivors) prove that radiation induces cancer. In human beings, these radiation-induced cancers may take 5 or more years to develop. Distinguishing radiation-induced cancer by its physical appearance is difficult because it does not appear different from cancers caused by other agents. Cancer from natural causes frequently occurs, and the number of cancers induced by radiation is small compared with the natural incidence of malignancies even at doses many times those encountered in diagnostic radiology. Therefore, cancer caused by low-level radiation is difficult to identify. Human evidence of radiation carcinogenesis comes from the observation of irradiated humans and from epidemiologic studies conducted many years after subjects were exposed to high doses of ionizing radiation. Examples of these data are listed in Box 6-3. An explanation of each example follows.

BOX 6-3

Human Evidence for Radiation Carcinogenesis

1. Radium watch-dial painters (1920s and 1930s)
2. Uranium miners (early years, and Navajo people of Arizona and New Mexico during the 1950s and 1960s)
3. Early medical radiation workers (1896-1910)
4. Patients injected with the contrast agent Thorotrast (1925-1945)
5. Infants treated with x-radiation to reduce an enlarged thymus gland (1940s and 1950s)
6. Children of the Marshall Islanders inadvertently subjected to high levels of fallout during an atomic bomb test in 1954
7. Japanese atomic bomb survivors, 1945
8. Evacuees from the Chernobyl nuclear power station disaster in 1986

Radium Watch-dial Painters During the early years of the last century (1920s and 1930s), a radium watch-dial painting industry flourished in some factories in New Jersey. Young, unprotected, and ill-informed girls employed in these factories hand painted the luminous numerals on watches and clocks with a radium-containing paint. The girls used sable brushes to apply the paint. To do the fine work required, some would place the paint-saturated brush tip on their lips to draw the bristles to a fine point. The girls who followed this procedure ingested large quantities of radium. Because it is chemically similar to calcium, the radium was incorporated into bone tissue. The accumulation of this toxic substance eventually caused development of osteoporosis (decalcification of bone), osteogenic sarcoma (bone cancer), and other malignancies such as carcinoma of the epithelial cells lining the nasopharynx and paranasal sinuses. The bones most frequently affected included the pelvis, femur, and mandible. Doses of 5 Gy (500 rads) or more are assumed to have induced the aforementioned malignancies. The number of head carcinomas attributed to the radium watch-dial painting industry, although small, is statistically significant. Of 1474 women in the industry, 61 were diagnosed with cancer of the paranasal sinuses and 21 with cancer of the mastoid air cells. Studies attribute the death of at least 18 of the radium watch-dial painters to radium poisoning.

Uranium Miners During the early years of the last century, people worked in European mines to extract pitchblende, a uranium ore. Uranium is a radioactive element with a very long half-life (the half-life of ^{238}U is 4.5 billion years); it decays through a series of radioactive nuclides by emitting alpha, beta, and gamma radiation. One of the most important members of its decay family is radium (atomic number [Z] = 88). Radium, itself radioactive, decays with a half-life of 1622 years to the radioactive element radon (Z = 86). Radon is a gas that decays with a half-life of 3.8 days by way of alpha particle emission. This gas emanates through tiny gaps in the rocks, creating an insidious airborne hazard to miners. Throughout many years of employment, some miners inhaled significant amounts of radon. Possessing high LET, alpha particles passing through a person's lungs have a high probability of producing a great deal of cellular damage. About 50% of the miners eventually succumbed to lung cancer.

During the 1950s and 1960s, at the height of the Cold War between the United States and Russia, the U.S. government needed fuel for nuclear weapons and plants. The Navajo people of Arizona and New Mexico mined uranium to meet this need. Because the government did not regulate working conditions in the mines to ensure safety from exposure—despite an awareness of risk—some 15,000 Navajo and whites who worked in the uranium mines sustained lethal doses of ionizing radiation by breathing radioactive dust and drinking radioactive water. Experts estimate that each miner unknowingly received an approximate equivalent dose of 10 Sv (1000 rem) or more.[12] As a result, an alarmingly high number of miners died from cancer and other respiratory diseases. Compounding this tragedy, the families of the miners also were affected. Because the miners had no knowledge of the adverse effects of ionizing radiation, they did not promptly change their work clothing on returning home. Because the clothing was contaminated by radioactive material, the miners' immediate families were extremely vulnerable to radiation-induced cancers.

Early Medical Radiation Workers A number of the first generation of radiation workers (radiologists, dentists, and technologists) were exposed to large amounts of ionizing radiation. This resulted in some severe radiation injuries. Many radiologists and dentists developed cancerous skin lesions on their hands as a result of occupational exposure (Fig. 6-14). When compared with their nonradiologist counterparts, many early radiologists showed a higher incidence of blood disorders such as aplastic anemia and leukemia. Because all worked without the benefit of protective devices and some received doses estimated at more than 1 Gy/year (100 rads/year), the occurrence of these radiation-induced injuries is understandable. Today, as a result of programs stressing radiation safety education and protective devices, radiation workers employed in medical imaging need not experience any adverse health effects as a consequence of their work. Studies of radiographers and physicians who began their careers in radiology after the 1940s show that these radiation workers have had no increase in adverse health effects as a result of their occupational exposure. This finding is attributed to increased knowledge and use of proper protective measures and devices.

Patients Injected with the Contrast Agent Thorotrast Between 1925 and 1945, Thorotrast was used as a contrast agent for diagnostic angiography. This medium contained a radioactive colloidal suspension that was approximately 25% thorium dioxide (ThO_2) by weight.[7] When administered by intravascular injection, this radioactive material emitted particles that were deposited in the patient's reticuloendothelial system. The liver and spleen became the recipients of this adverse substance. Following a latent period of 15 to 20 years, this high alpha-emitting contrast agent resulted in many cases of liver and spleen cancer as well as angiosarcomas and biliary duct carcinomas. When this agent was administered by extravascular injection, the tissue surrounding the injection site eventually became cancerous.

Infants Treated for Enlarged Thymus Gland During the 1940s and early 1950s, physicians diagnosed thymus gland enlargement in many infants suffering from respiratory distress. The thymus is located adjacent to the thyroid in the mediastinal cavity, which extends into the neck as far as the lower edge

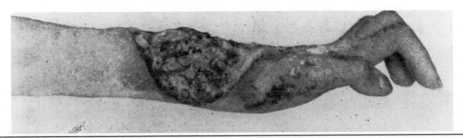

FIG. 6-14. Carcinoma of the distal arm and hand developing after an x-ray burn (in 1904). (From Allen CW: *Radiotherapy and phototherapy including radium and high frequency currents,* New York, 1904, Lea Brothers.)

of the thyroid gland. Functioning as a vital part of the immune mechanism, this gland plays a crucial role in the body's defense against infection. Shortly after birth the thymus gland in these infants responded to infection by enlarging. To reduce the size of the gland, physicians treated the infants with therapeutic doses (1.2 to 60 Gy, or 120 to 6000 rads) of x-radiation. Because the thyroid is adjacent to the thymus, the thyroid gland also received a substantial radiation dose. This resulted in the development, some 20 years later, of thyroid nodules and carcinomas in many persons whose thymus had been irradiated in infancy.

Children of the Marshall Islanders Thyroid cancer also occurred in the children of the Marshall Islanders who were inadvertently subjected to high levels of fallout during an atomic bomb test (code name BRAVO) on March 1, 1954. During the detonation of a 15-megaton thermonuclear device on Bikini Atoll, the wind shifted and carried the fallout over the neighboring islands. As a consequence of this exposure, the children received substantial absorbed doses to the thyroid from both external exposure and internal ingestion of radioiodine. Estimates indicate that inhabitants of Rongelap Atoll received a mean dose of radiation to the thyroid gland of 21 Gy (2100 rads), and the inhabitants of Utrik Atoll received 2.80 Gy (280 rads).[13,14] Hence a dose of 12 Gy (1200 rads) is considered to be representative of a population average dose for these two areas combined.

Japanese Atomic Bomb Survivors

Atomic bomb detonation on Hiroshima and Nagasaki On August 6, 1945, the United States dropped the first atomic bomb on the Japanese city of Hiroshima, marking the pivotal moment in the latter stages of World War II. Three days later, on August 9, 1945, a second bomb was dropped on the city of Nagasaki. Of the 300,000 people living in these two cities at the time of these bombings, approximately 88,000 people were killed and at least 70,000 more were injured. Many of those who died were killed by the heat and blast (Fig. 6-15). Many of those who survived became victims of radiation injuries. These individuals have been observed since that time for signs of stochastic late somatic effects of radiation.

Data obtained from epidemiologic studies Epidemiologic studies of approximately 100,000 Japanese survivors of the atomic bombings

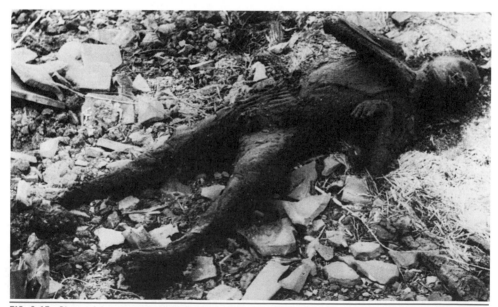

FIG. 6-15. Charred human remains found in the epicenter of Nagasaki after the detonation of the atomic bomb on August 9, 1945. (Courtesy Magnum Photos.)

at Hiroshima and Nagasaki indicate that ionizing radiation causes leukemia (proliferation of the white blood cells). According to estimates, atomic bomb survivors (*hibakusha*) exposed to radiation doses of about 1 Gy (100 rads) or more showed a significant increase in the incidence of leukemia. When compared with the spontaneous incidence of leukemia in the Japanese population at the time of the bomb, the incidence of leukemia in the irradiated population increased about 100-fold after the high dose of radiation was received. "Studies of the atomic bomb survivors in both Hiroshima and Nagasaki show a statistically significant increase in leukemia incidence in the exposed population compared with the nonexposed population. In the period 1950 to 1956, 117 new cases of leukemia were reported in the Japanese survivors; approximately 64 of these can be attributed to radiation exposure."[15]

Incidence of leukemia and occurrence rate of other radiation-induced malignancies The incidence of leukemia has slowly declined since the late 1940s and early 1950s. However, the occurrence rates of other radiation-induced malignancies have continued to escalate since the late 1950s and early 1960s. Among these are a variety of solid tumors such as thyroid, breast, lung, and bone cancers. As identified by Warren K. Sinclair, Fig. 6-16 demonstrates the nominal risk of malignancy from a dose of 0.01 Gy (1 rad) of uniform whole-body radiation.[16] The graph indicates that leukemia occurs approximately 2 years after the initial exposure, rises to its highest level between 7 and 10 years, and then declines to almost zero at about 30 years. Unlike leukemia, solid tumors take approximately 10 years to develop and generally increase in occurrence at the same rate that cancer increases as people age. Whether the risk for solid tumors continues to rise beyond 40 years or declines as with leukemia is still unknown. Follow-up studies of the atomic bomb survivors may eventually provide the answer.

Incidence of breast cancer in Japanese women In general, Japanese women have a lower natural incidence of breast cancer compared with American and Canadian women.[17] The female Japanese atomic bomb survivors provide strong evidence that ionizing radiation can induce breast cancer. The incidence of breast cancer in these women rises with radiation dose. It follows a linear, nonthreshold curve. Numerous studies of female survivors indicate a relative risk for breast cancer of 4:1 to as high as 10:1.

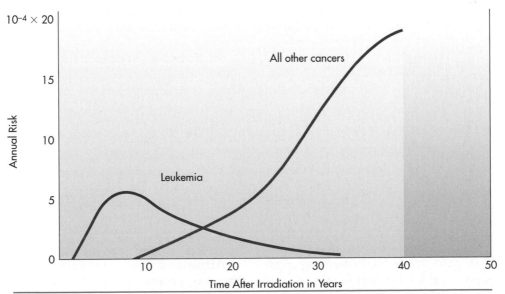

FIG. 6-16. Nominal risk of malignancy from a dose of 0.01 Gy (1 rad) of uniform whole-body radiation. (Modified from Sinclair WK: *J Radiat Oncol Biol Phys* 131(2):387-392, 1995.)

Effectiveness of ionizing radiation as a cancer-causing agent Although studies from Hiroshima and Nagasaki confirm that high doses of ionizing radiation cause cancer, radiation is not a highly effective cancer-causing agent. For example, follow-up studies of approximately 82,000 atomic bomb survivors from 1950 to 1978 reveal an excess of only 250 cancer deaths attributed to radiation exposure. Instead of the expected 4500 cancer deaths, 4750 actually occurred. This means that of about every 300 atomic bomb survivors, one died of a malignancy attributed to an average whole-body radiation dose of approximately 0.14 Sv (14 rem).

Radiation dose and radiation-induced leukemia Epidemiologic data about the Hiroshima atomic bomb survivors also indicate that a linear relationship exists between radiation dose and radiation-induced leukemia. In other words, the chance of contracting leukemia as a result of exposure to radiation is directly proportional to the magnitude of the radiation exposure. Available information of the kind necessary to establish the existence of a threshold dose-response relationship (i.e., whether a harmless dose exists) is inconclusive. Hence, radiation-induced leukemia is assumed to follow a linear, nonthreshold dose-response relationship compared with a population that has not been exposed to ionizing radiation.[7] Recent reevaluation of the quantity and type of radiation that was released in the cities of Hiroshima and Nagasaki provides a better foundation for radiation dose and damage assessment. Originally, neutrons were credited with the damage in Hiroshima. However, when recent studies revealed that the uranium-fueled bomb dropped on Hiroshima provided more gamma radiation exposure and less neutron exposure than previously believed, data on the survivors were updated to reflect this more accurate information. Researchers have established that gamma radiation and neutrons each provided about 50% of the radiation dose inflicted on the population of Hiroshima. On the other hand, the inhabitants of Nagasaki, who were exposed to a plutonium bomb, received only 10% of their exposure from neutrons and 90% from gamma radiation. Based on the revised atomic bomb data, radiation-induced leukemias and solid tumors in the survivors may be attributed predominantly to gamma radiation

exposure. The impact of the atomic bomb dosimetry revision is a significant increase in cancer risk estimates. The BEIR V Report provides a summary of the new estimates.

Evacuees from the Chernobyl Nuclear Disaster

Need for follow-up studies The 1986 nuclear power station accident at Chernobyl requires long-term follow-up studies to assess the magnitude and severity of late effects on the exposed population. Detailed observations investigating potential increases in the incidence of leukemia, thyroid problems, breast cancer, and other possible radiation-induced malignancies will continue.

Evacuation of people within 36 hours after the accident Within 36 hours of the nuclear catastrophe, 49,360 people residing at Pripyat, a city 2 miles from the plant, were evacuated. An additional 85,640 people, most of whom were living in a 10-mile (30-km) radial zone of Chernobyl, also were evacuated over a period of 14 days after the disaster. In general the 135,000 evacuees received an average equivalent dose of 0.12 Sv (12 rem) per person. Of the 135,000, approximately 24,000 people received an equivalent dose of about 0.45 Sv (45 rem). The remaining 111,000 people received from 0.03 to 0.06 Sv (3 to 6 rem).[4,5] If the evacuees are monitored for at least 30 years, important estimates of radiation-induced leukemias, thyroid cancers, and other malignancies may be obtained.

Worldwide effects of the accident The possibility of late effects occurring from the Chernobyl power station disaster is still a source of concern worldwide. Because winds carried the radioactive plume in several different directions during the 10 days after the accident, more than 20 countries received fallout as a consequence of the catastrophe. Approximately 400,000 people received some exposure to fallout. In February 1989, Dr. Richard Wilson, professor of physics at Harvard University in Cambridge, Massachusetts, estimated "that about 20,000 people throughout the world" will develop a radiation-induced malignancy from the Chernobyl accident.[18]

Attempts by physicians to prevent thyroid cancer in children ^{131}I is one of the radioactive materials that became airborne in the radioactive plume. [131]I concentrates in the thyroid gland and may cause cancer many years after the initial exposure. In an attempt to prevent thyroid cancer resulting from the accidental overdose of ^{131}I, physicians administered potassium iodide to children in Poland and other countries after the Chernobyl disaster. By offering a substitute for take-up by the thyroid gland, potassium iodide is intended to block effectively the gland's uptake of [131]I. The degree of effectiveness of this preventive treatment remains to be determined. In other accidentally exposed populations, thyroid cancer has occurred in some individuals at doses of 1 Gy (100 rads) or less. The approximate time for the appearance of such radiation-induced thyroid malignancies is usually between 10 and 20 years after exposure.

Incidence of thyroid cancer and breast cancer since the accident During the first 10 years following the Chernobyl disaster, the incidence of thyroid cancer increased dramatically among children living in the regions of Belarus, Ukraine, and Russia (Fig. 6-17), where the heaviest radioactive iodine contamination occurred. Thyroid cancer has been the "most pronounced health effect" of the radiation accident.[19] As of April 1996, more than 700 cases of thyroid cancer were diagnosed in children

residing in these areas. The number of new thyroid cancer cases identified since the Chernobyl incident is significantly higher than anticipated, and by 1998 a total of 1700 cases were diagnosed.[20] Radiation scientists from the western and eastern hemispheres are collaborating to determine the reason for this increase. Some possible explanations for the higher-than-expected number of thyroid cancers are (1) chronic iodine deficiency during the years preceding the accident in the children living in the regions contaminated and (2) genetic predisposition to developing thyroid malignancy after radiation exposure in some subgroups of the exposed population.[19] If the first theory is valid, the thyroid gland of these individuals would have assimilated isotopes of the radioactive material inhaled from a cloud or ingested from contaminated milk supplies. If the second theory is valid, some of the exposed individuals may have a disorder that prevents the mechanism normally used by healthy cells to initiate repair and mend the genetic damage.

Why early studies did not demonstrate a significant increase in the incidence of leukemia after the accident From the earlier discussion of the Japanese atomic bomb survivors, we have learned that radiation causes leukemia and that

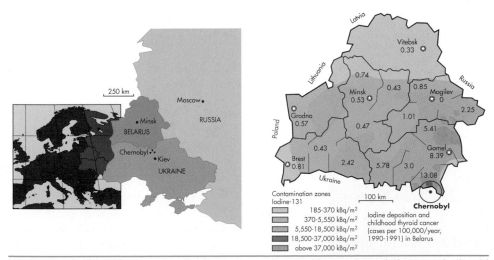

FIG. 6-17. In the first 10 years after the Chernobyl nuclear accident, a dramatic increase in thyroid cancer was seen among children living in the regions of Belarus, Ukraine, and Russia, where the heaviest contamination occurred. (From Abelin et al: *BMJ*, vol. 12, 1994.)

the disease follows a linear, nonthreshold dose-response curve. However, early studies of the Chernobyl victims did not demonstrate a significant increase in the incidence of leukemia, possibly because the radioactive iodine and cesium expelled into the environment during the accident may produce damaging health effects in different ways.[21] For example, ^{131}I has a relatively short half-life (measured in days) and is assimilated by the body and quickly distributed to the thyroid gland, thereby delivering an abrupt, acute dose to that organ. Radioactive cesium, on the other hand, has a longer life. It causes whole-body irradiation over time through its presence in the environment and food supply lines. This probably increases the incidence of childhood leukemia (Fig. 6-18). However, this increase is difficult to detect without very sensitive and reliable monitoring procedures.

Subsequent findings As stated in Chapter 1, later studies have begun to show some of the expected effects. Reports indicate that there has been about a 50% increase in leukemia cases in children and adults in the Gomel region since the Chernobyl disaster.[22,23] Although the World Health Organization (WHO) reported that it found no increase of leukemia in the populations hit hardest by fallout from Chernobyl by

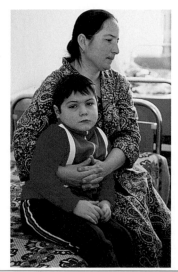

FIG. 6-18. Mother with son who is suffering from radiation-induced leukemia. The child is a victim of the 1986 nuclear power plant explosion at Chernobyl. (Courtesy Ken Graham Photography.)

1993,[24] in 1995 the WHO reported that nearly 700 cases of thyroid cancer among children and adolescents have been linked to the Chernobyl accident.[25] Also, in June 2001, the 3rd International Conference held in Kiev reported that there was a statistically significant rise in the number of leukemia cases in the Russian liquidators (cleanup workers) who worked during 1986 and 1987 at the Chernobyl power station complex.[23,26] Since the time of the Chernobyl accident, there has also been an increase in the incidence of breast cancer directly attributed to the radiation exposure.[23,27] If these findings continue to be substantiated, it will take more time before all the adverse health effects will be understood. Further investigation is necessary.

Need for continuing epidemiologic studies Continued studies may impart a great deal of information about the link between ionizing radiation and cancer. A more thorough understanding of the effect of low-level ionizing radiation also may be gained. However, because the actual levels of risk from the accident are still unknown because of the limited data provided by the Russians, the risk for development of radiation-induced malignancies is difficult to determine.

The ETHOS Project Since the accident at Chernobyl, the affected population continues to work toward reconstructing their overall quality of life. The rehabilitation process among those persons living in contaminated territories is ongoing. The goal of ventures such as the ETHOS Project (see Chapter 1), is to help the local population rebuild acceptable living conditions through their own active involvement in the reconstruction process.[28]

Life Span Shortening

Animal Studies Laboratory experiments on small animals have shown that the life span of animals that were exposed to nonlethal doses of ionizing radiation was shortened as a consequence of the exposure. When compared with a control group of unexposed small animals, the exposed animals died sooner than the unexposed animals. Radiation was then believed to have accelerated all causes of death. This reduction in the life cycle was termed *nonspecific life span shortening*. It was also believed that radiation accelerated the aging process, making the animals more susceptible to several diseases. In actuality, early demise of the experimental animals resulted from the induction of cancer.

Human Studies

American radiologists In humans, studies of the life span of American radiologists made by the Radiological Society of North America from 1945 to 1954 revealed that radiologists did have a shorter life span than other, nonradiologist physicians.[7] However, the process of evaluation of the information has been subject to considerable criticism, and the conclusions of the study are questionable. Further analysis of the epidemiologic studies showed that shortening of the life span in both animals and humans was the result of cancer and leukemia and not other "nonspecific" causes or accelerated aging.

American radiologic technologists Initiated in 1982 and currently still in progress, an extensive study of approximately 146,000 U.S. Radiologic Technologists (USRT) is evaluating potential radiation-related health effects resulting from long-term, repeated exposures to low-dose ionizing radiation. These effects include cancer incidence and other work-related conditions. This occupational epidemiologic study is a collaborative effort between the University of Minnesota School of Public Health, the National Cancer Institute, and the American Registry of Radiologic Technologists. The study involves a series of mail surveys to all participating technologists and telephone interviews with approximately 1200 retired technologists in the field before 1950. The interviews provide important information about work practices that were common in the early years prior to the time that personnel monitoring devices were routinely used.[29,30]

As reported in the Volume 2, Spring 2004 edition of the USRT Newsletter, among the 90,305 technologists who completed the first survey in the mid-1980s, there were 1283 deaths from cancer. A comparison was made between technologists who started working in the 1960s or later with those who began working before 1940. A slightly higher risk of dying from any type of cancer was found in technologists working prior to 1940. Technologists who began working after 1940 did not demonstrate any elevated risk. However, technologists entering the medical radiation industry before 1950 have demonstrated a somewhat higher risk of dying from leukemia compared with individuals

entering the workforce in 1950 or later. The risk of dying from breast cancer has also been studied in technologists working in the field before 1940, in those working between 1940 and 1950, and in those entering the field in 1960 or later. Technologists that began working before 1940 had the greatest risk of dying of breast cancer, followed by those who worked up to 1950. When the risk of dying of breast cancer is compared in women who began their careers in the 1950s with women employed from 1960 or later, the risk is only slightly higher for the women first employed in the 1950s. Improvements in radiologic technology, medical imaging equipment, and radiation safety are factors in cancer risk reduction. Readers interested in obtaining more information about this ongoing study can visit the website at www.radtechstudy.org or they can write to: U.S. Radiologic Technologist Study, University of Minnesota, Health Science Section, MMC 807, 420 Delaware Street S.E., Minneapolis, MN 55455.

Compared with others who started working in the 1960s or later, technologists who began working before 1940 had a slightly higher risk of dying from any type of cancer. The risks were not elevated in technologists who began working in subsequent decades. Radiologic technologists who began working before 1950 had a somewhat higher risk of dying from leukemia compared with technologists who started working in 1950 or later.

Cataractogenesis

The lens of the eye contains transparent fibers that transmit light. The lens focuses light on the retina so that in formation the image may be transmitted through the optic nerve (Fig. 6-19, *B*). The probability that a single dose of ionizing radiation of approximately 2 Gy (200 rads) will induce the formation of cataracts (opacity of the eye lens) is high (Fig. 6-19, *A*). This results in partial or complete loss of vision. Laboratory experiments with mice show that cataracts may be induced with doses as low as 0.1 Gy (10 rads). Highly ionizing neutron radiation is extremely efficient in inducing cataracts. A neutron dose as low as 0.01 Gy (1 rad) has been known to cause cataracts in mice. Radiation-induced cataracts in human beings follow a threshold, nonlinear dose-response relationship. Evidence of human radiation cataractogenesis

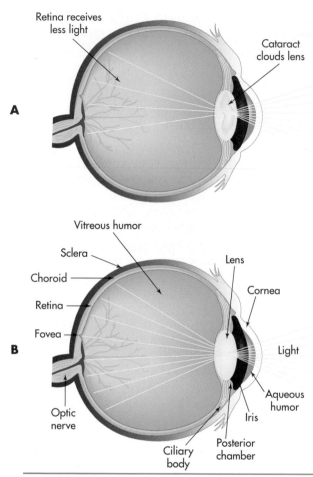

A

B

FIG. 6-19. **A,** Eye with cataract. **B,** Normal eye.

comes from observation of small groups of people who accidentally received substantial doses to the eyes. These groups include Japanese atomic bomb survivors, nuclear physicists working with cyclotrons (units that produce high-energy particles such as protons) between 1932 and 1960, and patients undergoing radiotherapy who received significantly high exposures to the eyes during treatment. The chance of radiation-induced cataracts occurring as a result of any diagnostic imaging procedures is very remote. However, in the realm of diagnostic radiology, fluoroscopic procedures do result in the highest radiation exposure to the lens of the eye. Occupational dose to this sensitive area can be substantially reduced when radiologists and radiographers wear protective eyewear while participating in

the examination (see Chapter 9 for further information). In patients, exposure to the lens and subsequent dose can be decreased by having them wear protective eye shields, provided that the use of such shields does not compromise the diagnostic value of the fluoroscopic examination.

Embryologic Effects (Birth Defects)

Stages of Gestation in Humans All life forms seem to be most vulnerable to radiation during the embryonic stage of development. The period of gestation during which the embryo-fetus is exposed to radiation governs the effects (death or congenital abnormality) of the radiation. Gestation in humans is divided into three stages: (1) preimplantation, which corresponds to 0 to 9 days after conception; (2) organogenesis, which corresponds to 10 days to 6 weeks after conception; and (3) the fetal stage, which corresponds to term (Fig. 6-20).

Embryonic Cell Radiosensitivity During the First Trimester of Pregnancy Because embryonic cells begin dividing and differentiating after conception, they are extremely radiosensitive and hence may easily be damaged by exposure to ionizing radiation. The first trimester seems to be the most crucial period as far as irradiation of the embryo-fetus is concerned because the embryo-fetus contains a large number of stem cells* during this period of gestation. Because the central nervous system and related sense organs contain many stem cells, they are extremely radiosensitive and are therefore susceptible to radiation-induced damage. Irradiation of the embryo during the first 8 weeks of development to equivalent doses in excess of 200 mSv (20 rem) frequently results in death or causes congenital abnormalities.

During the preimplantation stage, the fertilized ovum divides and forms a ball-like structure containing undifferentiated cells. If this structure is irradiated with a dose in the range of 0.05 to 0.15 Gy (5 to 15 rads), embryonic death will occur. Malformations

---

*It is in fact the utilization for medical research of these nonspecialized cells derived from embryos that would otherwise be discarded that has currently become the focus of much controversy between those who perceive a great potential for medical benefit and those who view these embryos as living entities that should not be used for research.

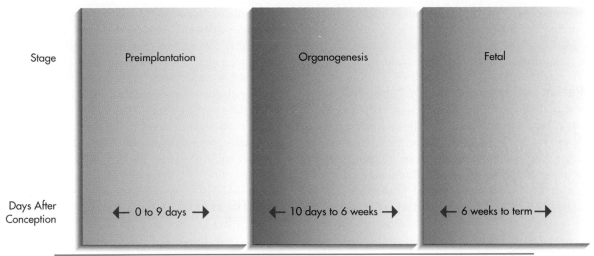

FIG. 6-20. Division of gestation in humans. (Data from Riegh R: *Am J Roentgenol* 89:182, 1963.)

resulting from radiation exposure do not occur at this stage. Because organogenesis occurs between 10 days to 6 weeks after conception, the developing fetus is most susceptible to radiation-induced congenital abnormalities during this period. This is actually the time when the undifferentiated cells are beginning to differentiate into organs. The central nervous system in the growing human fetus, however, remains undifferentiated and does not normally complete development until approximately the twelfth year of life. Abnormalities occurring as a consequence of irradiation during the period of organogenesis may include growth inhibition, mental retardation, microcephaly, genital deformities, and sense organ damage.

During the late stages of organogenesis, the presence of fatal abnormalities in the fetus will cause neonatal death (death at birth). High doses of radiation also will cause this to occur during the fetal stage (a growth period) of development. Skeletal damage from radiation exposure occurs most frequently during the period from week 3 to week 20 of development. The development of cancer or functional disorders during childhood are other possible effects of irradiation during the fetal stage.

Embryonic Cell Radiosensitivity During the Second and Third Trimesters of Pregnancy Fetal radiosensitivity decreases as gestation progresses. Hence, during the second and third trimesters, the developing fetus is less sensitive to ionizing radiation exposure. However, even in these later trimesters, congenital abnormalities and functional disorders such as sterility may be caused by radiation exposure. A great deal of the evidence for radiation-induced congenital abnormalities in human beings comes from more than four decades of follow-up studies of children exposed in utero during the atomic bomb detonations in Hiroshima and Nagasaki. Although the risk of radiation-induced leukemia is greater when the embryo-fetus is irradiated during the first trimester, leukemia also may be induced by exposure to radiation during the second and third trimesters. Although some studies of children irradiated in utero indicate an excess of cancer and leukemia deaths, studies of children exposed in utero during the atomic bomb detonations in Hiroshima and Nagasaki have not demonstrated significant rates of cancer and leukemia deaths.[31]

Embryonic Effects Resulting from the Chernobyl Nuclear Power Plant Accident Of the 135,000 evacuees from the 18-mile (30-km) radial zone of the Chernobyl nuclear power plant, approximately 2000 were pregnant women. Each received an average total-body equivalent dose of 0.43 Sv (43 rem). No obvious abnormalities were observed in the 300 live babies born by August of 1987. However, from 1986 through 1990, the Ministry of Health in

Ukraine recorded an increased number of miscarriages, premature births, and stillbirths.[22,23] Also recorded by the Ministry was an increase three times the normal rate of deformities and developmental abnormalities in newborns.[22,23]

Review of Fetal Effects by UNSCEAR Fetal effects such as mortality, induction of malformations, mental retardation, and childhood cancer were reviewed by the United Nations Scientific Committee on the Effects of Atomic Radiation (UNSCEAR).[32] This group proposed an upper-limit combined radiation risk for the aforementioned fetal effects of "3 chances per 1000 children for each rem of fetal dose."[33] If each effect was estimated individually, the estimate would be a little lower. Without radiation, these fetal effects have an estimated normal total risk of "60 chances per 1000 children (6%)."[33]

International Chernobyl Project In 1990, the International Chernobyl Project was initiated in response to a request for assistance from the former Soviet Union. The Director of the Radiation Effects Research Foundation in Hiroshima, Japan, led this project. The study compared seven contaminated Russian villages with six uncontaminated villages. By 1990, no significant increases in fetal and genetic abnormalities were seen in this population.[34] However, because of the relatively long latency period for radiogenic cancer, particularly solid tumors, researchers expect that more time will be required before the ultimate impact on the population of Russia is known. Estimates of as many as 500 excess cancers in the former Soviet Union during the next 50 to 60 years have been made.[35]

Effects of Low-Level Ionizing Radiation on the Embryo-Fetus The effects of low-level ionizing radiation on the embryo-fetus can only be estimated. Documentation of the effects of low-level radiation on the unborn irradiated in utero is insufficient because some types of abnormality occur in a small percentage (approximately 4%) of all live births in the U.S. In addition, no birth abnormalities unique to high levels of radiation have appeared. Abnormalities in this context are the same as those that occur naturally; however, if the exposure occurs during a period of major organogenesis, the abnormality may be more pronounced. Assessment of radiation-induced birth abnormalities from low-level exposure also may be dif-

ficult because human genes vary naturally or as a consequence of the environment.

Because the embryo-fetus is relatively sensitive to radiation, radiation workers should exercise caution and employ appropriate safety measures when performing diagnostic radiographic procedures that result in any dose to the unborn. Most diagnostic procedures result in equivalent doses less than 0.01 Sv (1 rem). Such doses are not usually considered dangerous to the unborn.

GENETIC EFFECTS

Cause of Genetic Mutations

Biologic effects of ionizing radiation on future generations are termed **genetic effects.** These effects occur as a result of radiation-induced damage to the DNA molecule in the sperm or ova of an adult. When these germ cell mutations occur, faulty genetic information is transmitted to the offspring. This faulty genetic information may manifest itself as various diseases or malformations.

Natural Spontaneous Mutations

Normally, mutations in genetic material occur spontaneously, without a known cause. Mutations in genes and DNA that occur at random as a natural phenomenon are called *spontaneous mutations*. Because these genetic alterations are permanent and heritable, they can be transmitted from one generation to the next. Spontaneous mutations in human genetic material cause a wide variety of disorders or diseases, including hemophilia, Huntington's chorea, Down syndrome (mongolism), Duchenne's muscular dystrophy, sickle cell anemia, cystic fibrosis, and hydrocephalus. A genetic disorder is present in approximately 10% of all live births in the United States.

Mutagens Responsible for Genetic Mutations

In each generation, some genetic mutations occur as part of the natural order of events. However, certain agents such as elevated temperatures, ionizing radiation, viruses, and chemicals can increase the frequency of mutation. These agents are called *mutagens,* and ionizing radiation is one of the more effective mutagens known. Any nonlethal radiation dose received by the germ cells can cause chromosome mutations that may be transmitted to successive generations.

Radiation Interaction with DNA Macromolecules

When radiation interacts with DNA macromolecules, it can modify the structure of these molecules by causing breaks in the chromosomes or change the amount of DNA belonging to a cell by causing a deletion or an alteration in the sequence of nitrogen bases. Such modifications change the cell's genetic information. A mutation of this type could eventually lead to genetic disease in subsequent generations.

Cellular Damage Repair by Enzymes

Enzymes attempt to repair cellular damage by mending structural breaks in chromosomes that have been hit by ionizing radiation. If repair is successful, the cell continues to function normally. If repair does not occur, the cell may suffer functional impairment or die.

Incapacities of Mutant Genes

Mutant genes cannot properly govern the cell's normal chemical reactions or properly control the sequence of amino acids in the formation of specific proteins. These incapacities result in various genetic diseases. For example, sickle cell anemia arises from the defective synthesis of the protein hemoglobin. About 300 amino acids combine to form the hemoglobin molecule. Sickle cell anemia is caused by the omission of only one vital amino acid.

Dominant or Recessive Point Mutations

Point mutations (genetic mutations at the molecular level) may be either dominant (probably expressed in the offspring) or recessive (probably not expressed for several generations). Radiation is thought to cause primarily recessive mutations, if any. For a recessive mutation to appear in the offspring, both parents must have the same genetic defect. This means that the defect must be located on the same part of a specific DNA base sequence in each parent.

Because this rarely occurs, the effects of recessive mutations are not likely to appear in a population. However, an increase in the number of individuals who receive radiation exposure increases the likelihood that two individuals having the same type of mutation will have offspring. Therefore imaging professionals should limit not only the amount of radiation received by an individual but also the radiation exposure of the entire population. Damage from recessive mutations sometimes manifests itself more subtly and may appear as allergies, a slight alteration in metabolism, decreased intelligence, and predisposition to certain diseases.

Ionizing Radiation as a Cause of Genetic Effects

The only concrete evidence showing that ionizing radiation causes genetic effects comes from extensive experimentation with fruit flies and mice at high radiation doses. The data on mice may be extrapolated to low doses and then applied to humans. The information obtained from the experiments indicates that genetic effects do not have a threshold dose—in other words, a dose of ionizing radiation at which genetic effects begin to occur and below which they cannot occur. Because this implies that even the smallest radiation dose could cause some genetic damage, there is no such thing as a "100% safe" gonadal radiation dose.

Radiation-Induced Genetic Effects in Humans

Existing data on radiation-induced genetic effects in humans are both contradictory and inconclusive. Some of the data accumulated come from observation of test groups of children conceived after one or both parents had been exposed to radiation resulting from the atomic bomb detonation in Hiroshima or Nagasaki. As of the third generation, no radiation-induced genetic effects are known. However, this does not mean that effects will not be seen in subsequent generations. J. F. Crow, a geneticist who spent many years experimenting with fruit flies, stated the following: "The most frequent mutations in man are not those leading to freaks or obvious hereditary diseases, but those causing minor impairments leading to higher embryonic death rates, lower life expectancy, increase in disease, or decreased fertility."[36]

In 2001, an UNSCEAR study on hereditary effects of radiation concluded that no radiation-induced genetic diseases have so far been demonstrated in human populations exposed to ionizing radiation.[23,37] However, several other studies after the Chernobyl accident contradict this conclusion. These studies indicate an increase in abnormalities, or at least in genetic mutations, as a result of the accident.[23] Interested readers wanting more information about these contradictory studies can contact the Chernobyl-Tschernobyl-Information web site under genetic effects. The web address is http:www.chernobyl.info/.

Currently, evidence of radiation-induced genetic effects has not been observed in persons employed in diagnostic imaging or in patients undergoing radiologic examinations. To minimize the possibility of genetic effects in those persons engaged in the practice of medical imaging and in patients, gonadal shielding must be effectively utilized and all radiation exposure must be maintained ALARA (as low as reasonably achievable).

Doubling Dose Concept

Animal studies of radiation-induced genetic effects have led to the development of the doubling dose concept. This dose measures the effectiveness of ionizing radiation in causing mutations. **Doubling dose** is the radiation dose that causes the number of spontaneous mutations occurring in a given generation to increase to two times their original number. For example, if 7% of the offspring in each generation are born with mutations in the absence of radiation other than background levels, the administration of the doubling dose to all members of the population would eventually increase the number of mutations to 14%. The radiation doubling equivalent dose for humans, as determined from studies of the offspring of the atomic bomb survivors of Hiroshima and Nagasaki, is estimated to have a mean value of 1.56 Sv (156 rem) based on the genetic indicators of untoward pregnancy outcome (e.g., stillbirths, major congenital abnormalities, death during the first postnatal week), childhood

mortality, and sex chromosome aneuploidy (possessing an abnormal number of chromosomes). For this reason, the administration of even low doses of radiation to the gonads must be strictly controlled to reduce the risk of genetic damage in future generations. This precaution will help preserve the biologic fitness of the human race.

SUMMARY

➤ Information obtained from a radiation dose response curve can be used to predict the risk of malignancy in human populations exposed to low levels of ionizing radiation.
   ■ Curves that graphically demonstrate radiation dose-response relationships can be either linear or nonlinear and depict either a threshold or a nonthreshold dose.
   ■ A linear, nonthreshold curve currently is being used for most types of cancer.
   ■ Risk associated with low-level radiation can be estimated with the linear-quadratic, nonthreshold curve.
   ■ Nonstochastic (deterministic) effects of significant radiation exposure may be graphically demonstrated through the use of a linear, threshold curve of radiation dose response.
   ■ High-dose cellular response may be demonstrated through the use of a sigmoid threshold curve.
➤ Acute radiation syndrome (ARS) occurs when the whole body is exposed to 6 Gy (600 rads) of ionizing radiation.
   ■ ARS can manifest itself as hematopoietic syndrome, gastrointestinal syndrome, and cerebrovascular syndrome.
   ■ ARS presents in four major response stages: prodromal, latent period, manifest illness, and recovery or death.
➤ LD (lethal dose) 50/30 signifies the whole-body dose of ionizing radiation that can be lethal to 50% of an exposed population within 30 days.
   ■ LD in humans is usually given as LD 50/60 and is estimated to be 3 to 4 Gy (300 to 400 rads).
   ■ When cells are exposed to sublethal doses of ionizing radiation, repair and recovery are possible.

- Surviving cells begin to repopulate.
- Approximately 90% of radiation-induced damage may be repaired over time; 10% is irreparable.

➤ Early somatic effects occur within a short period of time after exposure to ionizing radiation.
- These effects include nausea, fatigue, erythema, epilation, and blood/intestinal disorders.

➤ Late somatic effects occur after a period of months or years after irradiation.
- Late effects include carcinogenesis, cataractogenesis, and embryologic (birth) defects.
- Cancer is the most important late stochastic somatic effect caused by exposure to ionizing radiation.
- Effects directly related to dose received that occur months or years after radiation exposure are called *late nonstochastic(deterministic) somatic effects*.
- Effects that have no threshold, occur arbitrarily, are independent of dose, and occur months or years after exposure are called *late stochastic somatic effects*.

➤ Risk estimates are given in terms of *absolute risk* or *relative risk*.
- The absolute risk model predicts that a specific number of excess cancers will occur as a result of radiation exposure.
- The relative risk model predicts that the number of excess cancers rises as the natural incidence of cancer increases with advancing age in a population.
- Linear and linear-quadratic models are used for extrapolation of risk from high-dose to low-dose data.

➤ The first trimester of pregnancy is the most critical period for radiation exposure of the embryo-fetus.
- Radiation-induced congenital abnormalities can occur between 10 days and 6 weeks after conception.
- Skeletal abnormalities most frequently occur between weeks 3 and 20.
- Radiation exposure in the second and third trimesters can cause congenital abnormalities, functional disorders, and a predisposition to the development of childhood cancer.

➤ Genetic effects on ionizing radiation are biologic effects on generations yet unborn.
- Radiation-induced abnormalities are caused by unrepaired damage to DNA within ova or sperm.
- There is no 100% safe gonadal radiation dose; even the smallest radiation dose could cause some genetic damage.
- Doubling dose measures the effectiveness of ionizing radiation in causing mutations; it is the radiation dose that causes the number of spontaneous mutations in a given generation to increase to two times their original number.
- For humans, the doubling dose is estimated to have a mean value of 1.56 Sv (156 rem).

References

1. Straume T, Dobson RL: Implications of new Hiroshima and Nagasaki dose estimates: cancer risks and neutron RBE, *Health Phys* 41:666, 1981.
2. Webster EW: *Proceedings No. 3, Critical issues in setting radiation dose limits*, Washington, DC, 1982, NCRP.
3. Finch SC: Acute radiation syndrome, *JAMA* 258:666, 1987.
4. Gale RP: Immediate medical consequences of nuclear accidents: lessons from Chernobyl, *JAMA* 258:625, 1987.
5. Perry AR, Iglar AF: The accident at Chernobyl: radiation doses and effects, *Radiol Technol* 61:290, 1990.
6. Linnemann RE: Soviet medical response to Chernobyl nuclear accident, *JAMA* 258:639, 1987.
7. Bushong SC: *Radiologic science for technologists: physics, biology and protection*, ed 8, St. Louis, 2004, Mosby.
8. Fry RJM: Acute radiation effects. In Wagner LK et al, editors: *Radiation bioeffects and management: test and syllabus*, Reston, Va, 1991, American College of Radiology.
9. Hendee WR, editor: *Health effects of low-level radiation*, Norwalk, Conn, 1984, Appleton-Century-Crofts.
10. International Commission on Radiological Protection: Recommendations of the International Commission on Radiological Protection, ICRP Publication No. 60, *Ann ICRP* 21(1-3), 1991.
11. National Research Council, Commission of Life Sciences, Committee on Biological Effects on Ionizing Radiation (BEIR V), Board on Radiation Effects Research: *Health effects of exposure to low levels of ionizing radiations*, Washington, DC, 1989, National Academy Press.

12. Tilke B: Navajo miners battle long-term effects of radiation, *Adv Radiol Technol* 3:3, 1990.

13. Hamilton TE, vanBelle G, LoGerfo J: Thyroid neoplasia in Marshall Islanders exposed to nuclear fallout, *JAMA* 258:629, 1987.

14. Lessard E et al: Thyroid absorbed dose for people at Rongelap, Utrik, and Sifo on March 1, 1954, US Department of Energy publication (BNL) 51-882, Upton, NY, 1985, Brookhaven National Laboratory.

15. Travis EL: *Primer of medical radiobiology*, ed 2, Chicago, 1989, Year Book Medical Publishers, Inc.

16. Sinclair WK: Radiation protection recommendations on dose limits: the role of the NCRP and the ICRP and future developments, *J Radiation Oncology Biol Phys* 131(2):387-392, 1995.

17. Hall EJ: *Radiobiology for the radiologist*, ed 5, Philadelphia, 2000, Lippincott Williams & Wilkins.

18. WGBH Transcript: Bach to Chernobyl, *Nova* No. 1604, Boston, 1989 (television program originally broadcast on PBS on February 14, 1989).

19. Balter M: Children become the first victims of fallout, *Science* 272:357, 1996.

20. United Nations Scientific Committee on the Effects of Atomic Radiation (UNSCEAR): *2000 report to the General Assembly, with Scientific Annexes, UNSCEAR 2000: sources and effects of ionizing radiation*, New York, 2000, United Nations.

21. Williams N: Leukemia studies continue to draw a blank, *Science* 272:358, 1996.

22. Otto Hug Strahleninstit: Information, Ausgabe 9/2001 K, 2001.

23. Chernobyl Info. Available at: http://www.chernobyl.info/. Accessed June 30, 2004 and January 2, 2005.

24. Walker SJ: *Permissible dose: a history of radiation protection in the twentieth century*, Berkeley and Los Angeles, California, 2000, University of California Press.

25. Chernobyl Accident. Available at: http://www.worldnuclear.org/info/chernobyl/inf07print.htm. Accessed December 2, 2004.

26. Conclusions of 3rd International Conference: *Health effects of the Chernobyl accident, Intl J Radiation Med* 3:3-4, 2001.

27. European Commission, OCHA et al, International Conference: *Fifteen years after accident: Lessons learned*, Executive Summary, Kiev, April 2001.

28. Dubreuil GH, Lochard J, Girard P et al: Chernobyl post-accident management: the Ethos Project, *Health Physics* 77:361-372, 1999.

29. University of Minnesota, Health Studies Section, *U.S. Radiologic Technologists Study*, Vol 2, Minneapolis, Minn, Spring 2004.

30. *U.S. Radiologic Technologists Study*. Available at: www.radtechstudy.org. Accessed March 17, 2005.

31. Stewart A, Webb J, Hewitt D: A survey of childhood malignancies, *Br Med J* 1:1495, 1958.

32. United Nations Scientific Committee on the Effects of Atomic Radiation (UNSCEAR): *Biological effects of prenatal irradiation*, 35th Session of UNSCEAR, Vienna, April 1986, New York, 1986, United Nations.

33. Webster EW et al: *A primer on low-level ionizing radiation and its biological effects*, AAPM Report No. 18, New York, 1986, American Institute of Physics (published for the American Association of Physicists in Medicine).

34. Eijgenraam F: Chernobyl's cloud: a lighter shade of gray, *Science, News and Comment* 252:1245, 1991.

35. Goss LB: International team examines health in zones contaminated by Chernobyl, *Physics Today, Search and Discovery*, p 20, Aug 1991.

36. Crow JF: Genetic effects of radiation, *Bull Atomic Scientists* 14:19, 1958.

37. United Nations Scientific Committee on the Effects of Atomic Radiation (UNSCEAR): *Hereditary effects of radiation*, New York, 2001, United Nations.

GENERAL DISCUSSION QUESTIONS

1. How can the information obtained from a radiation dose-response curve be used?

2. What did the BEIR Committee's 1990 revised risk estimates for the atomic bomb survivors of Hiroshima and Nagasaki indicate?

3. What rationale is used when regulatory agencies establish radiation protection standards?

4. What type of diagnostic radiologic procedure could possibly cause a radiation dose sufficient to cause early deterministic effects?

5. Why is LD 50/60 a more accurate indicator of outcome for humans receiving large radiation exposures than LD 50/30?

6. What is the difference between late nonstochastic (deterministic) somatic effects and late stochastic (probabilistic) somatic effects of ionizing radiation?

7. What is the difference between the absolute risk model and the relative risk model used for estimating risk caused by a specific exposure to ionizing radiation?

8. Name five groups of humans exposed to high doses of ionizing radiation that prove radiation induces cancer and explain the circumstances that led to the exposure received by each group.
9. What is organogenesis and what are the consequences to the developing fetus if irradiated during this period?
10. Describe the concept of doubling dose.

REVIEW QUESTIONS

1. Cancer and genetic defects are examples of _____ effects.
   A. Stochastic
   B. Nonstochastic
   C. Birth
   D. Deterministic

2. Lethal dose of ionizing radiation for humans is usually given as:
   A. LD 50/30
   B. LD 50/60
   C. LD 50/90
   D. LD 50/120

3. Which of the following provide the foundation for the sigmoid, or "S-shaped" (nonlinear), threshold curve of radiation dose response?
   1. Data from human populations observed after acute high doses of radiation
   2. Data from human populations observed after chronic low doses of radiation
   3. Laboratory experiments on animals
   A. 1 only
   B. 2 only
   C. 3 only
   D. 1, 2, and 3

4. The linear, nonthreshold curve implies that biologic response is:
   A. Directly proportional to the dose
   B. Inversely proportional to the dose
   C. Insignificant in relation to dose
   D. Not able to be plotted on a dose-response curve

5. Acute radiation syndrome presents in four major response stages. In what order do these stages occur?
   A. Latent period, prodromal, manifest illness, recovery or death
   B. Manifest illness, prodromal, latent period, recovery or death
   C. Prodromal, latent period, manifest illness, recovery or death
   D. Manifest illness, latent period, prodromal, recovery or death

6. Radiation dose-response relationship is demonstrated graphically through the use of a curve that maps the observed effects of radiation exposure in relation to the dose of radiation received. Which of the following curves expresses a linear-quadratic, nonthreshold dose response?
   A. ∠
   B. ∠
   C. ∠
   D. ∠

7. During the 10 years immediately after the 1986 Chernobyl nuclear power station accident, which of the following was the *most pronounced* health effect observed?
   1. Dramatic increase in the incidence of childhood leukemia
   2. Dramatic increase in thyroid cancer in children living in the regions where the heaviest radioactive contamination occurred
   3. Major increase in the number of solid tumors in the general population of the former Soviet Union
   A. 1, 2, and 3
   B. 1 only
   C. 2 only
   D. 3 only

8. Early demise of the experimental animals exposed to nonlethal doses of ionizing radiation actually resulted from:
   A. Accelerated aging
   B. Hemorrhage
   C. Induction of cancer
   D. Respiratory distress

9. **Which of the following systems is the *most* radiosensitive vital organ system in human beings?**
   A. Cerebrovascular
   B. Gastrointestinal
   C. Hematopoietic
   D. Skeletal

10. **When cells are exposed to sublethal doses of ionizing radiation, approximately _____ of radiation-induced damage may be repaired over time, and about _____ is irreparable.**
    A. 25%, 75%
    B. 50%, 50%
    C. 75%, 25%
    D. 90%, 10%

Dose Limits for Exposure to Ionizing Radiation

KEY TERMS

action limits
agreement states
ALARA concept
annual occupational effective
  dose limit
collective effective dose
  (ColEfD)

cumulative effective dose
  (CumEfD) limit
effective dose
effective dose limit
effective dose (EfD) limiting
  system
equivalent dose (EqD)

International Commission on
  Radiological Protection
  (ICRP)
lifetime effective dose
National Council on Radiation
  Protection and Measurements
  (NCRP)

Continued

negligible individual dose (NID)
nonstochastic (deterministic)
   effects
Nuclear Regulatory Commission
   (NRC)

optimization
radiation hormesis
radiation-induced malignancy
radiation safety committee
   (RSC)

radiation safety officer (RSO)
risk
stochastic (probabilistic)
   effects
tissue weighting factor (W$_T$)

OBJECTIVES

After completing this chapter, the reader will be able to perform the following:

- List and describe the function of the four major organizations that share the responsibility for evaluating the relationship between radiation equivalent dose and induced biologic effects and five U.S. regulatory agencies responsible for enforcing established radiation effective dose limiting standards.
- Explain the function of the radiation safety committee (RSC) in a medical facility and describe the role of the radiation safety officer (RSO) by listing the various responsibilities he or she must fulfill.
- Describe effective dose limit and the effective dose limiting system.
- Explain the purpose of the Radiation Control for Health and Safety Act of 1968 and the Consumer Patient Health and Safety Act of 1981.
- List the important provisions of the code of standards for diagnostic x-ray equipment that began on August 1, 1974.
- Explain the ALARA concept.
- Describe current radiation protection philosophy and state the goal and objectives of radiation protection.
- Identify radiation-induced responses that warrant serious concern for radiation protection.
- Explain the concept of *risk* as it relates to the medical imaging industry.
- Identify the risk from exposure to ionizing radiation at low absorbed doses.
- Discuss current National Council on Radiation Protection and Measurements recommendations.
- Given appropriate data, calculate the cumulative effective dose for the whole body for a radiation worker.
- Explain the function of collective effective dose and list the unit used to express this quantity.
- Discuss the significance of action limits in health care facilities.
- Explain the concept of radiation hormesis.
- State the following in terms of International System (SI) units and traditional units:
  - a. Annual occupational effective dose limit and cumulative effective dose (CumEfD) limit for whole-body exposure excluding medical and natural background exposure, which are based on stochastic effects.
  - b. Annual occupational equivalent dose limits for tissues and organs such as lens of the eye, skin, hands, and feet, which are based on deterministic effects.
  - c. Annual effective dose limit for continuous (or frequent) exposure and for infrequent exposure of the general public from manmade sources other than medical and natural background, which are based on stochastic effects.

Continued

OBJECTIVES—*cont'd*

d. Annual equivalent dose limit for tissues and organs such as lens of the eye, skin, hands, and feet of members of the general public, which are based on deterministic effects.

e. Annual effective dose limit for an occupationally exposed student under the age of 18 years (excluding medical and natural background radiation exposure).

f. Occupational monthly equivalent dose limit to the embryo-fetus (excluding medical and natural background radiation) once the pregnancy is known.

Exposure of the general public, patients, and radiation workers to ionizing radiation must be limited to minimize the risk of harmful biologic effects. To this end, scientists have developed occupational and nonoccupational effective dose (EfD) limits and equivalent dose (EqD) limits for tissues and organs such as the lens of the eye, skin, hands, and feet. An **effective dose (EfD) limiting system,** a set of numeric dose limits that are based on calculations of the various risks of cancer and genetic effects to tissues or organs exposed to radiation, has been incorporated into Title 10 of the Code of Federal Regulations, Part 20, a document prepared and distributed by the U.S. Office of the Federal Register. The rules and regulations of the Nuclear Regulatory Commission (NRC) and fundamental radiation protection standards governing occupational radiation exposure are included in this document.

BASIS OF EFFECTIVE DOSE LIMITING SYSTEM

The concept of radiation exposure and associated risk of **radiation-induced malignancy,** cancerous neoplasms caused by exposure to ionizing radiation, is the basis of the effective dose limiting system. Information contained in the National Council on Radiation Protection and Measurements' Report No. 116 and the International Commission on Radiological Protection's Publication No. 60 serves as a resource for the revised recommendations. Future radiation pro-

tection standards are expected to continue to be based on risk.

Because medical imaging professionals share the responsibility for patient safety from radiation exposure and also are subject to such exposure in the performance of their duties, they must be familiar with previous, existing, and new guidelines. By keeping informed, they will be more conscious of good radiation safety practices. A radiographer may obtain the required knowledge by becoming familiar with the functions of the various advisory groups and regulatory agencies discussed in this chapter (Fig. 7-1).

RADIATION PROTECTION STANDARDS ORGANIZATIONS

The discussion that follows concerns the four major organizations responsible for evaluating the relationship between radiation equivalent dose (EqD) and induced biologic effects. In addition, the following organizations are concerned with formulating risk estimates of somatic and genetic effects after irradiation:

1. International Commission on Radiological Protection (ICRP)
2. National Council on Radiation Protection and Measurements (NCRP)
3. United Nations Scientific Committee on the Effects of Atomic Radiation (UNSCEAR)
4. National Academy of Sciences/National Research Council Committee on the Biological Effects of Ionizing Radiation (NAS/NRC-BEIR)

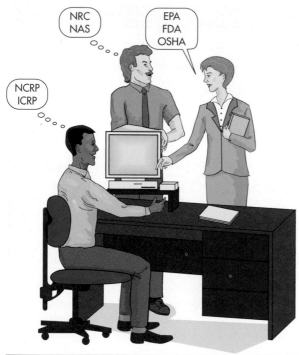

FIG. 7-1. The various advisory groups and regulatory agencies, usually referred to by abbreviations and acronyms, may be extremely confusing.

TABLE 7-1	
Summary of Radiation Protection Standards Organizations	
Organization	**Function**
ICRP	Evaluates information on biologic effects of radiation and provides radiation protection guidance through general recommendations on occupational and public dose limits
NCRP	Reviews regulations formulated by the ICRP and decides ways to include those recommendations in U.S. radiation protection criteria
UNSCEAR	Evaluates human and environmental ionizing radiation exposure and derives radiation risk assessments from epidemiologic data and research conclusions; provides information to organizations such as the ICRP for evaluation
NAS/NRC-BEIR	Reviews studies of biologic effects of ionizing radiation and risk assessment and provides the information to organizations such as the ICRP for evaluation

A summary of radiation standards organizations is presented in Table 7-1.

International Commission on Radiological Protection

The **International Commission on Radiological Protection (ICRP)** is considered the international authority regarding the safe use of sources of ionizing radiation. It is composed of a main commission with 12 active members, a chairman, and four standing committees, which include committees on radiation effects, on radiation exposure, on protection in medicine, and on the application of ICRP recommendations.[1] Since its inception in 1928, the ICRP has been the leading international organization responsible for providing clear and consistent radiation protection guidance through its recommendations on occupational and public dose limits. Originally,

these were published as reports in selected scholarly journals. Since 1959, the ICRP has had its own series of publications, and from 1977 onward, the scientific journal, the *Annals of the ICRP,* has published ICRP information. The information on which the recommendations are based is supplied by scientific papers published in scholarly journals and by organizations such as the United Nations Scientific Committee on the Effects of Atomic Radiation and the National Academy of Sciences/National Research Council Committee on the Biological Effects of Ionizing Radiation, which are discussed later in this chapter. The ICRP only makes recommendations; it does not function as an enforcement agency. Each nation must develop and enforce its own specific regulations.

National Council on Radiation Protection and Measurements

In the United States a nongovernmental, nonprofit, private corporation known as the **National Council on Radiation Protection and Measurements (NCRP),** chartered by Congress in 1964, reviews the recommendations formulated by the ICRP. The NCRP determines the way ICRP recommendations are incorporated into U.S. radiation protection criteria. The council implements this task by formulating general recommendations and publishing them in the form of various NCRP reports. These reports may be purchased from NCRP Publications in Bethesda, Maryland. A listing of current NCRP reports available for purchase at cost may be found at www.ncrp.com.

Because the NCRP is not an enforcement agency, enactment of its recommendations lies with federal and state agencies that have the power to enforce such standards after they have been established. To facilitate understanding of the function of the NCRP, the council's objectives are identified in Box 7-1. Governmental organizations (e.g., the Nuclear Regulatory Commission, the Environmental Protection Agency, and state governments) utilize the recommendations of the NCRP as the scientific basis of their radiation protection activities.[2] Nongovernmental groups desiring to improve their radiation safety practices and their promotion and disbursement of pertinent radiation protection materials look to this public service organization for direction.

BOX 7-1

Objectives of the National Council on Radiation Protection and Measurements

Objectives 4 to 7 are identified in the "charter" of the council (Public Law 88-376) as follows: "To:

4. Collect, analyze, develop and disseminate in the public interest information and recommendations about (a) protection against radiation (b) radiation measurements, quantities and units, particularly those concerned with radiation protection.
5. Provide a means by which organizations concerned with the scientific and related aspects of radiation protection and of radiation quantities, units and measurements may cooperate for effective utilization of their combined resources, and to stimulate the work of such organizations.
6. Develop basic concepts about radiation quantities, units and measurements, about the application of these concepts, and about radiation protection.
7. Cooperate with the International Commission on Radiological Protection, the International Commission on Radiation Units and Measurements, and other national and international organizations, government and private, concerned with radiation quantities, units and measurements and with radiation protection."

From National Council on Radiation Protection and Measurements (NCRP): *Report #116, limitation of exposure to ionizing radiation,* Bethesda, Md, 1993, NCRP.

United Nations Scientific Committee on the Effects of Atomic Radiation

The United Nations Scientific Committee on the Effects of Atomic Radiation (UNSCEAR), which was established in 1955, is another group that plays a prominent role in the formulation of radiation protection guidelines. This group evaluates human and environmental ionizing radiation exposures from a variety of sources, including radioactive materials, radiation-producing machines, and radiation accidents. The UNSCEAR uses epidemiologic data (e.g., information from follow-up studies of Japanese atomic bomb survivors), information acquired from the Radiation Effects Research Foundation (a group run by the government of Japan primarily for the purpose of studying the survivors), and research conclusions to derive radiation risk assessments for radiation-induced cancer and for genetic effects.

National Academy of Sciences/National Research Council Committee on the Biological Effects of Ionizing Radiation

The National Academy of Sciences/National Research Council Committee on the Biological Effects of Ionizing Radiation (NAS/NRC-BEIR) is another advisory group that reviews studies of biologic effects of ionizing radiation and risk assessment. This group formulated the 1990 BEIR V Report, *Health Effects of Exposure to Low Levels of Ionizing Radiation.* BEIR V supersedes four earlier BEIR reports that list studies of biologic effects and associated risk of groups of people who were either routinely or accidentally exposed to ionizing radiation. Such groups include early radiation workers, atomic bomb victims of Hiroshima and Nagasaki, and evacuees from the Chernobyl nuclear power station disaster.

As previously noted, recommendations for effective dose limits and equivalent dose limits are made by the ICRP, NCRP, UNSCEAR, and NAS/NRC-BEIR. Based on these recommendations, limits on radiation exposure are established by congressional act or state mandates. National and state agencies are charged with the responsibility of enforcing standards after they are established.

U.S. REGULATORY AGENCIES

After radiation protection standards have been determined, responsible agencies must enforce them for the protection of the general public, patients, and occupationally exposed personnel.

Regulatory agencies include the following:
1. Nuclear Regulatory Commission (NRC)
2. Agreement states
3. Environmental Protection Agency (EPA)
4. Food and Drug Administration (FDA)
5. Occupational Safety and Health Administration (OSHA)

A summary of the U.S. regulatory agencies is presented in Table 7-2.

Nuclear Regulatory Commission

The **Nuclear Regulatory Commission (NRC),** formerly known as the Atomic Energy Commission, is a federal agency that has the authority to control the possession, use, and production of atomic energy in the interest of national security. This agency also has the power to enforce radiation protection standards. However, the NRC does not regulate or inspect x-ray imaging facilities. The main function of the NRC is to oversee the nuclear energy industry. This agency

TABLE 7-2

Summary of U.S. Regulatory Agencies

Agency	Function
NRC	Oversees the nuclear energy industry, enforces radiation protection standards, publishes its rules and regulations in Title 10 of the U.S. Code of Federal Regulations, enters into written agreements with state governments permitting the state to license and regulate the use of radioisotopes and certain other material within that state
Agreement states	Enforces radiation protection regulations through their respective health departments
EPA	Facilitates the development and enforcement of regulations pertaining to the control of radiation in the environment
FDA	Conducts an ongoing product radiation control program, regulating the design and manufacture of electronic products, including x-ray equipment
OSHA	Functions as a monitoring agency in places of employment, predominantly in industry

supervises the design and working mechanics of nuclear power stations, the production of nuclear fuel, the handling of expended fuel, and the supervision of hazardous radioactive waste material. In addition, the NRC controls the manufacture and use of radioactive substances formed in nuclear reactors and used in research, nuclear medicine imaging procedures, therapeutic treatment (e.g., most commonly, prostate cancer radioactive seed implants and iodine-131 used for thyroid carcinoma), and industry. The NRC also licenses users of such radioactive materials and periodically makes unannounced inspections to determine whether these users are in compliance with the provisions of their license. It does not, however, regulate the usage of radioactive substances that are produced outside of a reactor by high-energy particle accelerators such as cyclotrons. A common example of a cyclotron-produced isotope that is used in nuclear medicine is thallium-201. It is regulated by the State Bureau of Radiation Protection.

The NRC writes standards that are presented as rules and regulations. The agency publishes these rules and regulations in Title 10 of the U.S. Code of Federal Regulations. The U.S. Office of the Federal Register prepares and distributes this document. Fundamental radiation protection standards governing occupational radiation exposure may be found in Part 20 of Title 10. Therefore, the abbreviation 10 CFR 20 is used.

The NRC has the authority to enter into written contracts with state governments. These agreements permit the contracting state to undertake the responsibility of licensing and regulating the use of radioisotopes and certain other radioactive materials within that state.

Agreement States

The majority of states in the United States have entered into "agreements" with the NRC to assume the responsibility of enforcing radiation protection regulations through their respective health departments. These states are known as **agreement states.** In nonagreement states, both the state and the NRC enforce radiation protection regulations by sending agents to health care facilities. Hospitals that use x-rays and radioactive materials are evaluated to determine whether they are in compliance with existing radiation safety regulations. Individual states also may legislate their own regulations regarding radiation safety. Inspection of nuclear reactors and assurance of adherence to federal radiation safety regulations in agreement or nonagreement states fall solely under the jurisdiction of the NRC.

Environmental Protection Agency

The U.S. Environmental Protection Agency (EPA) was established on December 2, 1970. It was created through the reorganization plan of former U.S. president Richard M. Nixon. The agency was created to bring several agencies under one organization that would be responsible for protecting the health of human beings and for safeguarding the natural environment.

The EPA facilitates the development and enforcement of regulations pertaining to the control of radiation in the environment. It directs federal agencies, oversees the general area of environmental monitoring, and has the authority for specific areas such as determining the action level for radon.

Food and Drug Administration

Under Public Law 90-602, the Radiation Control for Health and Safety Act of 1968, the U.S. Food and Drug Administration (FDA) conducts an ongoing products radiation control program, regulating the design and manufacture of electronic products, including diagnostic x-ray equipment. A more detailed explanation of the Radiation Control for Health and Safety Act of 1968 is given later in this chapter.

To determine the level of compliance with standards in a given x-ray facility, the FDA conducts onsite inspections of x-ray equipment, especially mammography units. Compliance with FDA standards ensures protection of occupationally and nonoccupationally exposed persons from faulty manufacturing.

Occupational Safety and Health Administration

The U.S. Occupational Safety and Health Administration (OSHA) functions as a monitoring agency in places of employment, predominantly in industry. OSHA regulates occupational exposure to radiation through Part 1910 of Title 29 of the U.S. Code of Federal Regulations (29 CFR 1910). It is responsible for regulations concerning an employee's "right to know" with regard to hazards that may be present in the workplace. A series of statutes passed by the individual states require that employees be made aware of the hazards in the workplace. The act covers hazardous substances, infectious agents, ionizing radiation, and nonionizing radiation. The act requires employers to evaluate their workplaces for hazardous agents and to provide training and written information to their employees. OSHA also regulates training programs in the workplace.

RADIATION SAFETY PROGRAM

Requirement

Facilities providing imaging services must have an effective and detailed radiation safety program to ensure adequate safety of patients and radiation workers. Implementation of an effective program begins with the administration of the facility. Individuals in executive positions must provide the resources necessary for creating and maintaining such a program. They can delegate operational funds in the budget, oversee the development of policies and procedures, and provide the equipment necessary for starting and for continuing the program.

Radiation Safety Committee and Radiation Safety Officer

The NRC mandates that a **radiation safety committee (RSC)** be established for the facility to assist in the development of the radiation safety program. This committee provides guidance for the program and facilitates its ongoing operation. A **radiation safety officer (RSO)** should be selected to oversee the program's daily operation and provide for its formal review each year. An RSO is normally a medical physicist, health physicist, radiologist, or other individual qualified through adequate training and experience. This person has been designated by a health care facility and approved by the NRC and the state to ensure that the facility follows internationally accepted guidelines for radiation protection.

Responsibilities of the Radiation Safety Officer

The RSO is responsible for developing an appropriate radiation safety program for the facility to ensure that all persons are adequately protected from radiation. To fulfill this responsibility, management of the facility must grant the RSO the authority necessary to implement and enforce the requirements of the radiation safety program. The RSO also is responsible for maintaining radiation-monitoring records for all personnel and for providing counseling for individuals who receive monitor readings in excess of allowable limits.

Required Training and Experience for a Radiation Safety Officer

The necessary training and experience for an RSO is described in sections 10 CFR 35.50 and 10 CFR 35.900 of the Code of Federal Regulations. The NRC publishes regulatory guides to accompany its rules. Although on a legal level health care facilities do not need to comply with the guide, they frequently choose to do so to facilitate the chances of a successful outcome of an NRC inspection or approval of license changes because the guide is actually the NRC's interpretation of how to implement its own rules.

A new proposed regulatory guidance for new Part 35 of the Code of Federal Regulations requires that RSOs must have adequate training and experience. The training and experience requirements for the RSO are described in 10 CFR 35.50 and 10 CFR 35.900 and allow for the following three training pathways:

1. Certification by one of the professional boards approved by the NRC
2. Didactic and work experience as described in detail in the regulations
3. Identification as an authorized user, authorized medical physicist, or authorized nuclear physicist on the license, with experience in the types of use for which the individual has RSO responsibilities

In addition, 10 CFR 35.24 requires that the licensee provide the RSO sufficient authority, organizational freedom, and management prerogative to do the following:

1. Identify radiation safety problems
2. Initiate, recommend, or provide corrective action
3. Stop unsafe operations involving by-product material
4. Verify implementation of corrective actions

Authority of the Radiation Safety Officer

The licensee must also establish, in writing, the authority, duties, and responsibilities of the RSO. The RSO is responsible for day-to-day supervision of the facility's radiation safety program. Therefore, the RSO must have independent authority to stop operations that he or she considers unsafe. This individual must be given sufficient time and resources and have sufficient commitment from management to fulfill certain duties and responsibilities to ensure that radioactive materials are used in a safe manner. The NRC requires the name of the RSO on the facility's license to ensure that licensee management has always identified a responsible, qualified person and that the named individual knows of his or her designation as RSO. Usually, the RSO is a full-time employee of the licensed facility; however, the NRC has authorized individuals who are not employed by the licensee (e.g., a consultant) to fill the role of an RSO or to provide support to the facility's RSO. Training for an RSO is covered in 10 CFR 35. It is the same in the revision as currently exists. A list of these requirements may be found in Appendix F.

EFFECTIVE DOSE LIMITING SYSTEM

The effective dose (EfD) limiting system is the current method for assessing radiation exposure and associated risk of biologic damage to radiation workers and the general public (Fig. 7-2). **Effective dose limit** concerns the upper boundary dose of ionizing radiation that results in a negligible risk of bodily injury or genetic damage. These limits may be expressed for whole-body exposure, partial-body exposure, and exposure of

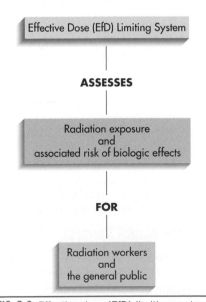

FIG. 7-2. Effective dose (EfD) limiting system.

individual organs. Separate limits are set for occupationally exposed individuals and for the general public. The sum of both the external and internal whole-body exposures is considered when effective dose limits are established. These upper limits are designed to minimize the risk to humans in terms of nonstochastic (deterministic) and stochastic (probabilistic) effects, and they do not include natural background and medical exposure. Nonstochastic and stochastic effects are discussed later in this chapter and also in Chapter 6.

Upper boundary radiation exposure limits for occupationally exposed persons are associated with risks that are similar to those encountered by employees in other industries such as manufacturing, trade, or government, which are generally considered to be reasonably safe. Radiation risks are derived from the complete injury caused by radiation exposure. The potential for terminal cancer, genetic imperfections induced by reproductive cell mutations, shortening of life span due to the induction of cancer, and the overall poorer quality of life are taken into account.

RADIATION CONTROL FOR HEALTH AND SAFETY ACT OF 1968

In 1968 the U.S. Congress passed the Radiation Control for Health and Safety Act (Public Law 90-602) to protect the public from the hazards of unnecessary radiation exposure resulting from electronic products such as microwave ovens and color televisions. Diagnostic x-ray equipment also was included. The act permitted the establishment of the Center for Devices and Radiological Health (CDRH). Until 1982 this organization was known as the Bureau of Radiological Health (BRH). The CDRH falls under the jurisdiction of the FDA. Essentially, it is responsible for conducting an ongoing electronic product radiation control program. This includes setting up standards for the manufacture, installation, assembly, and maintenance of machines for radiologic procedures. Further responsibilities include assessing the biologic effects of ionizing radiation, evaluating radiation emissions from electronic products in general, and conducting research to reduce radiation exposure.

Code of Standards for Diagnostic X-Ray Equipment

The code of standards for diagnostic x-ray equipment went into effect on August 1, 1974. This code applies to complete systems and major components manufactured after that date. Equipment in use before August 1, 1974, does not need to be modified or discarded. Some important provisions of the standards for diagnostic x-ray equipment are listed in Box 7-2.

Public Law 90-602 does not regulate the diagnostic x-ray user. It is strictly an equipment performance standard.

ALARA CONCEPT

In 1954 the National Committee on Radiation Protection (later to be known as the National Council on Radiation Protection and Measurements) put forth the principle that radiation exposures should be kept *"as low as reasonably achievable"* with consideration for economic and social factors. This principle, known as the **ALARA concept,** is accepted by all regulatory agencies. In 1987, the NCRP described the ALARA concept as "the continuation of good radiation protection programs and practices which traditionally have been effective in keeping the average and individual exposures for monitored workers well below the limit."[3] It also may be referred to as **optimization** in accordance with ICRP Publication No. 37 and Publication No. 55. Medical radiographers and radiologists share the responsibility to keep occupational and nonoccupational dose limits as low as possible. In practice this translates into effective and equivalent doses well below maximal allowable levels. This goal can usually be simply achieved through the employment of proper safety procedures performed by qualified personnel. Such procedures should be clearly described in a facility's radiation safety program. To define ALARA, health care facilities usually adopt investigation levels, defined as Level I and Level II. In the United States, these levels are traditionally one tenth to three tenths the applicable regulatory limits.

BOX 7-2

Provisions Included in the Standards for Diagnostic X-Ray Equipment

1. Automatic limitation of the radiographic beam to the image receptor regardless of image receptor size, a condition known as positive beam limitation.
2. Appropriate minimal permanent filtration of the x-ray beam to ensure an acceptable level of beam quality. Filtration provides significant reduction in the intensity of very "soft" x-rays that contribute only to added patient absorbed dose.
3. Ability of x-ray units to duplicate certain radiation exposures for any given combination of kilovolts at peak value (kVp), milliamperes (mA), and time to ensure both exposure reproducibility and linearity. *Reproducibility* is defined as consistency in output in radiation intensity for identical generator settings from one individual exposure to other subsequent exposures.* A variance of 5% or less is acceptable. *Exposure linearity* is defined as consistency in output radiation intensity at a selected kVp setting when changing from one milliamperage and time combination (mAs = mA × exposure time to another. *Linearity*, which is defined as the ratio of the difference in mR/mAs values between two successive generator stations to the sum of those mR/mAs values, must be less than 0.1).
4. Inclusion of beam limitation devices for spot films taken during fluoroscopy. Such devices should be located between the x-ray source and the patient.
5. Presence of "beam on" indicators to give visible warnings when x-ray exposures are in progress and both visual and audible signals when exposure has terminated.
6. Inclusion of manual backup timers for automatic (photo-timed) exposure control to ensure the termination of the exposure if the automatic timer fails.

---

*Mathematically, reproducibility is described by the coefficient of variation "C," which is equal to the standard deviation of at least five successive output measurements employing the same technique factors divided by the average or mean value of those measurements. The regulation requires that C must not exceed 0.05.

Model for the ALARA Concept

The ALARA concept presents an extremely conservative model with respect to the relationship between ionizing radiation and potential risk. The relationship is assumed to be completely linear (i.e., biologic effect

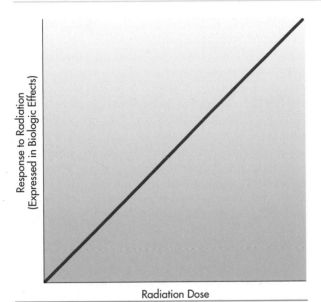

FIG. 7-3. Dose-response curve. Hypothetical linear (straight-line), nonthreshold curve for radiation dose-response relationship. The straight-line curve passing through the origin in this graph indicates both that the response to radiation (in terms of biologic effects) is directly proportional to the dose of radiation and that no known level of radiation dose exists below which absolutely no chance of sustaining biologic damage is evident.

and radiation dose are directly proportional) and without any threshold (Fig. 7-3). In the interest of safety, risk of injury should be overestimated rather than underestimated.

CONSUMER-PATIENT RADIATION HEALTH AND SAFETY ACT OF 1981

The Consumer-Patient Radiation Health and Safety Act of 1981 (Title IX of Public Law 97-35) (see Appendix G) provides federal legislation requiring the establishment of minimal standards for the accreditation of education programs for persons who administer radiologic procedures and the certification of such persons. The purpose of this federal act, which is under the directorship of the secretary of Health and Human Services, is to ensure that standard medical and dental radiologic procedures adhere to rigorous safety precautions and standards. Individual states are encouraged to enact similar statutes and administer certification

and accreditation programs based on the standards established therein. Because no legal penalty exists for noncompliance, many states, unfortunately, have not responded with appropriate legislation.

GOAL FOR RADIATION PROTECTION

NCRP Report No. 116, *Limitation of Exposure to Ionizing Radiation*, provides the most recent guidance on radiation protection. This report enunciates the goal of radiation protection, which reads as follows: "to prevent the occurrence of serious radiation-induced conditions (acute and chronic deterministic effects) in exposed persons and to reduce stochastic effects in exposed persons to a degree that is acceptable in relation to the benefits to the individual and to society from the activities that generate such exposures."[3] The whole essence of radiation protection is contained in the preceding statement.

RADIATION-INDUCED RESPONSES OF CONCERN IN RADIATION PROTECTION

Categories for Radiation-Induced Responses

Two all-inclusive categories encompass the radiation-induced responses of serious concern in radiation protection programs: (1) nonstochastic (deterministic) effects and (2) stochastic (probabilistic) effects.

Nonstochastic Effects

Nonstochastic (deterministic) effects are biologic somatic effects of ionizing radiation that can be directly related to the dose received. These cell-killing effects exhibit a threshold dose below which the effect does not normally occur and above which the severity of the biologic damage increases as the dose increases. For example, if a certain dose of radiation produces a skin burn, a higher dose of radiation will cause the skin burn to be more severe; however, a dose below the threshold level for skin burn will not demonstrate the effect. When radiation-induced biologic damage escalates, it does so because greater numbers of cells interact with the increased number of x-ray photons that are present at higher radiation doses. In general, nonstochastic effects occur only after large doses of radiation. Such radiation doses are usually much greater than those typically encountered by a patient in diagnostic radiology.*

Early and Late Nonstochastic Effects Deterministic effects may be early, such as (1) diffuse redness over an area of skin after irradiation (erythema), (2) a decrease in the white blood cell count, and (3) epilation, or loss of hair. Other, far more serious early consequences of radiation sickness can arise, such as (1) the hematopoietic syndrome, (2) gastrointestinal syndrome, and (3) cerebrovascular syndrome. These usually occur within a few hours or days after a very high level radiation exposure to a significant portion of the body. The aforementioned syndromes are collectively referred to as the *acute radiation syndrome*. (Radiation syndromes are discussed in detail in Chapter 6.) Late deterministic somatic effects also may occur months or years after high-level radiation exposure. They are classified as late effects and include cataract formation, fibrosis, organ atrophy, loss of parenchymal cells, reduced fertility, and sterility caused by a decrease in reproductive cells.

Early deterministic somatic effects such as erythema and late deterministic somatic effects such as cataract formation have a high probability of occurring when entrance radiation doses exceed 2 Gy (200 rads). The frequency of occurrence of high-dose deterministic effects is not proportional to the dose but rather follows a non-straight-line dose-effect curve that is sigmoidal (S-shaped) with a threshold (see Fig. 6-1, *B*).

Stochastic Effects

Stochastic (probabilistic) effects are mutational, nonthreshold, randomly occurring biologic somatic changes in which the chance of occurrence of the effect rather than the severity of the effect is proportional to the dose of ionizing radiation. This means that the effect occurs in an arbitrary manner (random in nature) and the severity of the effect is not dose

dependent. It is based on probabilities, with the chances of occurrence increasing with each radiation exposure. Examples of stochastic effects are cancer and genetic alterations. Stochastic effects may be demonstrated with the use of both the linear (see Fig. 6-2) and the linear-quadratic dose-response curves (see Fig. 6-3). A stochastic event is an all-or-none response, meaning that ionizing radiation could cause a disease process event such as cancer to occur within the general large population. Because these effects are random, determining which members of an exposed population will develop cancer is not possible before the radiation dose is received. Injury may result from exposure of a single cell or from damage in a sensitive substructure such as a gene. The assumption is that no minimal safe dose exists. The frequency of an occurrence in a population, however, does increase in proportion to the absorbed dose of ionizing radiation delivered to the entire population. Therefore, the net effect on the population group depends on the number of individuals irradiated as well as the mean dose that each individual receives.

Occurrence of Radiation-induced Malignancy Occurrence of radiation-induced cancer increases with absorbed dose to somatic cells, which include all cells in the human body except germ cells. However, the severity of the disease is not dose related. For example, if a cancer induced by 2 Gy (200 rads) of ionizing radiation and a cancer induced by 0.2 Gy (20 rads) of ionizing radiation are compared, the cancer induced by the larger absorbed dose is no worse than the cancer induced by the smaller absorbed dose, but the chance of cancer induction from the larger dose is greater.

Damage to Reproductive Cells When ionizing radiation damages reproductive cells, mutations may develop that could bring an injurious consequence in subsequent generations. An example of this is effects on offspring caused by irradiation of reproductive cells (sperm and ova) before conception. This effect is called mutagenesis.

Risk of Cancer Induction from High and Low Doses of Ionizing Radiation Although epidemiologic studies analyzing groups such as the Japanese atomic bomb survivors have provided sufficient evidence of the induction of cancers in humans from high radiation absorbed doses, no conclusive epidemiologic

---

*A significant exception to this is high-dose-rate fluoroscopic procedures. For these studies, entrance exposure rates as great as 20 R/min are not uncommon. A fluoroscopic exposure of 15 minutes then results in a patient entrance dose of approximately 3 Gy (300 rads). This represents a therapeutic dose level.

evidence suggests that low-level ionizing radiation exposures, such as those used in the most commonly performed diagnostic imaging procedures, can cause malignancies in humans. Although the sample sizes of the human population necessary to perform statistically valid studies to determine the carcinogenic potential of low absorbed doses of sparsely ionizing radiation are impracticable, radiation protection procedures must always be employed during diagnostic examinations. Currently, the risk of cancer induction from low absorbed doses of ionizing radiation can only be estimated by extrapolating (scaling down) from high-dose data, using either a linear or a linear quadratic model (see Figs. 6-2 and 6-3). With each model, the calculated risk from low-dose radiation is small compared with the risk for cancer, birth defects, and genetic mutations under normal circumstances. The fact that the latter occurs in considerable proportions in the human population makes obtaining precise estimates of the role of ionizing radiation alone in producing such effects extraordinarily difficult. Therefore, the identification of any stochastic occurrence increase in the general population exposed to small amounts of ionizing radiation is subject to considerable doubt. A summary of both stochastic (probabilistic) and nonstochastic (deterministic) effects is presented in Box 7-3.

BOX 7-3

Summary of Serious Radiation-Induced Responses of Concern

Nonstochastic (Deterministic) Effects	Stochastic (Probabilistic) Effects
Early Effects	Cancer
Erythema (diffuse redness over an area of skin after irradiation)	**Genetic Effects**
Blood changes (decrease of lymphocytes and platelets)	Mutagenesis (irradiation of the reproductive cells before conception)
Epilation (loss of hair)	
Acute radiation syndrome	
Hematopoietic syndrome	
Gastrointestinal syndrome	
Cerebrovascular syndrome	
Late Effects	
Cataract formation	
Fibrosis	
Organ atrophy	
Loss of parenchymal cells	
Reduced fertility	
Sterility	

OBJECTIVES OF RADIATION PROTECTION

Radiation protection has two explicit objectives:
1. To prevent any clinically important radiation-induced nonstochastic (deterministic) effect from occurring by adhering to dose limits that are beneath the threshold levels
2. To limit the risk of stochastic responses to a conservative level as weighted against societal needs, values, benefits acquired, and economic considerations

CURRENT RADIATION PROTECTION PHILOSOPHY

Both genetic and somatic responses to ionizing radiation were considered in developing the present effective dose limiting recommendations. Current radiation protection philosophy is based on the assumption that a linear, nonthreshold relationship exists between radiation dose and biologic response. This means that the chance of biologic damage and the amount of damage sustained are directly proportional to the amount of radiation absorbed, and no known level of radiation dose exists below which the probability of biologic damage is zero (see Fig. 7-3). Thus, even the most minuscule dose of radiation has the potential to cause some harm. The current philosophy also accepts the premise that ionizing radiation possesses a beneficial and a destructive potential. It proposes that, when employed in the healing arts for the welfare of the patient, the potential benefits of exposing the patient to ionizing radiation must far outweigh the potential risks involved.

RISK

Risk in the Medical Imaging Industry

In general terms, *risk* may be defined as the probability of injury, ailment, or death resulting from an activity. In the medical imaging industry, **risk** is viewed as the possibility of inducing a radiogenic cancer or genetic defect after irradiation. The way people look at probability and severity affects the perception of risk. As stated previously, no conclusive proof exists that low-level ionizing radiation causes a statistically significant increase in the threat of a malignancy. Although this risk may in fact be negligible, the subject is still highly controversial. (A discussion of risk estimates for both stochastic and nonstochastic effects is presented in Chapter 6.)

Revised Concepts of Radiation Exposure and Risk

Revised concepts of radiation exposure and risk have brought about the recent changes in NCRP recommendations for limits on exposure to ionizing radiation. Because many conflicting views exist on assessing the risk of cancer induction from low-level radiation exposure, the trend has been to create more rigorous radiation protection standards. The adoption of the effective dose (EfD) limiting system is a direct consequence of this conservatism. The benefit obtained from any diagnostic radiologic procedure must always be weighed against the risk that is taken. (Methods for assessing risk estimates for cancer induction are discussed in Chapter 6.)

Occupational Risk

Occupational risk associated with radiation exposure may be equated with occupational risk in other industries that are generally considered reasonably safe (refer to Chapter 9, p. 226). That risk is generally estimated to be a 2.5% chance of fatal accident over an entire career. The lifetime fatal risk in hazardous occupations such as logging and deep-sea fishing is many times greater.

To ensure that the hazard to radiation workers is no greater than the hazard to the general working public, the NCRP proposes that radiation protection programs for radiation workers should be designed to prevent individual workers from having a total external plus internal cumulative effective dose in excess of their age in years times 10 mSv (1 rem).[3] Consider the following situation: A worker at age 40 has been employed at a nuclear power plant for 10 years. He had previously been employed as a radiation worker in another industry, during the course of which he received a cumulative effective dose of 100 mSv (10 rem). Therefore, the radiation protection program for his current position should ensure that he has not accumulated a total effective dose greater than 300 mSv (30 rem) during 10 years of employment.

Vulnerability of the Embryo-Fetus to Radiation Exposure

The embryo-fetus in utero is particularly sensitive to radiation exposure. Epidemiologic studies of atomic bomb survivors exposed in utero have provided conclusive evidence of a dose-dependent increase in the incidence of severe mental retardation for fetal doses greater than approximately 0.4 Sv (40 rem). The greatest risk for radiation-induced mental retardation occurred when the embryo-fetus was exposed 8 to 15 weeks after conception.

BASIS FOR THE EFFECTIVE DOSE (EfD) LIMITING SYSTEM

Concept Underlying Radiation Protection

The essential concept underlying radiation protection is that any organ in the human body is vulnerable to damage from exposure to ionizing radiation. Even though some organs are known to be more sensitive to radiation than others, every organ is at some risk because of the assumed stochastic (probabilistic) nature of somatic or genetic radiation-induced effects.

The effective dose limiting system includes, for the determination of **equivalent dose (EqD)** for tissues and organs, all radiation-vulnerable human organs that can contribute to potential risk, rather than only those human organs considered critical. In earlier recommendations such as NCRP Report No. 39 (released in 1971), critical organs such as the gonads, blood-forming organs such as red bone marrow, and lung tissue were identified.[4]

Tissue Weighting Factor (W$_T$)

Although the tissue weighting factor was discussed in Chapter 3, a brief discussion of this factor follows to facilitate greater understanding of its importance as it relates to the effective dose limiting system. The effective dose limiting system is an attempt to equate the various risks of cancer and genetic effects to the tissues or organs that were exposed to radiation. Because various tissues and organs do not have the same degree of sensitivity to these effects, the system employed must compensate for the differences in risk from one organ to another. Therefore, a **tissue weighting factor (W$_T$)** is used. This factor "indicates the ratio of the risk of stochastic effects attributable to irradiation of a given organ or tissue (*T*) to the total risk when the whole body is uniformly irradiated."[5] Organ or tissue weighting factors recommended by the ICRP in Report No. 60 (released in 1991) and adopted by the NCRP in Report No. 116 (released in 1993) are reproduced in Box 7-4.

BOX 7-4

Organ or Tissue Weighting Factors (W$_T$) for Calculating Effective Dose

0.01	0.12
Bone surface	Red bone marrow
Skin	Colon
	Lung
0.05	Stomach
Bladder	**0.20**
Breast	
Liver	Gonads
Esophagus	
Thyroid	
Remainder*†	

From National Council on Radiation Protection and Measurements (NCRP): *Report #116, limitation of exposure to ionizing radiation,* Bethesda, Md, 1993, NCRP.
*The remainder takes into account the following additional tissues and organs: adrenals, brain, small intestine, large intestine, kidney, muscle, pancreas, spleen, thymus, and uterus.
†In extraordinary circumstances in which one of the remainder tissues or organs receives an equivalent dose in excess of the highest dose in any of the 12 organs for which a weighting factor (W$_T$) is specified, a W$_T$ of 0.025 should be applied to that tissue or organ and a W$_T$ of 0.025 to the average dose in the other remainder tissues or organs.

CURRENT NCRP RECOMMENDATIONS

NCRP Reports

The NCRP reiterates and updates its position on radiation protection standards and publishes recommendations on these standards in the form of reports. Recommendations contained in NCRP Report No. 116 now supersede those contained in NCRP Report No. 91 and No. 39. A summary of some important issues and changes follows.

Annual Occupational Effective Dose Limit

An **annual occupational effective dose limit** of 50 mSv (5 rem) (not including medical and natural background exposure) has been established for the whole body, with an added recommendation that the lifetime effective dose in mSv should not exceed 10 times the occupationally exposed person's age in years.

Cumulative Effective Dose (CumEfD) Limit

A radiation worker's **lifetime effective dose** must be limited to his or her age in years times 10 mSv (years times 1 rem). This is called the **cumulative effective dose (CumEfD) limit** and pertains to the whole body. Adhering to this limit ensures that the lifetime risk for these workers remains acceptable. Effective dose limits, however, do not include radiation exposure from natural background radiation or exposure acquired as a consequence of a worker undergoing medical imaging procedures. The limits do include the possibility of both internal and external exposure. The **effective dose** is therefore the sum or total of both the internal and external equivalent doses (EqD).

The following example demonstrates the application of the CumEfD limit for the whole body. In the example, EqD represents the CumEfD.

EXAMPLE: Determine the CumEfD limit to the whole body of an occupationally exposed person who is 37 years old.

ANSWER: In International System (SI) units:

$$EqD = 10\,mSv \times age\,(in\,years)$$
$$EqD = 10\,mSv \times 37$$
$$EqD = 370\,mSV$$

To determine the CumEfD limit of the same individual in rem, the equation is expressed in traditional units in the following manner:

$$EqD = age\,in\,rem$$
$$EqD = 37\,rem$$

This represents the CumEfD for the whole body that the occupationally exposed person may receive as a consequence of age.

Medical imaging personnel almost never receive equivalent doses that are close to the annual effective dose limit. If a radiation safety program is well structured and properly maintained, occupational exposure will not remotely approach 50 mSv (5 rem) in any given year.

Collective Effective Dose (ColEfD)

The **collective effective dose (ColEfD)** has been designated for use in the description of population or group exposure from low doses of different sources of ionizing radiation. Collective effective dose is determined as the product of the average effective dose for an individual belonging to the exposed population or group and the number of persons exposed. The person-sievert (previously referred to as man-rem) is the unit of choice to express this quantity. If 1000 people are exposed to low doses of different sources of ionizing radiation and receive an average effective dose of 0.5 mSv (50 millirem [mrem]), the collective effective dose is 500 person-millisieverts, which equals 0.5 person-sievert (50 man-rem).

ICRP Recommendation for Downward Revision of the Annual Effective Dose Limit

Levels of ionizing radiation formerly considered acceptable by the ICRP have been revised downward.

In 1991 the ICRP recommended the reduction of the annual effective dose limit for occupationally exposed persons from 50 mSv (5 rem) to 20 mSv (2 rem) as a result of new information obtained from the Japanese atomic bomb survivors in which the risk of radiation from the atomic bomb detonations was estimated to be approximately three to four times greater (more damaging) than previously estimated.[6] The NCRP is still considering the possibility of reducing exposure standards because of (1) the revised risk estimates derived from the recent reevaluations of dosimetric studies on the atomic bomb survivors of Hiroshima and Nagasaki[6] and (2) the appearance, as a result of longer follow-up time, of increased numbers of solid tumors in the survivor population. In the future, the annual whole-body effective dose limit for occupationally exposed persons in the United States may be limited to 10 to 20 mSv (1 or 2 rem) per year.* Of course, such a change will necessitate further evaluation of actual risk for persons employed in radiation industries. In the United States, lowering of the current limits is the responsibility of the NRC, individual states, and the FDA.

Limits for Nonoccupationally Exposed Individuals

In addition to limits for occupationally exposed individuals, the NCRP also sets limits for nonoccupationally exposed individuals who are not undergoing medical examinations. An example would be a spouse, parent, or guardian accompanying a patient to radiology. A limit also has been set for individual members of the general public not occupationally exposed. The NCRP-recommended annual effective dose limit is 1 mSv (0.1 rem) for continuous or frequent exposures from artificial sources other than medical irradiation and natural background and a limit of 5 mSv (0.5 rem) annually for infrequent exposure.[3] The annual effective dose nonoccupational limit set for individual members of the general public is designed to

---

*Manual 60 of the ICRP (Oxford, 1991, Pergamon Press) contains a recommendation for lowering the allowable occupational level of exposure to ionizing radiation from 50 mSv per year (5 rem per year) to 20 mSv per year (2 rem per year) averaged over defined periods of 5 years. This lower limit is not enforced in the United States.

limit that exposure "to reasonable levels of risk comparable with risks from other common sources, i.e., about 10^{-4} to 10^{-6} annually."[3] The 5-mSv (0.5 rem) annual limit for infrequent exposure is made because "annual exposures in excess of the 1 mSv recommendation, usually to a small group of people, need not be regarded as especially significant to the group as a whole provided it does not occur often to the same groups and that the average exposure to individuals in these groups does not exceed an average annual effective dose of about 1 mSv."[3]

Limits for Pregnant Female Radiation Workers

To reduce exposure for pregnant female radiation workers and control the exposure to the unborn during potentially sensitive periods of gestation, the NCRP now recommends a monthly equivalent dose limit not exceeding 0.5 mSv (0.05 rem) per month to the embryo-fetus and a limit during the entire pregnancy not to exceed 5.0 mSv (0.50 rem) after declaration of the pregnancy. The alert reader will note that the monthly limit is more stringent, as 9 months at 0.5 mSv will automatically result in an equivalent dose of less than 4.5 mSv, which is below the limit for the duration of pregnancy of 5.0 mSv. Nevertheless, both limits are in place to reflect the fact that not all pregnant workers are monitored monthly and to reflect the fact that personnel dosimetry does not result in exact measures of equivalent dose, just approximations based on the badge readings. This equivalent dose limit excludes both medical and natural background radiation and is designed to restrict significantly the total lifetime risk of leukemia and other malignancies in persons exposed in utero.[3] Deterministic effects such as small head size and mental retardation are expected to be negligible if the equivalent dose remains below the established limit.

Limits for Education and Training Purposes

For education and training purposes, the same dose limits should apply to students of radiography in general and to those individuals under 18 years of age. The dose limit is the same for kindergarten through 12th-grade students attending science demonstrations involving ionizing radiation as it is for radiologic technologists under the age of 18. The limit for any education and training exposures of individuals under the age of 18 is an effective dose of 1 mSv (0.1 rem) annually. However, occasional exposure for the purpose of education and training is permitted, provided that special care is taken to ensure that the annual effective dose limit of 1 mSv (0.1 rem) is not exceeded.

Limits for Tissues and Organs Exposed Selectively or Together with Other Organs

Nonstochastic limits or occupational dose limits for deterministic effects for tissues and organs exposed selectively or together with other organs have been set to prevent excessive doses to those organs and tissues. They include the following: 150 mSv (15 rem) to the crystalline lens of the eyes and 500 mSv (50 rem) for localized areas of the skin, the hands, and feet.[3] Although the established annual dose limit for localized areas of skin provides adequate protection for that organ against stochastic effects, it will actually require an additional limit to prevent deterministic effects.

Negligible Individual Dose (NID)

To provide a low-exposure cutoff level so that regulatory agencies may dismiss a level of individual risk as negligible risk, an annual **negligible individual dose (NID)** of 0.01 mSv/yr (1 mrem/yr) per source or practice has been set. This means that below this effective dose level, a reduction of individual exposure is unnecessary.

ACTION LIMITS

Health care facilities go to great lengths to avoid having personnel even approach effective dose limits. In a well-designed and well-run facility, radiologic technologists' badge readings should be well below a tenth of the maximum effective dose limits, even for those technologists who receive the most exposure. Health care facilities, such as hospitals, set their own internal **action limits.** These limits are set at levels far below the actual limits, typically a tenth of the limit, but at levels that are not routinely exceeded by personnel. They are meant to trigger an investigation that should uncover the reason for any unusually high exposure. Some reasons for unusual readings include badges that were exposed to unusual amounts of heat, as from being left on a car's dashboard in the summer or by accidentally going through a clothes dryer. Sometimes work habits, such as where the technologist stands during interventional radiography or computed tomography procedures, can be modified. In any case, the RSO is meant to be an active participant along with the radiology department manager in an ongoing program that prevents personnel from receiving anywhere near the maximum allowed exposures.

RADIATION HORMESIS

In Report No. 5 of the National Academy of Science on the Biological Effects of Ionizing Radiation (BEIR V), conclusions regarding the adverse effects on health from low levels of ionizing radiation are based on extrapolations from radiation equivalent doses greater than 0.5 Sv (50 rem). Such radiation levels are significantly greater than ordinary background radiation levels (3.3 mSv or 350 mrem per year). BEIR V espouses the linear "no threshold" view of the Japanese atomic bomb lifetime survival study (LSS) data. However, studies from the Radiation Effects Research Council in Hiroshima have indicated an apparent threshold dosage in the atomic bomb LSS data that is approximately between 0.2 and 0.5 Sv (20 to 50 rem). This lower value corresponds to the amount of natural radiation that average U.S. residents receive in their lifetimes. What is curious is that the lifetime survival data appear to indicate that Japanese atomic bomb survivors with moderate radiation exposure of 5 mSv to 50 mSv, or 0.5 rem to 5 rem, the equivalent of 1.5 to 15 years of natural radiation, have a reduced cancer death rate compared with a normally exposed control population. These data contradict the predictions of the BEIR V report and, if substantiated, seem to cast doubt on the BEIR V conclusion that any amount of radiation is potentially harmful. The reverse might actually be true, at least for moderate amounts of radiation exposure. More specifically, in seven Western states that have background radiation levels higher than other states by about 1 mSv per year (100 mrem per year), residents experience about 15% fewer cancer deaths per 1000 individuals than the U.S. average. A study was conducted in China from 1972 to 1975 of two stable populations of about 70,000 persons, each of whose annual background radiation levels differed by about 2 mSv (200 mrem). This study disclosed a cancer rate in the more exposed population of only about 50% of that of the other group. Other intriguing studies exist. These suggest a potential **radiation hormesis** effect, which is a beneficial consequence of radiation for populations continuously exposed to moderately high levels of radiation. During the course of human evolution over millions of years, advantageous genetic mutations caused by radiation exposure may have occurred, resembling those that allow lower animals today to demonstrate radiation hormesis. Therefore, to assume risk from very small amounts of radiation exposure (two or three times normal background levels) may be incorrect. However, until the radiation hormesis theory is proven, the medical radiation industry will continue to follow the principle of ALARA (as low as reasonably achievable) for radiation protection purposes.

OCCUPATIONAL AND NONOCCUPATIONAL DOSE LIMITS

Effective Dose Limits for Radiation Workers and the Population as a Whole

For the protection of radiation workers and the population as a whole, effective dose limits (Table 7-3) have been established as guidelines. All medical imaging personnel should be familiar with current NCRP recommendations. For this group the most important item is the 50 mSv (5 rem) per year whole-body occupational dose limit. This annual upper boundary is designed to limit the stochastic (probabilistic) effects of radiation. It takes into account the equivalent dose in all radiation-sensitive organs found in the body.

Special Limits for Selected Areas

Because the tissue weighting factors (see Box 7-3) used for calculating effective dose are so small for some organs, an organ that is associated with a low weighting factor may receive an unreasonably large dose while the effective dose remains within the allowable total limit. Therefore, special limits are set for the crystalline lens of the eye and localized areas of the skin, hands, and feet to prevent nonstochastic effects.

TABLE 7-3

Summary of the National Council on Radiation Protection and Measurements (NCRP) Recommendations*† (NCRP Report No. 116)

A. Occupational exposures‡		
1. Effective dose limits		
a. Annual	50 mSv	(5 rem)
b. Cumulative	10 mSv × age	1 rem × age
2. Equivalent dose annual limits for tissues and organs		
a. Lens of eye	150 mSv	(15 rem)
b. Localized areas of the skin, hands, and feet	500 mSv	(50 rem)
B. Guidance for emergency occupational exposure‡ (see Section 14, NCRP #116)		
C. Public exposures (annual)		
1. Effective dose limit, continuous or frequent exposure‡	1 mSv	(0.1 rem)
2. Effective dose limit, infrequent exposure‡	5 mSv	(0.5 rem)
3. Equivalent dose limits for tissues and organs‡		
a. Lens of eye	15 mSv	(1.5 rem)
b. Localized areas of the skin, hands, and feet	50 mSv	(5 rem)
4. Remedial action for natural sources		
a. Effective dose (excluding radon)	>5 mSv	(>0.5 rem)
b. Exposure to radon and its decay products§	>0.007 Jhm⁻³	(>2 WLM)
D. Education and training exposures (annual)‡		
1. Effective dose limit	1 mSv	(0.1 rem)
2. Equivalent dose limit for tissues and organs		
a. Lens of eye	15 mSv	(1.5 rem)
b. Localized areas of the skin, hands, and feet	50 mSv	(5 rem)
E. Embryo-fetus exposures‡		
1. Equivalent dose limit		
a. Monthly	0.5 mSv	(0.05 rem)
b. Entire gestation	5.0 mSv	(0.50 rem)
F. Negligible individual dose (annual)‡	0.01 mSv	(0.001 rem)

*Excluding medical exposures.
†See Tables 4.2 and 5.1 in NCRP Report #116 for recommendations on radiation weighting factors and tissue weighting factors, respectively.
‡Sum of external and internal exposures, excluding doses from natural sources.
§WLM stands for working level month and refers to a cumulative exposure for a working month (170 hours). As applied to radon and its daughter products, 1 WLM represents the cumulative exposure experienced in a 170-hour period resulting from a radon concentration of 100 pCi/L. The occupational limit for miners is 4 WLM per year, which results in an equivalent dose of approximately 0.15 Sv (15 rem) per year.

SUMMARY

➤ Effective dose limiting system:
- Adherence to occupational and nonoccupational effective dose limits helps prevent harmful biologic effects of radiation exposure.
- The concept of radiation exposure and associated risk of radiation-induced malignancy is the basis of the effective dose-limiting system.

- The sum of both external and internal whole-body exposures is considered when establishing effective dose limit.
- Accounting for tissue weighting factors is important because various tissues and organs do not have the same degree of sensitivity.
- Different biologic threats posed by different types of ionizing radiation must be taken into consideration even when absorbed dose is the same.

➤ Effective dose limit:

- The NCRP has established an annual occupational effective dose limit of 50 mSv (5 rem) and a lifetime effective dose that does not exceed 10 times the occupationally exposed person's age in years.
- Collective effective dose is used in the description of population/group exposure from low doses of different sources of ionizing radiation.
- Internal action limits are established by health care facilities to trigger an investigation to uncover the reasons for any unusual high exposures received by individual staff members.

➤ Radiation hormesis is the hypothesis that a positive effect exists for certain populations that are continuously exposed to moderate levels of radiation.

➤ Major organizations involved in regulating radiation exposure:

- The UNSCEAR and the NAS/NRC-BEIR supply information to the ICRP.
- The ICRP makes recommendations on occupational and public dose limits.
- The NCRP reviews ICRP recommendations and implements them into U.S. radiation protection policy.
- The NRC is the watchdog of the nuclear energy industry; it controls the manufacture and use of radioactive substances.
- The EPA develops and enforces regulations pertaining to the control of environmental radiation.
- The FDA regulates the design and manufacture of products used in the radiation industry.
- OSHA monitors the workplace and regulates occupational exposure to radiation.

➤ Individual health care facilities establish an RSC and designate an RSO.

- The RSO is responsible for developing a radiation safety program for the health care facility; he or she maintains personnel radiation-monitoring records and provides counseling in radiation safety.

➤ The ALARA concept (optimization) states that radiation exposure should be kept "as low as reasonably achievable."

➤ Serious radiation-induced responses may be classified as having either nonstochastic or stochastic effects.

- Nonstochastic effects are those biologic somatic effects of ionizing radiation that exhibit a threshold dose below which the effect does not normally occur and above which the severity of the biologic damage increases as the dose increases.
- Stochastic effects are nonthreshold, randomly occurring biologic somatic changes in which the chance of occurrence of the effect rather than the severity of the effect is proportional to the dose of ionizing radiation.

References

1. International Commission on Radiological Protection: *ICRP: Structure and organization.* Retrieved from the Internet March 7, 2001, www.icrp.org/newpage.htm.
2. National Council on Radiation Protection and Measurements: *Background information.* Retrieved from the Internet March 8, 2001, www.ncrp.com/info.html.
3. National Council on Radiation Protection and Measurements (NCRP): *Report #116, limitation of exposure to ionizing radiation,* Bethesda, Md, 1993, NCRP.
4. National Council on Radiation Protection and Measurements (NCRP): *Report #39, basic radiation protection criteria,* Washington, DC, 1971, NCRP.
5. National Council on Radiation Protection and Measurements (NCRP): *Report #91, recommendations on limits for exposure to ionizing radiation,* Bethesda, Md, 1987, NCRP.
6. Committee on Biological Effects of Ionizing Radiation, National Research Council, Commission of Life Sciences, Board of Radiation Research: *Health effects of exposure to low levels of ionizing radiation (BEIR V Report,* Washington, DC, 1989, National Academy Press.

GENERAL DISCUSSION QUESTIONS

1. Why must radiation exposure of the general public, patients, and radiation workers be limited?
2. What is the basis of the effective dose limiting system?
3. Why must health care facilities have an effective and detailed radiation safety program?
4. Describe the responsibilities of a radiation safety officer.
5. What authority must a radiation safety officer have?
6. Describe the effective dose limiting system.

7. What responsibilities do the Center for Devices and Radiological Health (CDRH) fulfill?
8. What is the goal of radiation protection according to NCRP Report #116?
9. What is the difference between nonstochastic and stochastic effects of ionizing radiation?
10. Describe current NCRP dose limiting recommendations.

REVIEW QUESTIONS

1. **Which of the following agencies is responsible for enforcing radiation safety standards?**
   A. ICRP
   B. NRC
   C. NCRP
   D. UNSCEAR

2. **Determine the cumulative effective dose (CumEfD) to the whole body of an occupationally exposed person who is 27 years old.**
   A. 2700 mSv
   B. 270 mSv
   C. 27 mSv
   D. 2.7 mSv

3. **Biologic effects such as cataracts that result from exposure to ionizing radiation appear to have which of the following?**
   A. Circular dose-response threshold relationship
   B. Linear, nonthreshold dose pattern
   C. Sigmoid threshold dose-response curve
   D. Sigmoid nonthreshold dose-response relationship

4. **For radiation workers, such as medical imaging personnel, occupational risk may be equated with occupational risk in which of the following?**
   A. Other industries that are generally considered reasonably safe
   B. Somewhat hazardous industries
   C. Hazardous industries
   D. Extremely hazardous industries

5. **Revised estimates derived from recent reevaluations of dosimetric studies on the atomic bomb survivors of Hiroshima and Nagasaki indicate which of the following?**
   A. A decrease in the number of solid tumors in the survivor population
   B. An increase in the number of solid tumors in the survivor population
   C. That low-level radiation causes cancer
   D. That the risk of radiation-induced cancer is nonexistent

6. **When exposed to radiation as part of their educational experience, 18-year-old students should *not* exceed an effective dose limit of _____ annually.**
   A. 0.5 mSv (0.05 rem)
   B. 1 mSv (0.1 rem)
   C. 5 mSv (0.5 rem)
   D. 50 mSv (5 rem)

7. **Which of the following groups has provided sufficient evidence of the induction of stochastic effects in humans resulting from high radiation absorbed doses?**
   A. Japanese atomic bomb survivors
   B. General population of the United States
   C. Population of occupationally exposed radiographers in the United States
   D. The 2 million people living within 50 miles of the Three Mile Island nuclear power plant after the accident on March 28, 1979

8. **Responsibilities of a medical facility's radiation safety officer (RSO) include which of the following?**
   1. **Developing an appropriate radiation safety program**
   2. **Maintaining radiation monitoring records for all personnel**
   3. **Repairing all broken or defective imaging equipment**
   A. 1 and 2 only
   B. 1 and 3 only
   C. 2 and 3 only
   D. 1, 2, and 3

9. **To reduce exposure for pregnant female imaging professionals and control the exposure to the unborn during potentially sensitive periods of gestation, the NCRP now recommends a monthly equivalent dose limit not exceeding _____ per month to the embryo-fetus and a limit during the entire pregnancy not to exceed _____ after declaration of a pregnancy.**
   A. 0.5 mSv (0.05 rem), 5.0 mSv (0.50 rem)
   B. 5 mSv (0.5 rem), 7.0 mSv (0.70 rem)
   C. 150 mSv (15 rem), 300 mSv (30 rem)
   D. 250 mSv (25 rem), 500 mSv (50 rem)

10. **Which of the following is the annual occupational effective dose that applies to radiographers during routine operations?**
   A. 5 mSv (0.5 rem)
   B. 50 mSv (5 rem)
   C. 250 mSv (25 rem)
   D. 750 mSv (75 rem)

8 Protection of the Patient during Diagnostic X-Ray Procedures

Continued

CHAPTER OUTLINE

KEY TERMS

air gap technique
bone marrow dose
computed radiography (CR)
cumulative timer
digital radiography (DR)
entrance skin exposure (ESE)
entrance skin exposure rates
filtration
genetically significant dose
  (GSD)
gonadal dose

half-value layer (HVL)
high-level-control fluoroscopy
  (HLCF)
image matrix
off-focus, or stem, radiation
positive beam limitation (PBL)
primary protective barrier
quantum mottle
radiographic grid
rare-earth screens
scattered radiation

skin dose
source-to-image receptor
  distance (SID)
source-to-skin distance (SSD)
thermoluminescent dosimeters
  (TLDs)
useful beam (primary beam or
  umbra)
x-ray beam limitation devices

OBJECTIVES

After completing this chapter, the reader will be able to perform the following:

- Explain the meaning of a holistic approach to patient care and recognize the need for effective communication between imaging department personnel and the patient.
- Explain how voluntary motion can be eliminated or at least minimized and how involuntary motion can be compensated for during a diagnostic radiographic procedure.
- List the various x-ray beam-limiting devices and describe each.
- Explain the importance of luminance of the collimator light source, state the requirements for good coincidence between the radiographic beam and the localizing light beam when using a variable rectangular collimator, and explain the function of the collimator's positive beam limitation (PBL) feature.
- Explain the function of x-ray beam filtration in diagnostic radiology, list two types of filtration used to adequately filter the beam, describe half-value layer (HVL), and give examples of HVLs required for selective peak kilovoltages.
- Explain the need for protective shielding during diagnostic imaging procedures, state the reason for using gonadal shielding or other specific area shielding, and compare the various types of shields available for use.
- Explain the function of a compensating filter when radiographing a body part that varies in thickness and list two types of such filters.
- Discuss the need to use appropriate radiographic technical exposure factors for all radiologic procedures and explain how these factors may be adjusted to reduce patient dose.
- Explain how adequate immobilization, the use of high-speed screen-film combinations, and correct film processing techniques reduce radiographic exposure for the patient.
- Explain the way radiographic grids increase patient dose and compare the use of an air gap technique for certain examinations such as a cross-table lateral projection of the cervical spine with the use of a midratio grid (8:1).
- State the reason for reducing the number of repeat radiographs when film serves as the image receptor and describe the benefits of repeat analysis programs.
- Explain the way patient exposure may be reduced during routine fluoroscopic procedures, C-arm fluoroscopic procedures, high-dose (high-level-control [HLC]) fluoroscopy interventional procedures, cineradiographic procedures, and digital fluoroscopic procedures.

Continued

OBJECTIVES—cont'd

- Explain the process of digital radiography and computed radiography and discuss why it is imperative that patients having digital imaging procedures not be overexposed initially.
- List four ways to indicate the amount of radiation received by a patient from diagnostic imaging procedures and explain each.
- Discuss the value of mammography for the detection of breast cancer and state the maximum dose to the glandular tissue of a 4.5-cm compressed breast using a screen-film system.
- Compare the patient dose received from a succession of adjacent computed tomography (CT) scans with the patient dose received from an ordinary series of diagnostic radiographs of the adult cranium.
- Describe special precautions employed in radiography to protect the pregnant or potentially pregnant patient and explain the reason children require special radiation protection when undergoing diagnostic radiologic procedures.

During a diagnostic x-ray procedure, a holistic approach to patient care is essential. This means treating the whole person rather than just the area of concern. Holistic patient care must begin with effective communication between the radiographer and patient. *Effective communication* is "an interaction that produces a satisfying result through an exchange of information."[1] This type of dialogue alleviates the patient's uneasiness and increases the likelihood for cooperation and successful completion of the procedure. To take care of all patients appropriately, the reader should develop easily understandable communication skills.

Radiographers must limit the patient's exposure to ionizing radiation by employing appropriate radiation reduction techniques and by utilizing protective devices that minimize radiation exposure. Patient exposure can be substantially reduced by using proper body or part immobilization, motion reduction techniques, appropriate beam limitation devices and adequate filtration of the x-ray beam, and gonadal or other specific area shielding. Selection of suitable technical exposure factors used in conjunction with either high-speed film-screen combinations or computer-generated digital images, correct radiographic film processing techniques or appropriate digital image processing, and

the elimination of repeat radiographic exposures can also contribute significantly to limiting patient exposure. Hence, this chapter provides an overview of the tools and techniques that radiographers use to minimize the patient's exposure to radiation during diagnostic x-ray procedures.

EFFECTIVE COMMUNICATION

Verbal Messages and Body Language

When verbal messages and unconscious actions or body language, or nonverbal messages, are understood as intended, communication between the radiographer and patient is effective. Good communication encourages closeness, reduces anxiety and emotional stress, enhances the professional image of the radiographer as a person who cares about the patient's well-being, and increases the chance for successfully completing the x-ray examination. Everyone within the imaging department should always behave as compassionate professionals. Words and actions must demonstrate understanding and respect for human dignity and individuality.

Importance of Clear, Concise Instructions

Patient protection during a diagnostic x-ray procedure should begin with clear, concise instructions (Fig. 8-1). When patients understand the procedure and their responsibilities, they can more fully cooperate. When health care professionals do not thoroughly explain procedures, patients fear the unknown and become anxious, especially during lengthy examinations. To alleviate the problem, the radiographer must take adequate time to explain the procedure in simple terms that the patient can understand. Patients should also be given the opportunity to ask questions. The radiographer must listen attentively to these questions and answer them truthfully in an appropriate tone of voice

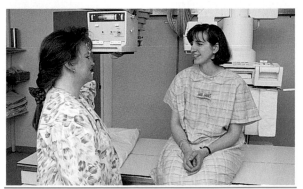

FIG. 8-1. Clear, concise instructions promote effective communication between the radiographer and the patient.

and in accordance with ethical guidelines. This creates a sense of trust between the patient and the radiographer and encourages further communication.

Appropriate Communication for Procedures That Will Cause Pain or Discomfort

If the radiographic procedure (e.g., angiocatheterization, or other study requiring an injection of a contrast medium [e.g., an intravenous urogram]) will cause pain, discomfort, or any strange sensations, the patient must be informed before the procedure begins (Fig. 8-2). However, to prevent the patient from imagining more pain or discomfort than the procedure will actually cause, the radiographer should try not to overemphasize this aspect of the examination.

Repeat Radiographic Exposures That Result from Poor Communication

Repeat radiographic exposures can sometimes be attributed to poor communication between the radiographer and the patient. Inadequate or misinterpreted instructions may prevent the patient from being able to cooperate. For example, during an interventional radiographic examination that creates some thermal discomfort, patients could move abruptly because they are surprised or want to inform the technologist or physician that something seems to be wrong. Such a movement usually results in a

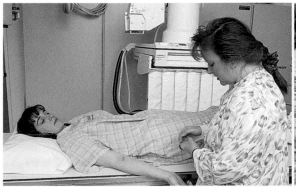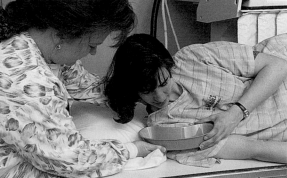

FIG. 8-2. Before the procedure begins, inform the patient of any pain, discomfort, or strange sensations that he or she will experience during the procedure.

repeat exposure. Effective communication between radiographer and patient will prevent this problem from occurring.

IMMOBILIZATION

Need for Patient Immobilization

If a patient moves during a radiographic exposure, the radiographic image will be blurred. Because blurred images have little or no diagnostic value, a repeat examination is necessary, although it results in additional radiation exposure for the patient. Proper body or part immobilization and the use of motion reduction techniques can eliminate or at least minimize patient motion.

Types of Patient Motion

Two types of patient motion exist: voluntary and involuntary. Motion controlled by will is classified as *voluntary motion*. When there is a lack of control, voluntary motion results. Lack of control may be attributed to the patient's age, breathing patterns or problems, general anxiety, physical or mental discomfort, excitability, fear of the examination or of an unfavorable prognosis, or mental instability. To eliminate voluntary patient movement during radiography, the radiographer must gain the cooperation of the patient or adequately immobilize that individual during the radiographic exposure (Fig. 8-3). A variety of suitable restraining devices are available to immobilize either the whole body or the individual body part to be radiographed. These radiographic aids should be used whenever necessary.

Involuntary motion, caused by muscle groups such as those associated with the digestive organs or the heart, cannot be willfully controlled. Other clinical manifestations such as chills, tremors, spasms, or pain also cause involuntary motion. Shortening the length of exposure time with an appropriate increase in milliamperes (mA) to maintain sufficient milliampere-seconds (mAs) for useful radiographic density and utilizing very high speed imaging receptors can compensate for this type of motion.

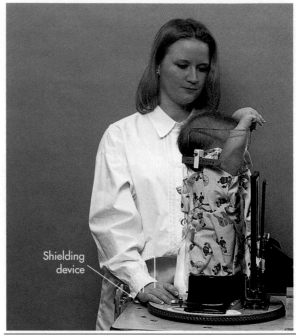

FIG. 8-3. Adequate immobilization during radiographic examinations eliminates or at least minimizes voluntary motion. This restraint has a shield *(left)* that may be adjusted to protect the child's reproductive organs from radiation exposure.

X-RAY BEAM LIMITATION DEVICES

Types of X-Ray Beam Limitation Devices

Basic **x-ray beam limitation devices** include aperture diaphragms, cones and cylinders, and collimators. These devices confine the **useful beam (primary beam or umbra)** before it enters the area of clinical interest, thereby limiting the quantity of body tissue irradiated. This also reduces the amount of **scattered radiation** in the tissue, preventing unnecessary exposure to tissues not under examination. Scattered radiation is all the radiation that arises from the interaction of an x-ray beam with the atoms of any object in the path of the beam.

Aperture Diaphragm

An aperture diaphragm is the simplest of all beam-limitation devices. It consists of a flat piece of lead with a hole of designated size and shape cut in its center. The dimensions of the hole determine the size and shape of the radiographic beam. Different film sizes and different source-to-image receptor distances require aperture diaphragms of various sizes to accommodate them. Diaphragm openings are rectangular, square, or round, with the rectangular shape being most common. Aperture diaphragms are used in trauma radiographic imaging systems, x-ray units designed specifically for chest radiography, and dental radiographic units.

Placed directly below the window of the x-ray tube, the aperture diaphragm confines the primary radiographic beam to dimensions suitable for covering a given size image receptor at a specified **source-to-image receptor distance (SID)** (i.e., the distance from the anode focal spot to the radiographic image receptor) (Fig. 8-4). Because an aperture diaphragm limits field size and thus the area of the body irradiated, the amount of scattered radiation produced decreases.

Cones

Flared Metal Tubes and Straight Cylinders

Radiographic cones are circular metal tubes that attach to the x-ray tube housing or variable rectangu-lar collimator to limit the x-ray beam to a predetermined size and shape. The design of this collimating device is simple, consisting of either a flared metal tube with the diameter of the upper end smaller than the diameter of the lower end, or a straight cylinder with the diameter the same at both the upper and lower ends (Fig. 8-5). Although the length and diameter of the cones vary, it is primarily the lower rim of the cone that governs beam limitation. Sharper size restriction is achieved when the cone or cylinder is longer. Field size at selected SIDs should be indicated on the cone.

Extension Cylinders Spot, or very small field, radiography is best accomplished through the use of extension cylinders, which are cylindrical metal tubes with a 10- to 20-inch metal extension at the far end of the barrel (Fig. 8-6). The use of this extension piece further limits the size of the useful beam.

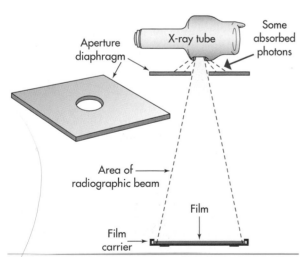

FIG. 8-4. An aperture diaphragm, a flat piece of lead with a hole of designated size and shape cut in its center, is placed directly below the window of the x-ray tube to confine the primary radiographic beam dimensions suitable to cover a given size of film at a specified source-to-image receptor distance.

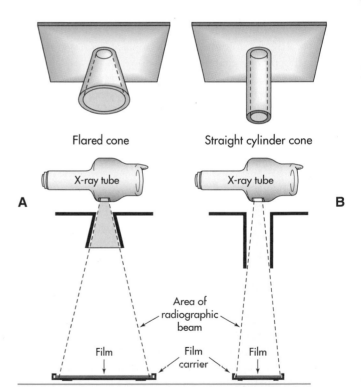

FIG. 8-5. Radiographic cones are circular metal tubes that attach to the x-ray tube housing or variable rectangular colli-mator to limit the radiographic beam to a predetermined size and shape. **A,** Cone fashioned in the form of a flared metal tube. **B,** Cone fashioned in the form of a straight cylinder.

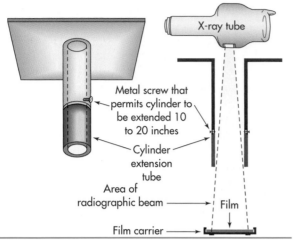

FIG. 8-6. Extension cylinder used for spot or very small field radiography.

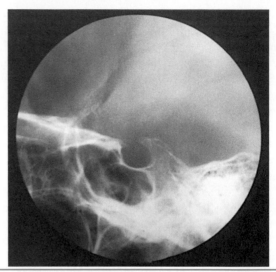

FIG. 8-7. Coned-down lateral projection of the sella turcica. (From Ballinger PW, Frank ED: *Merrill's atlas of radiographic positions and radiologic procedures,* ed 10, St Louis, 2003, Mosby.)

Light-Localizing Variable-Aperture Rectangular Collimators Light-localizing variable-aperture rectangular collimators have replaced cones for most radiographic examinations. However, cones are still sometimes used for radiographic examinations of the head (e.g., coned-down lateral projection of the sella turcica [Fig. 8-7] or projections of the paranasal sinuses [Fig. 8-8]), vertebral column, and chest.

Beam-Defining Cones Used in Dental Radiography Beam-defining cones are widely used in dental radiography. Because dental x-ray equipment is usually less bulky than general-purpose equipment, a one-piece beam limitation device, such as a cone made of plastic, is convenient. Some dental cones are lined with lead. By using lead-lined cones instead of the conventional plastic cones, dentists reduce patient exposure by eliminating the source of secondary radiation (the plastic cone itself).[2]

Collimators

Construction The collimator is the most versatile device for defining the size and shape of the radiographic beam. The light-localizing variable-aperture rectangular collimator (Fig. 8-9, A) is the type of collimator most often used with multipurpose x-ray units. It is box shaped and contains the radiographic beam-defining system (Fig. 8-9, B). This system consists of two sets of adjustable lead shutters mounted within the

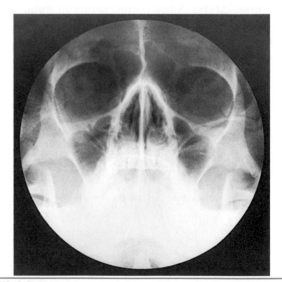

FIG. 8-8. Coned-down parietoacanthial projection of the maxillary sinuses. (From Ballinger PW, Frank ED: *Merrill's atlas of radiographic positions and radiologic procedures,* ed 10, St Louis, 2003, Mosby.)

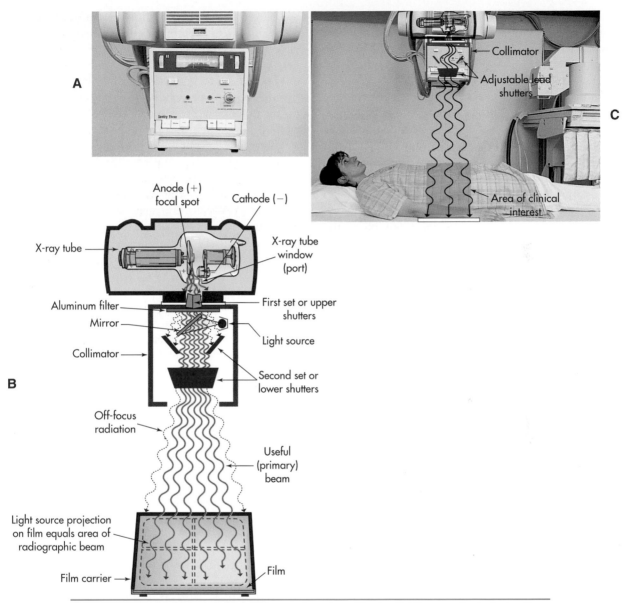

FIG. 8-9. **A,** Light-localizing variable-aperture rectangular collimator. **B,** Diagram of a typical collimator demonstrating radiographic beam-defining system: *1,* anode focal spot; *2,* x-ray tube window; *3,* first set or upper shutters; *4,* aluminum filter; *5,* mirror; *6,* light source; *7,* second set or lower shutters. The metal shutters collimate the radiographic beam so that it is no larger than the image receptor. **C,** Collimator containing the radiographic beam-defining system, which establishes the parameters (margins) of the beam. Adjustable lead shutters limit the cross-sectional area of the beam and confine it to the area of clinical interest.

device at different levels, a light source to illuminate the x-ray field and permit it to be centered over the area of clinical interest, and a mirror to deflect the light beam toward the object to be radiographed.

The first set of shutters, the upper shutters, are mounted as close as possible to the tube window to reduce the amount of **off-focus, or stem, radiation** (x-rays emitted from parts of the tube other than the focal spot), coming from the primary beam and exiting at various angles from the x-ray tube window. This radiation can never be completely eliminated because the metal shutters cannot be placed immediately beneath the actual focal spot of the x-ray tube, but placing the first set, or upper shutters, as close as possible to the tube window can reduce it significantly. This practice reduces patient exposure resulting from off-focus radiation.

The second set of collimator shutters, the lower shutters, are mounted below the level of the light source and mirror and function to confine further the radiographic beam to the area of clinical interest (Fig. 8-9, B and C). This set of shutters consists of two pairs of lead plates oriented at right angles to each other. Each set may be adjusted independently so that a variety of rectangular shapes can be selected. In this way the field is not limited to the circular or square shapes that sometimes irradiate areas of the patient not requiring imaging.

Skin Sparing To minimize skin exposure to electrons produced by photon interaction with the collimator, the patient's skin surface should be at least 15 cm below the collimator. Some collimator housings contain "spacer bars," which project down from the housing to prevent the collimators from being closer than 15 cm to the patient.

Luminance *Luminance* is a scientific term referring to the brightness of a surface. Specifically, luminance quantifies the intensity of a light source (i.e., the amount of light per unit area coming from its surface). Luminance is determined by measuring the concentration of light over a particular field of view. This may be understood by examining the units used to describe luminance. The primary unit is the candela per square meter, known more simply as the *nit*. One candela corresponds to 3.8 million billion photons per second being emitted from a light source through a conelike field of view. A good analogy is the sound intensity

emerging from a drill sergeant with a megaphone held to his lips. With appropriate dimensions, the megaphone's larger opening corresponds to the conelike field of view associated with the candela. Luminance of the collimator light source must be adequate to permit the localizing light beam to outline the margins of the radiographic beam adequately on the patient's anatomy. If the light field were not sufficiently bright, a radiographer might improperly position the x-ray field on a patient or at the very least have great difficulty accurately centering the x-ray beam, especially in the case of a dark-skinned patient. With insufficient brightness, the x-ray unit may fail a state inspection. The luminance must be high enough so that a calibrated light meter reading taken at a distance of 40 inches will be at least 15 "foot-candles" when averaged over the four quadrants of a 10-inch-by-10-inch field size. A foot-candle is approximately equivalent to 10.76 nit (the unit of luminance). Therefore, a distance of 15 foot-candles corresponds to a collimator light source with a luminance of about 161 nit or 161 candela per square meter. In summary, if the luminance of the collimator light source is adequate, the localizing light beam will adequately outline the margins of the radiographic beam on the area of interest on all patients.

Coincidence between the Radiographic Beam and the Localizing Light Beam Also when using a light-localizing variable aperture rectangular collimator, good coincidence (i.e., both physical size and alignment) between the radiographic beam and the localizing light beam is essential to eliminate collimator cutoff of the body structures being radiographed. Both alignment and length and width dimensions of the radiographic and light beams must correspond to within 2% of the SID. As an example, 40 inches, which is equal to 101.6 cm, is the most commonly used SID in radiography. At this SID, the maximal allowable difference in either length or width dimensions of the projected light field in relation to the radiographic beam at the level of the image receptor must be no more than 2% of 40 inches (0.8 inch) or 2% of 101.6 cm, or approximately 100 cm (2 cm).

Positive Beam Limitation (PBL) In the collimator system described earlier, the radiographer could inadvertently use an image receptor size much smaller than the size of the radiation field. Thus, areas of the patient would be irradiated that would not be recorded on the image receptor. Either the radiation field size should be smaller (if the additional anatomy is not of diagnostic interest) or the image receptor should be larger (if the anatomy is indeed of diagnostic interest). To prevent such a mismatch, radiographic collimators that are part of fixed radiographic equipment manufactured in the United States generally include a feature called **positive beam limitation (PBL).** The PBL feature consists of electronic sensors in the cassette holder that send signals to the collimator housing. When PBL is activated, the collimators are automatically adjusted so that the radiation field matches the size of the image receptor. If special conditions require the radiographer to have complete control of the system, the PBL feature may be deactivated by turning a key. However, in such a circumstance a warning light is automatically lit to indicate that the PBL system has been deactivated.

The PBL system illustrates an important principle of patient protection during radiographic procedures. The radiographer must ensure that collimation is adequate by *collimating the radiographic beam so that it is no larger than the image receptor* (Fig. 8-10, A-C). The regulatory standard requires an accuracy by 2% of the SID with PBL.

FILTRATION

Purpose of Radiographic Beam Filtration

Filtration of the radiographic beam reduces exposure to the patient's skin and superficial tissue by absorbing most of the lower-energy photons (long-wavelength or soft x-rays) from the heterogeneous beam (Fig. 8-11). This increases the mean energy, or "quality," of the x-ray beam. This change is also referred to as "hardening" the beam.

Effect of Filtration on the Absorbed Dose to the Patient

Because filtration absorbs some of the photons in a radiographic beam, it decreases the overall intensity (quantity or amount) of radiation. The remaining photons, however, are as a whole more penetrating and therefore less likely to be absorbed in body tissue. Hence, the absorbed dose to the patient decreases when the correct amount and type of filtration are placed in the path of the radiographic beam. If adequate filtration were not present, very-low-energy photons (20 keV or lower) would enter the patient and be almost totally absorbed in the body, increasing the patient's radiation dose but contributing nothing to the image process. They should be removed from the radiographic beam through the process of filtration. Filter material used for this purpose includes elements that are built in or added to the x-ray tube.

Types of Filtration

Two types of filtration are available:
1. Inherent filtration
2. Added filtration

Inherent filtration includes the glass envelope encasing the x-ray tube, the insulating oil surrounding the tube, and the glass window in the tube housing. This inherent material amounts to approximately 0.5-mm aluminum equivalent, meaning that the built-in material provides the same amount of filtration as a 0.5-mm thickness of aluminum. The light-localizing variable-aperture rectangular collimator provides an additional 1-mm aluminum equivalent. The reflective surface of the collimator mirror provides most of this aluminum equivalent.

Added filtration usually consists of sheets of aluminum (or the equivalent) of appropriate thickness. This additional filtration is located outside the glass window of the tube housing above the collimator shutters. It is readily accessible to service personnel and may be changed as the x-ray tube ages. The inherent and added filtration combine to equal the required amount of *total* filtration necessary to filter the useful beam adequately (Box 8-1).

BOX 8-1

Total Filtration

Total filtration= Inherent filtration plus added filtration

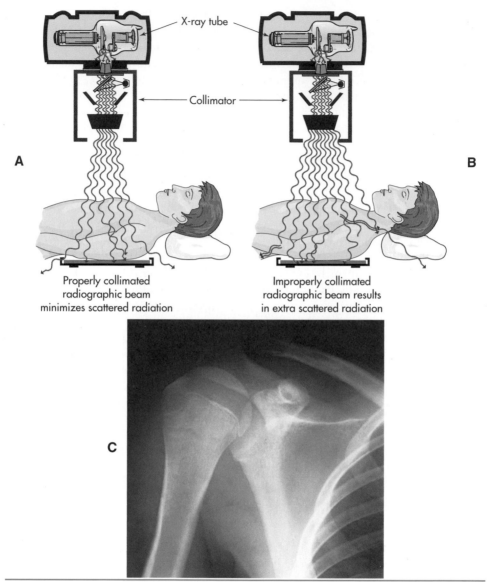

FIG. 8-10. Collimate the radiographic beam so that it is no larger than the image receptor. Limiting the beam to the area of clinical interest decreases the amount of tissue irradiated and minimizes patient exposure by reducing the amount of scattered and absorbed radiation. **A,** Good collimation. **B,** Poor collimation. **C,** AP radiograph of the shoulder demonstrating good collimation.

Requirement for Total Filtration

The peak kilovoltage of a given x-ray unit determines the total amount of filtration required. *Total filtration* of 2.5-mm aluminum equivalent for fixed x-ray units operating above 70 kVp is the regulatory standard (Fig.

8-12).[3] Because such fixed x-ray equipment comes from the manufacturer with inherent filtration of 0.5-mm aluminum equivalent, and because 1-mm aluminum equivalent is attributed to the collimator components, the manufacturer needs only to place an additional 1-mm aluminum equivalent filter between the tube housing and collimator to meet the requirement for minimum total filtration.

Stationary (fixed) radiographic equipment requires total filtration of 1.5-mm aluminum equivalent for x-ray units operating from 50 to 70 kVp, while fixed units operating below 50 kVp only require 0.5-mm aluminum equivalent.[3] Mobile diagnostic units and fluoroscopic equipment require a minimum of 2.5-mm aluminum equivalent total permanent filtration. A summary of required minimum total filtration may be found in Box 8-2.

Filtration for Mammographic Equipment

Appropriate filtration also is necessary for mammographic equipment, which produces photons with an energy range of 17 to 20 keV. Metallic elements such

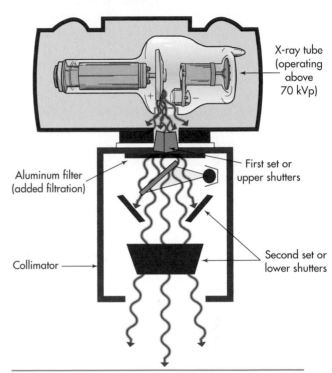

FIG. 8-12. A minimum of 2.5-mm aluminum equivalent total filtration is required for fixed radiographic units operating above 70 kVp.

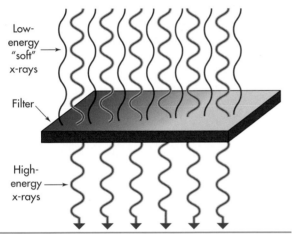

FIG. 8-11. Filtration removes low-energy photons (long-wavelength or "soft" x-rays) from the beam by absorbing them and permits higher energy photons to pass through. This reduces the amount of radiation that the patient receives.

BOX 8-2

Summary of Required Minimum Total Filtration

Stationary (Fixed) Radiographic Equipment

Tube Potential Minimum Total Filtration Required (kVp)	Minimum Total Filtration Required Specified in mm Al. Eq.*
Above 70	2.5 mm
50-70	1.5 mm
Below 50	0.5 mm

Mobile Diagnostic Units and Fluoroscopic Equipment

Mobile diagnostic units and fluoroscopic equipment require a minimum of 2.5 mm Al Eq. total permanent filtration.

*Modified from National Council on Radiation Protection and Measurements: *Medical x-ray, electron beam and gamma-ray protection for energies up to 50 MeV (equipment design, performance, and use)*. Report No. 102, Bethesda, Md, 1989, NCRP.

as molybdenum (Z = 42) and rhodium (Z = 45) are commonly employed as filters. When the x-ray tube target is made of molybdenum, either a 0.03-mm molybdenum filter or a 0.025-mm rhodium filter may be selected.[4] For rhodium x-ray tube targets, rhodium filters are used. These filtration materials facilitate adequate contrast in the radiographic image over the clinical extent of compressed breast thickness by preferentially selecting a particular range or window of energies from the x-ray spectrum emerging from the x-ray tube target. Molybdenum filters allow a lower energy window (17 to 20 keV) than rhodium filters (20 to 23 keV) (Fig. 8-13). Molybdenum filters are therefore suitable for small and average breast thickness, while rhodium filters are better for larger or dense breasts (i.e., compression thickness of 6 cm and

greater). The intelligent use of such materials has the effect of reducing the mean glandular dose in firm breast tissue. Maintaining and enhancing subject contrast is important in mammography. Beryllium (Z = 4) takes the place of glass in the window of the low-kVp-producing mammographic x-ray tube to accommodate this need. This light, strong metal permits the relatively soft characteristic radiation important for enhancing contrast to exit the tube without undergoing any significant attenuation.

Filtration for General Diagnostic Radiology

In general diagnostic radiology, aluminum (atomic number 13) is the metal most widely selected as a filter

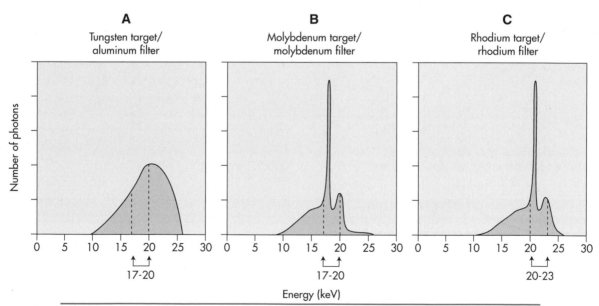

FIG. 8-13. A and **B,** X-ray emission spectrums for tungsten and molybdenum anodes. Note that tungsten produces a high volume of x-ray photons above the 17- to 20-keV range considered ideal for mammography. These photons merely degrade the quality of the recorded image. The molybdenum anode produces few x-ray photons above the ideal energy range, initiating a higher contrast image on the finished radiograph. **C,** A rhodium anode produces a higher average energy x-ray beam than does the molybdenum anode. The energy range for rhodium-produced photons is 20 to 23 keV. Photons from this energy range provide better penetration of larger, denser breasts. (From Ballinger PW, Frank ED: *Merrill's atlas of radiographic positions and radiologic procedures,* ed 9, St Louis, 1999, Mosby.)

material because it effectively removes low-energy (soft) x-rays from a polyenergetic (heterogeneous) x-ray beam without severely decreasing the x-ray beam intensity. Also, aluminum is lightweight, sturdy, relatively inexpensive, and readily available. In compliance with the Radiation Control for Health and Safety Act of 1968, a diagnostic x-ray beam must always be adequately filtered. This means that a sufficient quantity of low-energy photons has been removed from a beam produced at a given peak kilovoltage. The **half-value layer (HVL)** of the beam must be measured to verify this. HVL may be defined as the thickness of a designated absorber (customarily a metal such as aluminum) required to decrease the intensity (quantity or amount) of the primary beam by 50% of its initial value. A radiologic physicist should obtain this measurement at least once a year and also after an x-ray tube is replaced or repairs have been made on the diagnostic x-ray tube housing or collimation system. For diagnostic x-ray beams, the HVL is expressed in millimeters of aluminum. Because HVL is a measure of beam quality or effective energy of the x-ray beam, a certain minimal HVL is required at a given peak kilovoltage. Examples of required HVLs for selected peak kilovoltages are listed in Table 8-1.

TABLE 8-1

HVL Required by the Radiation Control for Health and Safety Act of 1968 and Detailed by the Bureau of Radiological Health* in 1980

Peak Kilovoltage	Minimum Required HVL in Millimeters of Aluminum
30	0.3
40	0.4
50	1.2
60	1.3
70	1.5
80	2.3
90	2.5
100	2.7
110	3.0
120	3.2

*The Bureau of Radiological Health changed its name to the Center for Devices and Radiological Health in 1982.

PROTECTIVE SHIELDING

Need for Protective Shielding

The potential for radiation exposure to radiosensitive body organs or tissues requires the use of protective shielding (a structure or device made of certain materials such as concrete, lead, or lead-impregnated material that will adequately attenuate ionizing radiation) to reduce or eliminate a radiation dose that would otherwise result in biologic damage. The lens of the eye, the breasts, and the reproductive organs should be shielded from the useful beam whenever possible. These areas may be selectively shielded through the use of specific area shielding, which is the use of lead or lead-impregnated material to protect selected body areas (e.g., reproductive organs) from exposure to ionizing radiation.

Gonadal Shielding

Use of Gonadal Shielding Devices

Gonadal shielding devices are used during diagnostic x-ray procedures to protect the reproductive organs from exposure to the useful beam when they are in or within approximately 5 cm of a properly collimated beam. Gonadal shielding is used unless it will compromise the diagnostic value of the examination. Gonadal shielding should be a secondary protective measure, not a substitute for an adequately collimated beam. Adequate collimation of the radiographic beam to include only the anatomy of interest (Fig. 8-14, A and B) must always be the first step in gonadal protection.

Dose Reduction from the Use of Gonadal Shielding for Females and Males

As a consequence of their anatomic location, the female reproductive organs receive about three times more exposure during a given radiographic procedure involving the pelvic region than do the male reproductive organs. However, gonadal exposure for both men and women may be greatly reduced through the application of appropriate shielding. For female patients, the use of a flat contact shield (containing 1 mm of lead) placed over the reproductive organs reduces exposure by about 50% (Fig. 8-15, A). Primary

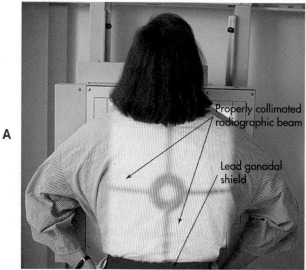

A

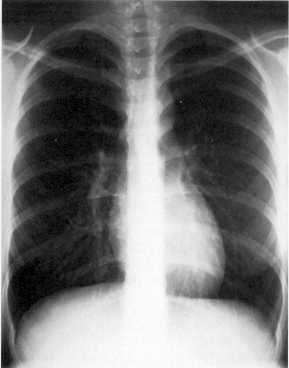

B

FIG. 8-14. **A,** Adequate and precise collimation of the radiographic beam must always be the first step in gonadal protection. **B,** When the gonads are not in the area of clinical interest, precise collimation of the radiographic beam reduces gonadal exposure.

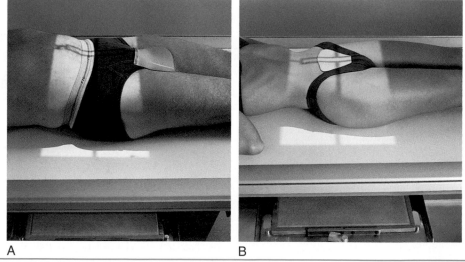

A   B

FIG. 8-15. **A,** Contact shield correctly placed over the reproductive organs of a female patient. **B,** Contact shield correctly placed over the reproductive organs of a male patient. (From Ballinger PW, Frank ED: *Merrill's atlas of radiographic positions and radiologic procedures,* ed 10, St Louis, 2003, Mosby.)

beam exposure for male patients may be reduced as much as 90% to 95% when the gonads are covered with a contact shield (also containing 1 mm of lead) (Fig. 8-15, B). Gonadal shielding should always be used whenever it will not obscure necessary clinical information. Every imaging department should establish a written shielding protocol for each of its radiologic procedures. This reduces the cumulative population gonad dose.

Placement of Gonadal Shielding Devices

When a gonadal shield is used during a radiographic exposure, it must be correctly placed directly over the patient's reproductive organs to provide protection, as shown in Fig. 8-15, A and B. External anatomical landmarks on the patient can be used to guide placement of a testicular or ovarian shield. For example, when a male patient is in the supine position, the symphysis pubis can be used to guide shield placement over the testes. For protection of the ovaries of a female patient, the shield should be placed approximately 1 inch medial to each palpable anterior superior iliac spine. If gonadal shields are not placed correctly, the reproductive organs will not be protected. Furthermore, if not placed correctly, the shield can obscure anatomical structures that may need to be included in the image. The loss of this essential anatomic information in the image can result in a repeat projection. If the projection is repeated, patient dose will increase as a consequence. For this reason gonadal shields must be correctly placed over the patient's reproductive organs before any exposure is made.

Types of Gonadal Shielding Devices

The following four basic types of gonadal shielding devices are used:
1. Flat contact shields
2. Shadow shields
3. Shaped contact shields
4. Clear lead

Flat Contact Shields Flat contact shields are made of lead strips or lead-impregnated materials. These shields may be placed directly over the patient's reproductive organs (Fig. 8-16) or secured to the patient with tape. These shields are most effective when used as protective devices for patients having anteroposte-

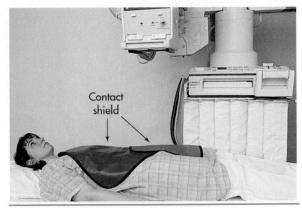

FIG. 8-16. An uncontoured, flat contact shield of lead-impregnated material may be placed over the patient's gonads to provide protection from x-radiation during a radiographic procedure.

rior (AP) or posteroanterior (PA) radiographs while in a recumbent position. Flat contact shields are not suited for nonrecumbent positions or projections other than AP or PA. If the flat contact shield is used during a fluoroscopic examination, it must be placed under the patient to be effective because the x-ray tube is located under the radiographic table.

Shadow Shields Shadow shields (Fig. 8-17, A) are made of a radiopaque material. Suspended from above the radiographic beam-defining system, these shields hang over the area of clinical interest to cast a shadow in the primary beam over the patient's reproductive organs (Fig. 8-17, B and C). The clear lead filter illustrated in Fig. 8-18 functions as a shadow shield and is used to shield breasts and gonads. The beam-defining light casts the shadow of the shield over the anatomy. The beam-defining light must be accurately positioned to ensure correct placement of the shadow shield. When the shield is correctly positioned, it provides protection from the radiographic beam as efficiently as does the contact shield. If the shield is not correctly positioned, a repeat examination may be necessary, resulting in an additional radiation exposure that will increase patient dose. The shadow shield is not suitable for use during fluoroscopy because no localizing light field exists and the field of view is usually moved about during a study. However, the shadow shield can be used effectively to provide gonadal protection in a sterile field or when examining incapacitated patients.

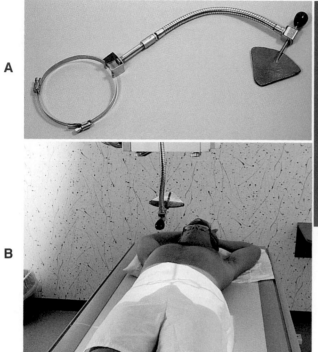

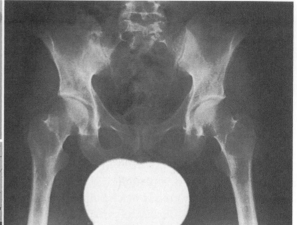

FIG. 8-17. **A,** Shadow shield components. **B,** A shadow shield suspended above the radiographic beam-defining system casts a shadow over the protected body area, the gonads. **C,** The radiographic image demonstrates effective gonadal shielding resulting from the use of a shadow shield. (Courtesy Fluke Biomedical.)

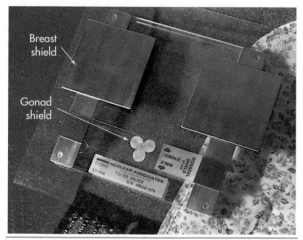

FIG. 8-18. Lead filter with breast and gonad shielding device. This shield functions as a shadow shield. (Courtesy Fluke Biomedical.)

Shadow shields have the advantage of reducing patient embarrassment by generally eliminating the need for the radiographer to palpate the patient's anatomy in the area of the reproductive organs before placing the shield in the appropriate position.

Shaped Contact Shields Shaped contact shields are made of radiopaque material contoured to enclose the male reproductive organs. Disposable or washable athletic supporters or jockey-style briefs function as carriers for these shields. The carriers each contain a pouch into which the shield is placed (Fig. 8-19). The cuplike shape of the shield permits it to be placed comfortably over the scrotum and penis whether the patient is in a recumbent or a nonrecumbent position. To ensure privacy and reduce embarrassment, the patient can don the garment containing the shield in the confines of the dressing room.

Because the carrier securely holds the shaped contact shield in place, AP, oblique, and lateral pro-

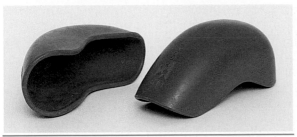

FIG. 8-19. Shaped-contact shields (cuplike in shape) may be held in place with a suitable carrier.

jections may be obtained with maximal gonadal protection. This shield is also suitable for use during fluoroscopic examinations. Shaped contact shields are not recommended for PA projections because the shield covers the anterior surface of the reproductive organs and the x-ray beam enters from the posterior surface; therefore, the shield does not protect the gonads.

Clear Lead Shields   Some of the basic gonadal shielding devices such as the previously described shaped contact shield and first-generation shadow shield are being replaced by clear lead gonad and breast shielding (see Fig. 8-18). These shields are made of transparent lead-plastic material impregnated with approximately 30% lead by weight. Examples of gonad and breast shielding are provided in Fig. 8-20, which demonstrates a full-spinal scoliosis examination. Along with the clear lead gonad and breast shields, a lightweight, fully transparent clear lead filter is incorporated to provide uniform density throughout the spinal canal (Fig. 8-20, A).

Specific Area Shielding

Need for Specific Area Shielding

Radiosensitive organs and tissues other than the reproductive organs may be selectively shielded from the primary beam during a diagnostic radiographic examination. Contact lens shields for the lens of the eye can reduce or eliminate exposure to that highly sensitive area. Particularly sensitive breast tissue may be shielded by using a clear lead shadow shield (see Fig. 8-18). This shielding is of vital importance in providing protection during juvenile scoliosis examina-

tions. Radiation dose to the breast of a young patient may be further reduced by performing the scoliosis examination with the radiographic beam entering the posterior surface of the patient's body instead of the anterior surface. The use of the PA projection results in a lower radiation dose to the anterior body surface, thereby significantly reducing the dose to the patient's breasts.

Benefit of Specific Area Shielding

In summary, effective shielding programs can be established in any health care facility by providing the appropriate shields. Patients with the potential to reproduce should be shielded during x-ray procedures whenever the diagnostic value of the examination is not compromised. This action minimizes the number of potentially deleterious x-ray–induced mutations expressed in future generations. Specific area shielding for selected body areas other than the gonads significantly reduces radiation exposure to those areas and should be used whenever possible.

COMPENSATING FILTERS

Dose reduction and uniform radiographic imaging of body parts that vary considerably in thickness or tissue composition may be accomplished by use of compensating filters constructed of aluminum, lead-acrylic, or other suitable materials. These devices partially attenuate x-rays that are directed toward the thinner, or less dense, area while permitting more x-radiation to strike the thicker, or more dense, area. For example, the *wedge filter* (Fig. 8-21) may be used to provide uniform density when radiographing the foot in the dorsoplantar projection. For this examination, the wedge is attached to the lower rim of the collimator and positioned with its thickest part toward the toes and its thinnest toward the heel. The *trough*, or *bilateral wedge, filter*, which is used in some dedicated chest radiographic units, is another example of a compensating filter. This filter is thin in the center to permit adequate x-ray penetration of the mediastinum and thick laterally to reduce exposure to the aerated lungs. With this device, a radiographic image with uniform average density is obtained.

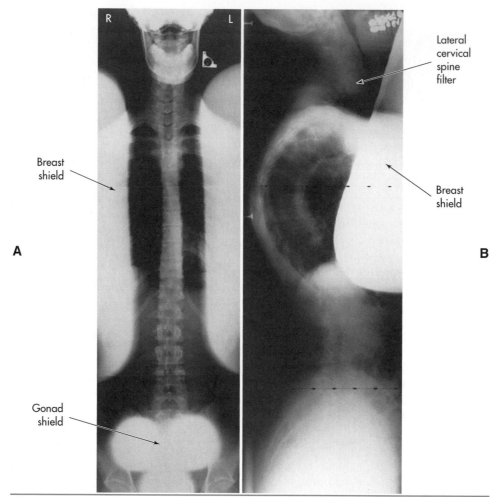

FIG. 8-20. A, AP radiograph of a full-spine scoliosis examination demonstrating lead filter with breast and gonad shields. **B,** Lateral radiograph of full-spine scoliosis examination with lateral cervical filter and breast shield. (Courtesy Fluke Biomedical.)

TECHNICAL EXPOSURE FACTORS

Selection of Appropriate Technical Exposure Factors

Selection of appropriate technical exposure factors for each x-ray examination is essential to ensure a diagnostic image with minimal patient dose. The technique chosen must ensure sufficient penetration of the area of clinical interest, adequate radiographic density

(exposure), and an adequate amount of radiographic contrast between adjacent tissue densities. The appropriate technical factors are determined by considerations such as those listed in Box 8-3.

Use of Standardized Technique Charts

To ensure uniform selection of technical x-ray exposure factors, efficient imaging departments use standardized technique charts for each x-ray unit. The

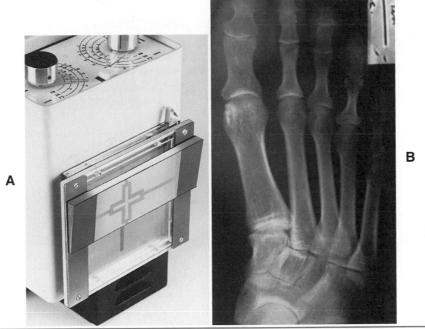

FIG. 8-21. **A,** Wedge-shaped lead-acrylic compensating filter used to provide uniform density for **(B)** a dorsoplantar projection of the foot.

BOX 8-3

Technical Exposure Factor Considerations

1. Mass per unit volume of tissue of the area of clinical interest
2. Effective atomic numbers and electron densities of the tissues involved
3. Film-screen combination or other type of image receptor
4. Source-to-image distance (SID)
5. Type and quantity of filtration employed
6. Type of x-ray generator used (single phase, three phase, or high frequency)
7. Balance of radiographic density and contrast required

radiographer is responsible for consulting this chart before making each radiographic exposure to ensure a diagnostic image with minimal patient dose. Neglecting to use standardized technique charts necessitates estimating the technical exposure factors, which may result in poor quality images, repeat examinations, and additional, unnecessary exposure for the patient.

Use of High kVp and Low mAs Exposure Factors to Reduce Dose to the Patient

Technical exposure factors that minimize the radiation dose to the patient should be selected whenever possible. The use of higher kilovoltage (kVp) and lower milliamperage and exposure time in seconds (mAs)* reduces patient dose (Fig. 8-22, A and B). However, this technical exposure factor combination produces a poorer quality image. As kVp increases and mAs decreases, radiographic contrast is reduced. Consequently, the amount of diagnostically useful information in the recorded image is reduced. The radiographer must achieve a balance in

---

*Milliampere seconds (mAs) is the product of x-ray electron tube current and the amount of time in seconds that the x-ray beam is on.

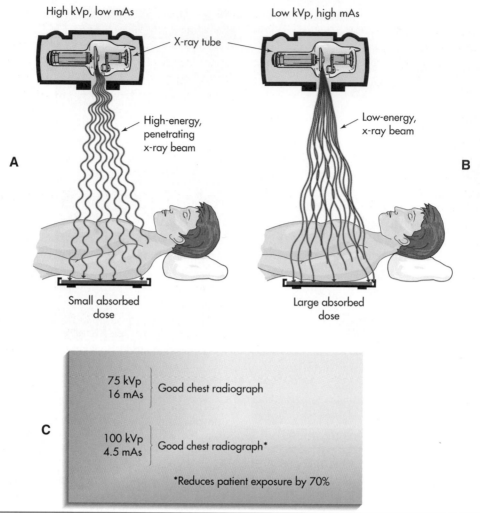

FIG. 8-22. The use of higher kilovoltage (kVp) and lower milliamperage and exposure time in seconds (mAs) reduces patient dose. **A,** The use of high kVp and low mAs results in a high-energy, penetrating x-ray beam and a small patient absorbed dose. **B,** The use of low kVp and high mAs results in a low-energy x-ray beam, the majority of which the patient will easily absorb. **C,** Example of a higher-kVp, lower-mAs technique resulting in a 70% reduction in patient exposure without significantly compromising radiographic quality.

technical radiographic exposure factors to ensure the presence of adequate information in the recorded image and minimize patient dose. To achieve this balance, the radiographer must select the highest practical kVp and the lowest mAs that will yield sufficient information for each radiographic examination (Fig. 8-22, C).

RADIOGRAPHIC FILM PROCESSING

Need for Correct Radiographic Film Processing

When screen-film image receptor systems are used, correct radiographic film processing enhances image quality by making diagnostic information visible on the finished radiograph. Poorly processed radiographs offer inadequate diagnostic information, leading to repeat examinations and unnecessary patient exposure.

Quality Control Program

To ensure standardization in film-processing techniques, it is absolutely essential that every imaging department establish a *quality control program* that includes monitoring and maintenance of all processors in the facility. Such a program ensures the production of quality diagnostic radiographs. A number of excellent reviews have been written on this subject. These reviews include step-by-step procedures for performance, monitoring, and quality control.[5-8]

SCREEN-FILM COMBINATIONS

Value of Intensifying Screens in Patient Dose Reduction

X-ray film, most of which is double-emulsion x-ray film (i.e., emulsion coated on both sides of the film), responds strongly to the light emitted by intensifying screens. Intensifying screens enhance the action of x-rays on film by converting x-ray energy into visible light. About 95% of the radiographic density of the recorded image results from the visible light photons emitted by the intensifying screens. Because a single x-ray photon can produce 80 to 95 light photons, this conversion drastically enhances the film exposure process and permits radiographic exposure time to be substantially reduced. This leads to a sizable reduction in patient dose. At the time of this writing, when screen-film image receptors are used, intensifying screens used in conjunction with matching radiographic film are predominantly **rare-earth screens.** These screens are made with rare-earth phosphors, namely, gadolinium, lanthanum, and yttrium. The rare-earth elements used in these screens have high atomic numbers ranging from 57 to 71. Consequently, because they have high atomic numbers, the screens facilitate higher x-ray absorption of the incident x-ray

beam. Therefore, they can convert the x-ray energy to light more efficiently (by 15% to 20%). Rare-earth screens are noticeably faster than the calcium tungstate screens that were used until the 1970s. Rare-earth screens also place less thermal stress on the x-ray tube, increasing its life span. In addition, when rare-earth screens are used, radiation shielding requirements for the x-ray room are decreased because a general reduction of x-radiation in the environment occurs.

Effect of Faster Screen-Film Systems on Patient Dose

To reiterate, film speed and the use of intensifying screens significantly influence radiographic exposure time. While rare-earth screens and matching film combinations with relative speeds from 200 to 1200 are available, 400-speed systems are considered standard for general radiography at the time of this writing. When the speed of screen-film systems doubles, for example when changing from a 200-speed system to a 400-speed system, patient radiation exposure is reduced by approximately 50%. When the amount of silver halide crystals (approximately 95% of which are silver bromide) contained in radiographic film emulsion is increased, the speed of the film is increased. This means that less radiation is required to obtain an image. As radiographic exposure decreases, patient dose decreases. One manufacturer has developed an 800-speed medical film that can be used with regular intensifying screens. The use of such a film can reduce the patient's radiation exposure by as much as 50%.[9]

It is essential that screen-film systems be matched correctly. If they are not correctly matched or compatible, patient dose can increase.

Effect of Kilovoltage on Screen Speed and Patient Dose

Kilovoltage also affects screen speed. As kilovoltage increases, screen speed increases, which reduces the patient dose. The selection of peak kilovoltage and the screen-film combination are two of the most important technical considerations in the amount of patient dose.

Selection of Film-Based Image Receptor Systems

Although the use of high-speed film-screen image receptor systems with calcium tungstate intensifying screens that were used until the 1970s significantly reduced patient dose, a loss of radiographic quality was also possible because the recorded image may have had poorer resolution. As a result, the use of these image receptor systems was not practical for all radiography. When compared with slower speed rare-earth film-screen image receptor systems, faster speed rare-earth film-screen image receptor systems can demonstrate an effect referred to as **quantum mottle.** These faint blotches (image noise) can degrade the radiographic image and be annoying to the radiologist interpreting the image. Therefore, higher speed rare-earth systems may not be suitable for all radiography either. To be able to select the appropriate film-based image receptor system for a given radiographic examination, the radiographer must be aware of the capabilities and limitations of the different systems available. Manufacturers or distributors supply product information about these various film-based image receptor systems, which can be obtained by contacting the appropriate source.

Summary of Benefits of Rare-Earth Intensifying Screens

As mentioned previously, rare-earth intensifying screens are more efficient than calcium tungstate intensifying screens in converting x-ray energy into light photons. Made of rare-earth phosphors, namely, gadolinium, lanthanum, or yttrium, these screens absorb approximately five times more x-ray energy than the previously used calcium tungstate screens; hence, they emit considerably more light. This significantly reduces the radiographic exposure required to obtain an image of acceptable quality. An additional benefit of rare-earth screens is that high resolution (the ability of a system to make two adjacent objects visually distinguishable) of the recorded image remains constant. This ensures radiographic quality. Higher-speed rare-earth systems do, however, produce quantum mottle (faint blotches) in the recorded image, causing some degradation of the image. Therefore, they may not be suitable for all radiography.

X-ray tube life span is increased because rare-earth screens place less thermal stress on the tube. Also, since x-radiation in the environment is reduced when rare-earth screens are used, radiation shielding requirements for the room decrease.

Use of Carbon Fiber as a Front Material in a Radiographic Cassette

The use of carbon fiber as a front material in a cassette that holds radiographic film and intensifying screens is a recent technologic advancement. When compared with the traditional material in the front of a cassette (aluminum or cardboard), the cassette front containing the carbon fiber absorbs approximately half as much radiation. This lowers the patient dose, because lower radiographic techniques are required to produce the recorded image. In addition, since lower radiographic techniques are employed when using cassettes with carbon fiber front material, the life of the x-ray tube may also be prolonged.

Use of Asymmetric Film Emulsion and Intensifying Screen Combinations

Another recent technologic advancement is the use of asymmetric film emulsion and intensifying screen combinations. With this system, the front screen and film emulsion (the side that faces the x-ray tube) is slower than the back screen and film emulsion, which contains a faster system. This screen-film combination results in a recorded image with greater uniformity and a decrease in patient exposure.

RADIOGRAPHIC GRIDS

Construction, Purpose, Technical Value, and Impact of a Radiographic Grid on Patient Dose

A **radiographic grid** (Fig. 8-23) is a device made of parallel radiopaque strips alternated with low-attenuation strips of aluminum, plastic, or wood. It is placed between the patient and the radiographic image receptor to remove scattered x-ray photons that emerge from the patient before they reach the film or other

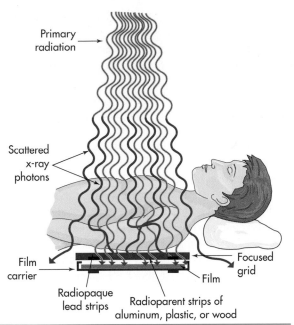

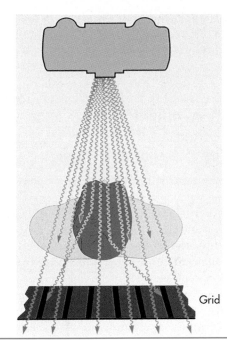

FIG. 8-23. Radiographic grids remove scattered x-ray photons that emerge from the object being radiographed before this scattered radiation reaches the image receptor and decreases radiographic quality.

FIG. 8-24. The radiographic grid acts as a sieve to block the passage of photons that have been scattered at some angle from their original path. (From *Mosby's radiographic instructional series: radiobiology and radiation protection,* St Louis, 1999, Mosby.)

image receptor. This significantly improves radiographic contrast and visibility of detail. Generally, this device is used when the thickness of the body part to be radiographed is greater than 10 cm. Although the use of a grid increases patient dose, the benefit obtained in terms of the improved quality of the recorded image, making available a greater quantity of diagnostic information, is a fair compromise. Because several different types of grids are available, care must be taken to ensure that the correct type is used for a particular examination, or else a repeat may be necessary, which would negate the benefit of increased image quality.

Summarizing the Function of a Radiographic Grid

To summarize, when x-rays pass through an object, some of the photons are scattered away from their original path as a result of coherent and Compton scattering processes. Radiographic quality is highest when

these scattered photons are not recorded on the image. If scattered photons are recorded, a general darkening of the image occurs, which detracts from the viewer's ability to distinguish between the different structures of the object being radiographed. Thus, only those photons that have passed through matter with no deviation from their original path should be recorded. To minimize the influence of scattered photons, a grid is inserted between the patient and the image receptor. It is designed to act as a sieve to block the passage of photons that have been scattered at some angle from their original path (Fig. 8-24).

Grid Ratio and Patient Dose

As previously noted, grids are made of parallel radiopaque lead strips alternated with low-attenuation strips of aluminum, plastic, or wood. Because some fraction of the image receptor is covered with lead, mAs must be increased to compensate for the use of the grid. Hence, patient dose increases whenever a grid is used, and because more lead is contained in higher ratio grids (e.g., 16:1), patient dose increases as grid ratio increases.

AIR GAP TECHNIQUE

Reduction of Scattered Radiation

The **air gap technique** is an alternative procedure to the use of a radiographic grid for reducing scattered radiation during certain examinations (e.g., cross-table lateral projection of the cervical spine, areas of chest radiography, and selected special procedures such as cerebral angiography in which some degree of magnification is acceptable). This technique removes scatter radiation by using an increased object-to-image receptor distance (OID). If magnification is not desired, a complementary increase in SID may be made. To perform an air gap technique, the image receptor is placed 6 to 10 inches from the patient while the x-ray tube is placed approximately 10 to 12 feet away from

the image receptor. The scattered x-rays produced in the patient (the source of the scatter) are disseminated in many directions at acute angles to the primary beam when the radiographic exposure is made. Because of this and the increased distance between the anatomy being imaged and the image receptor, a higher percentage of the scattered x-rays produced are then less likely to strike the image receptor (Fig. 8-25). This air gap method results in an adequate grid-type scatter cleanup effect. In general, the use of an air gap technique requires the selection of technical exposure factors that are comparable to those used with an 8:1 ratio grid. Therefore, when patient dose is compared with a nongrid technique, it is higher. When compared with the patient dose resulting from the use of a midratio grid (8:1), the dose from an air gap technique is about the same as with the midratio grid.

High-kVp Radiography

In high-kVp radiography that employs kVps of 90 or above, air gap techniques are for the most part inef-

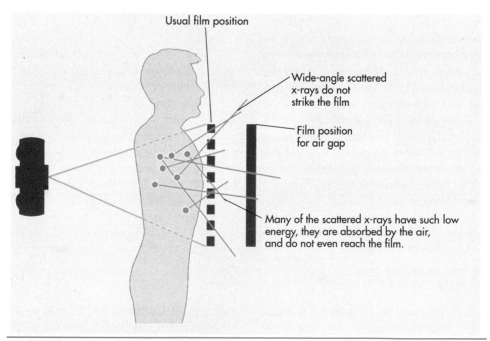

FIG. 8-25. The air gap technique. (From *Mosby's radiographic instructional series: radiobiology and radiation protection,* St Louis, 1999, Mosby.)

fective. However, some facilities that perform chest radiography using peak kilovoltages between 120 and 140 do successfully use air gap techniques. When scattered x-rays are directed more in a side-to-side fashion such as those produced at less than 90 kVp, air gap techniques are more efficient.

REPEAT RADIOGRAPHS WHEN FILM SERVES AS THE IMAGE RECEPTOR

Consequence of Repeat Radiographs

The *repeat radiograph* refers to any radiograph that must be performed more than once because of human or mechanical error during the production of the initial radiograph. This additional exposure increases patient dose. The patient's skin and possibly the gonads receive a "double dose" whenever a repeat examination occurs. For this reason, repeat radiographs must be minimized. An occasional repeat radiograph is permissible when recommended by the radiologist for the purpose of obtaining additional diagnostic information. However, repeat exposures resulting from carelessness or poor judgment on the part of the radiographer must be eliminated. The radiographer must correctly position the patient and select the appropriate technical radiographic exposure factors that will ensure the production of optimal images for each initial examination.

Benefit of a Repeat Analysis Program

Health care facilities using radiographic film can benefit significantly by implementing and maintaining a *repeat analysis program*. By determining the number of repeats and the reasons for producing unacceptable radiographs, existing problems and conditions in an imaging department will be identified. Many categories may be established for discarded radiographs. These categories are listed in Box 8-4.

The benefits of an aggressive repeat analysis program in an imaging department are listed in Box 8-5. In addition to these benefits, the program should reduce an imaging department's film volume. A quality control radiographer or other designated person reviews discarded radiographs with co-workers

---

BOX 8-4

Categories for Discarded Radiographs

1. Radiographs too dark or too light because of inappropriate selection of technical exposure factors
2. Incorrect patient positioning
3. Incorrect centering of the radiographic beam
4. Patient motion during the radiographic exposure
5. Improper collimation of the radiographic beam
6. Presence of external foreign bodies
7. Processing artifacts

BOX 8-5

Benefits of a Repeat Analysis Program

1. The program increases awareness among staff and student radiographers of the need to produce optimal quality recorded images.
2. Radiographers generally become more careful in producing their radiographic images because they are aware that the images are being reviewed.
3. When the repeat analysis program identifies problems or concerns, in-service education programs covering these specific topics may be designed for imaging personnel.

---

to point out the causes of various repeats. At the very least, this practice should lead to an improvement in technical skills.

UNNECESSARY RADIOLOGIC PROCEDURES

Benefit versus Risk

As discussed in Chapter 1, the responsibility for ordering a radiologic examination lies with the referring physician. In making this decision, the physician must determine whether the benefit to the patient in terms of medical information gained sufficiently justifies subjecting the patient to the risk of the absorbed radiation resulting from the procedure.

Nonessential Radiologic Examinations

Some radiographic examinations are performed in the absence of definite medical indications. This unnecessarily exposes the patient to radiation because there is virtually no benefit for the patient in terms of useful information gained from the procedure. Examples of nonessential radiologic examinations are described in Box 8-6.

MINIMAL SOURCE-SKIN DISTANCE (SSD) FOR MOBILE RADIOGRAPHY

Requirement

Mobile radiographic units require special precautions to ensure patient safety. When operating the unit, the radiographer must use a source-skin distance (SSD) of

at least 12 inches (30 cm) (Fig. 8-26). The 12-inch distance limits the effects of the inverse square falloff of radiation intensity with distance. This falloff is more pronounced the shorter the SSD. In practice, longer distances (e.g., 40 inches from x-ray source to image receptor) are generally used.

Effect of SSD on Patient Entrance Exposure

When the SSD is small, patient entrance exposure is significantly greater than exit exposure. By increasing SSD, the radiographer maintains a more uniform distribution of exposure throughout the patient.

Use of Mobile Units

Mobile (portable) units should be used to perform radiographic procedures only on patients who cannot be transported to a fixed radiographic installation (an

---

BOX 8-6

Unnecessary Radiologic Procedures

1. A chest x-ray examination on scheduled admission to the hospital. This examination should not be performed without clinical indications of chest disease or another important concern that justifies exposing the patient to ionizing radiation. This includes presurgical patients. A panel of physicians appointed by the Food and Drug Administration (FDA)[10] concluded that a chest x-ray examination is not necessary for every presurgical patient. Patients admitted for treatment of pulmonary problems or diseases, however, may benefit from a preadmission chest x-ray examination.
2. A chest x-ray examination as part of a preemployment physical. Very little information about previous illness or injury can be gained through this examination, and it is unlikely to be useful to the employer.
3. Lumbar spine examinations as part of a preemployment physical. As with the preemployment chest x-ray examination, this examination provides very little information about previous illness or injury that would be useful to an employer.
4. Chest x-rays or other unjustified x-ray examinations as part of a routine health checkup. Radiologic procedures should not be performed unless a

patient exhibits symptoms that merit radiologic investigation.
5. Chest x-ray examination for mass screening for tuberculosis (TB). Such examinations are of little value for most people. Testing for TB may be done with more efficient procedures. However, Bushong indicates that some x-ray screening is still acceptable. This applies to high-risk groups such as members of the medical and paramedical community, people working in fields such as education and food preparation, and selected groups of workers such as miners and workers dealing with material such as asbestos, beryllium, glass, and silica.[5]
6. Whole-body multislice spiral CT screening. Patients may elect to undergo this type of CT procedure for screening purposes without an order from a referring physician. They may simply locate a facility that offers this service to the general public. At the time of this writing, the disease detection rate simply does not justify the relatively high radiation dose received by the patient from this procedure. Until there is evidence of a significant disease detection rate, this whole-body multislice spiral CT screening procedure should not be done.[5]

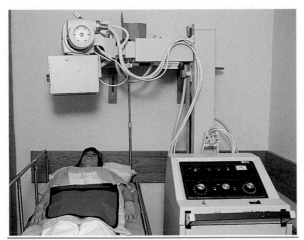

FIG. 8-26. Mobile radiographic examinations require a minimal source-skin distance of 12 inches (30 cm). The 12-inch distance limits the effects of the inverse square falloff of radiation intensity with distance.

x-ray room). Mobile units are not designed to replace specially designated rooms.

DIGITAL IMAGING

Use of the Computer

The computer is a device that electronically processes independent groups of information. Since the 1970s, the use of computers has virtually revolutionized the medical industry. In particular, computers have had a major impact on imaging. They are now used extensively in almost all imaging modalities. The primary examples of this are computed tomography (CT), computed radiography (CR) and digital radiography (DR), digital fluoroscopy (DF), nuclear medicine imaging (NM), magnetic resonance imaging (MRI), and ultrasound (US).

Conventional Radiography: Analog Image

In conventional radiography, after x-rays pass through an anatomical area of clinical interest, they form an invisible, or latent, image of that area on radiographic film. This temporary image produced conventionally by ionizing radiation must then be chemically processed to make the unseen image visible. The finished radiograph that results from this process is an "analog image." Conventional radiography permits the production of optimal quality images that make possible adequate visualization and demonstration of various anatomical structures. However, there are some disadvantages to the use of this technology in addition to the waiting time it takes for the chemical processing of these film-based images. Radiographic film must be physically handled by authorized personnel and then stored in a centralized file. Manually retrieving radiographs is often time consuming and requires adequate personnel power. As a consequence of human error, film jackets containing patient radiographs may be misfiled or misplaced, making these records unavailable at a time when a physician may need them for patient care.

Digital Radiography (DR)

The information contained in a conventional radiograph consists of various shades of gray that represent the amount of x-ray penetration through various biologic tissues. As stated earlier, the latent imaged produced by conventional means must be chemically processed to make the unseen image visible. With **digital radiography (DR),** the latent image formed by x-ray photons on a radiation detector is actually an electronic latent image.[5] Because this image is produced by a computer representation of anatomical information, it is called a digital image.[11] The numeric values of the digital image are aligned in a fixed number of rows and columns that form individual miniature square boxes, each of which corresponds to a particular place in the image. These individual boxes collectively constitute the **image matrix.** Each miniature square box in this matrix is called a picture element, or *pixel.* The pixels collectively represent the information contained in a volume of tissue.[12] The size of the pixels determines the sharpness of the image. Resolution (detail) is sharper when pixels are smaller.

The numerical value in each miniature square box that makes up the image matrix can be converted into a visual brightness, or density level, that can be seen on a video display monitor. Matrix size also affects detail of the image. Detail is better when the size of the matrix is larger because a larger matrix contains smaller pixels. When compared with the resolution of an optimal quality image produced on radiographic film, the resolution of the digital image is actually somewhat less. However, the digital image is diagnostic and permits adequate visualization of anatomic structures because it has better image contrast, and the radiographic density and contrast in the image can be manipulated to improve its overall quality. The image receptors used in digital radiography convert the energy of x-rays into electrical signals. The image receptor is divided into small detector elements that make up the picture elements, or pixels, of the digital image. There are various types of digital radiography image receptors. Some use a scintillator, such as amorphous silicon, to convert the x-ray energy into visible light. The visible light is then converted into electrical signals by an array of transistors or an array of charge-coupled devices, such as those found in video cameras. Other systems use a photoconductor, such as amorphous selenium, to convert the x-ray energy directly into electrical signals that are then read by an array of transistors. In these systems, the number and size of small transistors or charge-coupled devices determine the number and size of pixels in the digital image. Advances in materials technology have resulted in pixel sizes as small as 50 micrometers, which approaches the resolution of film-screen imaging systems (Fig. 8-27).

DR images can be accessed at several workstations at the same time, making image viewing very convenient for physicians providing patient care. Patient information and reports can be included in the patient's DR imaging file along with records from other imaging modalities.[13]

Computed Radiography (CR)

Process

When the invisible, or latent, image generated in conventional radiography is produced in a digital format using computer technology,[14] the process is called **computed radiography (CR).** Computed radiography involves the use of conventional radiographic equipment, traditional patient positioning performed by a radiographer, and the selection and use of standard technical exposure factors. The unseen radiographic image is actually produced in a rectangular, closed cassette containing a photostimulable phosphor (europium activated barium fluorohalide is the most commonly employed phosphor[5]) imaging plate as the image receptor. This reusable imaging plate is utilized instead of radiographic film in a light-tight, closed cassette that resembles that found in conventional radiography. The CR cassette may be referred to as a *filmless cassette.* When the enclosed phosphor is exposed to x-rays, it becomes energized. An image reading unit is

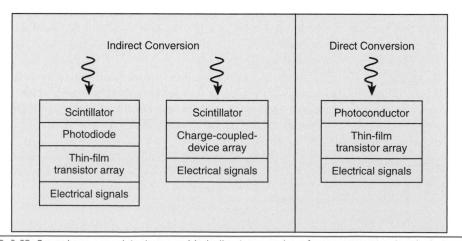

FIG. 8-27. Some large area detectors provide indirect conversion of x-ray energy to electrical charge through intermediate steps involving photodiodes or charge-coupled devices. Other area detectors provide direct conversion of x-ray energy to electrical charge through the use of a photoconductor. (From Hendee WR, Ritenour ER: *Medical image physics*, ed 4, Chicago, 2002, Wiley & Sons.)

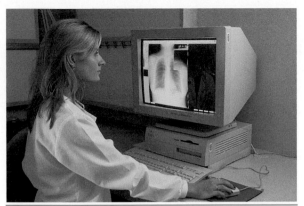

FIG. 8-28. The radiographer at the monitor uses the mouse to adjust the CR image of the body part to the proper size, density, and contrast before electronically sending the image for reading. (From Ballinger PW, Frank ED: *Merrill's atlas of radiographic positions and radiologic procedures,* ed 10, vol 1, St Louis, 2003, Mosby.)

used to scan the photostimulable phosphor imaging plate with a helium-neon laser beam. This results in the emission of violet light that is changed into an electronic signal by a device called a photomultiplier tube. A computer then converts the electronic signal into a digitized image of the anatomic area or part and stores the digital image for visual display on a monitor. If desired, the image can be printed on a laser film when hard copy is needed. While the digital image is displayed on a monitor, the radiographer can adjust it to the correct size, radiographic density, and contrast by manipulating the computer mouse[14] (Fig. 8-28). After adjustments have been completed, the image can be electronically sent for reading.

Avoiding Overexposure of the Patient

Although the radiographer can manipulate the CR image of the patient's anatomy of interest to adjust image size, radiographic density, and contrast, this technologic flexibility does not excuse overexposing the patient. Even with sophisticated digital technology, it is still the radiographer's responsibility to determine and use correct technical exposure factors the first time a patient is x-rayed to minimize radiation exposure. If patients are overexposed by radiographers who claim the rationale that computerized images can be manipulated later on to produce a diagnostic quality image, thereby avoiding the possibility of repeat expo-

sures, patients are actually receiving higher radiation doses than are necessary to produce those initial images. Therefore, the routine practice of overexposing patients to possibly avoid repeat radiographic exposures is unethical and unacceptable. For this reason, radiographers must exercise good judgment in selecting correct technical exposure factors the first time. This good practice conforms with ALARA (as low as reasonably achievable) protection guidelines.

CR Phosphor Sensitivity

The sensitivity of the phosphor used in computed radiography has been described as approximately equal to a 200-speed screen-film combination.[5] Phosphor sensitivity, however, can be significantly greater under certain conditions.

Kilovoltage

As in conventional radiography, kilovoltage controls radiographic contrast. However, CR imaging has greater kilovoltage flexibility than does conventional screen-film radiography. Therefore, a radiographer can select an appropriate kVp setting from a broader range of settings than are suitable for a particular radiographic projection.[14] An acceptable range of kVp that is adequate for penetration of the anatomy of interest should always be used. Kilovoltage above or below this acceptable range should not be used. Technique charts indicating optimal kVp for all CR projections should be available in the x-ray room near the operating console for the radiographer.

X-Ray Beam Collimation

For the computer to correctly form a CR image, the body area or part being radiographed must be positioned in or near the center of the CR cassette. In the event that two separate exposures are to be obtained on a divided cassette, only one half of the cassette should be exposed at a time while the other half of the cassette is covered with lead. The x-ray beam must be carefully collimated to the anatomy of interest so that noncollimated radiation does not reach areas of the imaging plate that should not be exposed to ionizing radiation. If noncollimated radiation reaches those areas, the resultant radiographic image may be too dark or too light, and consequently it may be of little diagnostic value.

Use of Radiographic Grids

When compared with conventional screen-film systems, the photostimulable phosphor in the CR imaging plate is much more sensitive to scatter radiation before and after it is sensitized through exposure to a radiographic beam. Because of this increased sensitivity, a radiographic grid may be used more frequently during CR imaging. For chest radiography, Carlton and Adler advocate the use of a grid for optimum images when chest measurements exceed 24 to 26 cm.[15] Some CR imaging manufactures recommend the use of a grid for certain radiographic projections that require the use of relatively high kVp. Grid selection depends on several factors, for example, the size of the anatomy to be radiographed, kVp selected, the amount of scatter removal preferred, and grid frequency (lines per cm or inch).[15]

FLUOROSCOPIC PROCEDURES

Patient Radiation Exposure Rate

Fluoroscopy is the process in which an x-ray examination is performed that demonstrates dynamic, or active, motion of selected anatomic structures (e.g., a stomach filled with barium sulfate and air during an upper gastrointestinal series) by producing a temporary image of those structures on a television monitor working in conjunction with an image intensification system under low-light conditions. Fluoroscopic procedures (Fig. 8-29) produce the greatest patient radiation exposure rate in diagnostic radiology. In view of this fact, the physician should carefully evaluate the need for a fluoroscopic examination to ascertain whether the potential benefit to the patient in terms of information gained outweighs the potentially adverse somatic or genetic effects of the examination. If the fluoroscopic procedure is necessary, every precaution must be taken to *minimize patient exposure time*.

Fluoroscopic Imaging Systems

Traditionally, fluoroscopic imaging systems have the x-ray tube positioned under the x-ray examination

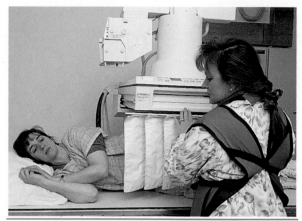

FIG. 8-29. Fluoroscopic procedures produce the largest patient radiation exposure rate in diagnostic radiology.

table and the image intensifier and spot film system (or in significantly older fluoroscopic equipment, an image receptor called a fluoroscopic screen) mounted on a C-arm and centered and suspended over the x-ray examination table. The C-arm design keeps the x-ray tube and the image receptor in constant alignment. Other equipment configurations are possible; for example, the unit can be arranged so that the x-ray tube can be placed over the x-ray examination table while the image receptor lies beneath the x-ray examination table. A fluoroscopic imaging system can also be set up as a remote control facility, permitting the equipment operator to remain outside of the fluoroscopic room. In the interest of patient and personnel safety, radiologists and assisting radiologic technologists have a responsibility to become fully knowledgeable regarding the safe operation of the equipment they use.

Image Intensification Fluoroscopy

Benefits

Image intensification fluoroscopy (Fig. 8-30) involves the use of an image intensifier (II) to increase the brightness of the real-time image produced on a fluorescent screen during fluoroscopy. It is used in virtually all state-of-the-art fluoroscopic equipment. Image intensification fluoroscopy has three significant benefits. These benefits are listed in Box 8-7.

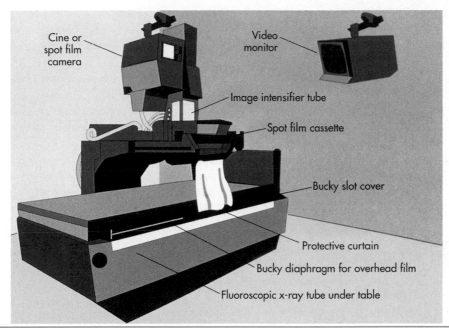

FIG. 8-30. Image intensification fluoroscopy unit. The x-ray tube used in this unit is mounted beneath the unit's radiographic table that supports the patient. The image intensifier and other image detection devices are then drawn forward and placed over the patient on the table to perform the examination. Other fluoroscopic equipment arrangements are possible. (From *Mosby's radiographic instructional series: radiobiology and radiation protection,* St Louis, 1999, Mosby.)

BOX 8-7

Benefits of Image Intensification Fluoroscopy

1. Increased image brightness
2. Saving of time for the radiologist
3. Patient dose reduction

Brightness of the Fluoroscopic Image

The x-ray image intensification system converts the x-ray image pattern into a corresponding amplified visible light pattern. Overall brightness of the fluoroscopic image increases to roughly 10,000 times the brightness of the image on the discontinued nonimage intensifier fluoroscopic systems operating* under the

same conditions. This dramatic increase in image brightness greatly improved the radiologist's perception of the fluoroscopic image.

Use of Photopic or Cone Vision to View Fluoroscopic Image

Because an image intensification system permits viewing of the fluoroscopic image at ordinary brightness levels (regular white light), the radiologist makes use of photopic, or cone, vision (daytime vision) when viewing the image through this system. With cone vision, the radiologist does not need to adapt to the darkness (by wearing of red goggles for up to 30 minutes), which was required before a nonimage intensification fluoroscopic examination in order for radiologists to use scotopic, or rod, vision

---

*A preimage intensification fluoroscopic operating system is an earlier system in which the fluoroscopic tube, mounted beneath the radiographic table as with most modern fluoroscopic systems, produces x-rays that pass through the table top and the patient before

striking a zinc-cadmium sulfide (ZnCdS) fluoroscopic screen that phosphoresces and produces a very dim image of the anatomy of interest, yielding poor visibility of detail of those structures by the radiologist.

(night vision) to view the dim fluoroscopic image. This saves considerable time. Cone vision also significantly improves visual acuity, thereby permitting the radiologist to better discriminate between small structures.

Milliamperage Required and Effect on Patient Dose

Because an image intensification system greatly increases brightness, image intensification fluoroscopy requires less milliamperage than does old-fashioned fluoroscopy (about 1.5 to 2 mA is used for many procedures with image intensification systems, whereas 3 to 5 mA was usually required for preimage intensification fluoroscopy). The consequent decrease in exposure rate can result in a sizable dose reduction for the patient.

Multifield, or Magnification, Image Intensifier Tubes

Multifield, or magnification, image intensifier tubes are found in the majority of image intensifiers. They are also found in digital fluoroscopic units (see the discussion on digital fluoroscopy presented later in this chapter). Multifield image intensification tubes vary in size, but the 30- to 15-centimeter (12- to 6-inch) diameter model is the most common commercial tube used in general-purpose image intensification fluoroscopic units. When the normal viewing mode (30-centimeter) is used, photoelectrons from the entire surface of a cesium iodide (CsI) input phosphor (i.e., where the x-ray photons passing through the patient first strike the image intensifier assembly) are accelerated to a zinc cadmium sulfide output phosphor. However, when magnification in the fluoroscopic image is needed and the viewing mode is changed to the 15-centimeter mode (or even less, e.g., 4.5 inch or 11 cm, in many new systems), the voltage on the electrostatic focusing lenses increases, thereby causing the focal point of the electrons to move to a greater distance away from the output phosphor.[5] As a result, only electrons from the central part of the 15-centimeter diameter of the input phosphor actually reach the output phosphor of the image intensifier. The change in the focal point of the electrons decreases the field of view with a corresponding increase in magnification of the image. The quality of the magnified image, as viewed on a television monitor, is somewhat degraded. This decrease in image clarity occurs because of a decrease in minification gain (i.e., increase in brightness resulting from minification of the image) caused by a lesser number of photoelectrons available to strike the output phosphor on the image intensifier. Thus, the resultant image is dimmer. Because it is necessary and desirable to maintain a constant level of brightness on the television monitor, fluoroscopic mA increases automatically. However, this increase in tube mA increases the dose to the patient.

Intermittent, or Pulsed, Fluoroscopy

Effect on Patient Dose

Intermittent, or pulsed, fluoroscopy involves manual or automatic periodic activation of the fluoroscopic tube by the fluoroscopist rather than lengthy continuous activation. This practice significantly decreases patient dose, especially in long procedures, and helps extend the life of the tube. Many systems include a *last-image-hold* feature that allows the fluoroscopist to see the most recent image without exposing the patient to another pulse of radiation. This feature also reduces patient dose.

Limiting Fluoroscopic Field Size

Benefit of Fluoroscopic Field Size Limitation

The radiologist must limit the size of the fluoroscopic field to include only the area of clinical interest by adequately collimating the x-ray beam. Adequate collimation involves adjusting the lead shutters placed between the fluoroscopic tube and the patient. When fluoroscopic field size is limited, patient area or integral dose decreases substantially.

Fluoroscopic Beam Length and Width Limitation

Primary beam length and width must be confined within the image receptor boundary. Regardless of the distance from the x-ray source to the image receptor, the useful beam ideally should not extend outside the image receptor. Visible borders should appear on the image monitor.

Technical Exposure Factors

Selection of Technical Exposure Factors for Adult Patients

The fluoroscopist must select technical exposure factors that will minimize patient dose during manual fluoroscopic procedures. Increases in peak kilovoltage and filtration reduce the patient radiation exposure rate. Most fluoroscopic examinations performed with image intensification systems employ a range of from 75 to 110 kVp for adult patients, depending on the area of the body being examined. This peak kilovoltage range produces the correct level of fluoroscopic image brightness. Lower peak kilovoltage, when used for greater diameter regions, increases patient dose because a lesser penetrating x-ray beam employed necessitates the use of a higher milliamperage (a larger quantity of x-ray photons in the beam) to obtain adequate image brightness. Besides using the correct kilovoltage, the operator can further limit excessive entrance exposure of the patient by ensuring that the x-ray **source-to-skin distance (SSD)** is not less than 15 inches (38 cm) for stationary (fixed) fluoroscopes and not less than 12 inches (30 cm) for mobile fluoroscopes. A 12-inch (30-cm) minimal distance is required, but a 15-inch (38 cm) minimal distance is preferred for all image intensification systems. On the other hand, the position of the input phosphor surface of the image intensifier should be maintained as close as is practical to the patient to also reduce the patient's entrance exposure rate.

Selection of Technical Exposure Factors for Children

Technical exposure factors for fluoroscopic procedures for children necessitate a decrease in peak kilovoltage by as much as 25%. The peak kilovoltage chosen should depend on part thickness just as it does in radiography. In addition to lowering technical exposure factors, maintaining source-to-skin distance (SSD) and minimizing the height of the image intensifier entrance surface above the patient, as described earlier, further limits excessive entrance exposure of the pediatric patient.

Filtration

Purpose and Requirements

The function of a filter in fluoroscopy, as in radiographic procedures, is to reduce the patient's skin dose. Adequate layers of aluminum equivalent material placed in the path of the useful beam remove the more harmful lower energy photons from the beam by absorbing them. A minimum of 2.5-mm total aluminum equivalent filtration must be permanently installed in the path of the useful beam of the fluoroscopic unit. With image intensification systems, a total aluminum equivalent filtration of 3.0 mm or greater may be preferred. Patient dose decreases by one fourth during fluoroscopic procedures when aluminum filtration increases from 1-mm aluminum to 3-mm aluminum. Although this increase in filtration causes a slight loss of fluoroscopic image brightness, increasing peak kilovoltage somewhat may compensate.

Half-Value Layer (HVL)

As in radiography, when filtration of the x-ray beam is questionable, the HVL of the beam must be measured. In standard image intensification fluoroscopy, an x-ray beam HVL of 3- to 4-mm aluminum is considered acceptable when peak kilovoltage ranges from 80 to 100.

Source-to-Skin Distance (SSD)

Requirement

In accordance with National Council on Radiation Protection (NCRP) regulations, the source-to-skin distance must be no less than 15 inches (38 cm) for stationary (fixed) fluoroscopes and no less than 12 inches (30 cm) for mobile fluoroscopes.[16] As discussed earlier, this standard ensures that the patient's entrance surface is not excessively exposed. Maintaining an appropriate source-to-skin distance reduces the radiographer's exposure as well.

Cumulative Timing Device

A **cumulative timer** must be provided and used with each fluoroscopic unit. This re-settable device times the x-ray beam-on time and sounds an audible alarm or temporarily interrupts the exposure after the fluoroscope has been activated for 5 minutes. It makes the radiologist aware of the length of time the patient receives exposure for each fluoroscopic examination. When the fluoroscope is activated for shorter periods, the patient, radiologist, and radiographer receive less exposure. Total fluoroscopic beam-on time should be documented for every fluoroscopic procedure.

Exposure Rate Limitation

Current federal standards limit **entrance skin exposure rates** of general-purpose intensified fluoroscopic units to a maximum of 10 roentgens (R) per minute (10 × 2.58 × 10⁻⁴ coulomb [C]/kg/min), whereas non-image intensification units may not exceed 5 R per minute (5 × 2.58 × 10⁻⁴ C/kg/min). Measured at tabletop with the image intensifier entrance surface at a prescribed 12 inches above, these standards have been imposed to give consideration to the cumulative small doses of radiation the patient receives over a lifetime. Fluoroscopic units equipped with high-level control (HLC) may permit a skin entrance exposure rate as great as 20 R per minute (20 × 2.58 × 10⁻⁴ C/kg/min). Because fluoroscopic procedures can result in the largest patient doses in diagnostic x-ray imaging, sometimes reaching the level of therapeutic doses, fluoroscopic exposure rates and fluoroscopic exposure times must be kept within established limits.

Primary Protective Barrier

A **primary protective barrier** of 2-mm lead equivalent is required for an image intensifier unit. The image intensifier assembly itself provides this barrier. The assembly must be joined with the x-ray tube, which is commonly located underneath the tabletop and interlocked so that the fluoroscopic x-ray tube cannot be activated when the image intensifier is in the parked position.

Fluoroscopic Exposure Control Switch

The fluoroscopic exposure control switch (e.g., the foot pedal) must be of the dead-man type (i.e., only

continuous pressure applied by the operator [usually a radiologist] can keep the switch activated and the fluoroscopic tube emitting x-radiation). This means that the exposure automatically terminates if the person operating the switch becomes incapacitated (e.g., suffers a heart attack).

MOBILE C-ARM FLUOROSCOPY

A mobile C-arm fluoroscopic unit is a portable x-ray unit that is C-shaped. It has an x-ray tube attached to one end of its arm and an image intensifier attached to the other end. C-arm fluoroscopes (Fig. 8-31) are frequently used in the operating room for orthopedic procedures (e.g., pinning of a fractured hip). They are also used for cardiac imaging, interventional procedures, and other potentially lengthy cases. The use of C-arm fluoroscopy in procedures such as these carries the potential for a relatively large patient radiation dose. C-arm fluoroscope operators, if standing close to the patient, could also receive a significant increase in occupational exposure during such cases (see Chapter 9 for discussion on C-arm operator protection). For this reason, equipment operators must have appropriate education and training to ensure that they will be able to follow guidelines for safe C-arm operation and also meet radiation safety protocols essential to patient and personnel safety.

Mobile fluoroscopic units are required to have a minimal source-to-end of collimator assembly distance of 12 inches (30 cm). Some type of spacer or collimator extension is usually installed to prevent any part of the patient from getting closer than 12 inches from the tube target. During C-arm fluoroscopic procedures, the patient-image intensifier distance should be as short as possible (Fig. 8-32). This reduces patient entrance dose. Also for dose reduction purposes, it is preferable to position the C-arm so that the x-ray tube is under the patient. With the x-ray tube in this position scatter radiation is less intense (Fig. 8-33). When the x-ray tube is positioned over the patient, scatter radiation becomes more intense, and patient dose increases correspondingly.

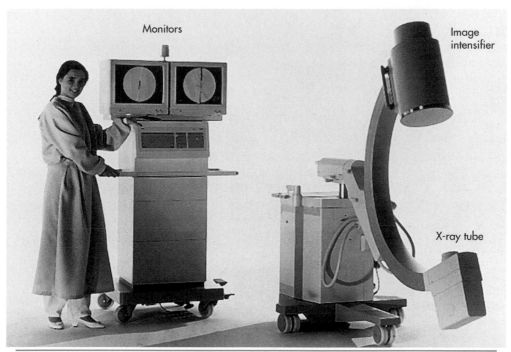

FIG. 8-31. C-arm fluoroscope and monitor. (From *Mosby's radiographic instructional series: radiobiology and radiation protection*, St. Louis, 1999, Mosby.)

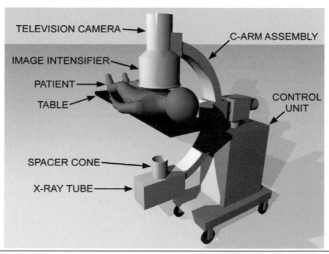

FIG. 8-32. To reduce patient entrance dose during C-arm fluoroscopy, patient-image intensifier distance should be as short as possible. (Courtesy Mark Rzeszotarski.)

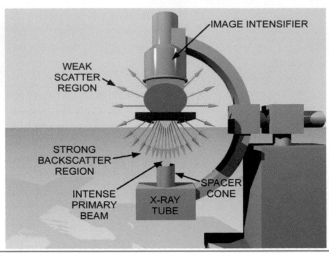

FIG. 8-33. To reduce scattered radiation during C-arm fluoroscopy, position the C-arm so that the x-ray tube is under the patient whenever possible. (Courtesy Mark Rzeszotarski.)

CINEFLUOROGRAPHY

Film Size

The techniques to reduce patient dose during fluoroscopy also apply to dose reduction during cinefluorography. In cinefluorography, or cine, a movie camera that uses either 16-mm film or 35-mm film is used to record the image of the output phosphor of the image intensifier. Since patient exposure is greater when 16-mm film is used, 35-mm film is most frequently used in the United States.

High Dose Rate Procedures

Dose-reduction techniques are especially important in cine because cine procedures can result in the highest patient doses of all diagnostic procedures. The high dose resulting from cine is caused by a relatively high inherent dose rate and the length of the procedure, particularly in cardiology, which involves cardiac imaging procedures such as heart catheterization, and in neuroradiology. Thus, a percentage decrease in cine dose yields a greater actual dose reduction than the same percentage decrease in noncine procedures.

Filming Frame Rate

Cinematic, or cine, cameras have filming frame rates of 7.5, 15, 30, and 60 frames per second.[5] Filming frame rate affects patient radiation dose. When the frame rate is higher, so is the radiation dose. Swallow function studies and cardiac imaging procedures require higher frame rates because they are dynamic function studies. When compared with patients undergoing procedures that use lower frame rates, patients undergoing more rapid dynamic function studies such as heart catheterization receive higher radiation doses.

Inference of Patient Dose from Tabletop Exposure Levels

Patient dose may be inferred from tabletop exposure levels. The amount of exposure varies with a number of operator-adjustable parameters. Typical cine tabletop exposure is approximately 25 mR per frame for 6- to 7-inch image intensification mode. This translates to 45 R per minute if a frame rate of 30 frames per second is used. Thus, any limitation of beam-on time is significant as long as the efficacy of the procedure is not compromised. Patient exposure increases when a smaller viewing mode (6 inches, compared with 9 inches) or a lower speed cine film is used. Exposure also increases if the frame rate is increased. For example, switching from a 9-inch to a 6-inch field of view approximately doubles the tabletop exposure rate. Increasing the frame rate from 30 frames per second to 60 frames per second doubles the exposure rate as well. If both adjustments are made at the same time, the resulting exposure rate goes up by a factor of 4. Other characteristics such as the image intensifier input phosphor exposure level set by the vendor, grid factor, and source-to-skin distance play a role in determining the typical dose levels for a system.

Collimation

Collimating to the anatomic area of interest has the same effect in cine as in ordinary fluoroscopy. Collimation decreases the integral dose (product of dose and volume of tissue irradiated) while increasing image quality by limiting scatter.

Dose Reduction Techniques

The radiologist or cardiologist can reduce exposure during cine procedures by shortening the time of the cine run and using fluoroscopy, when possible, to locate the catheter. When fluoroscopy is used, intermittent exposures to verify location and movement of the catheter between exposures can limit total fluoroscopy time as well. Some optional equipment features such as the last-frame-hold feature, in which the most recent fluoroscopic image remains in view as a guide to the radiologist when the x-ray beam is off, also promote lower patient dose by decreasing the total fluoroscopic beam-on time.

Patient Dose Determined by Procedure

The typical dose delivered to the patient depends on the procedure. In selective coronary arteriography, most radiation exposure is from the cine. In other procedures, although the dose rate is lower, the dose from fluoroscopy may exceed the dose from cine if the total fluoroscopy time is longer. This is often the case in percutaneous transluminal angioplasty.

DIGITAL FLUOROSCOPY

Use of Pulsed Progressive System for Dose Reduction

Various methods are used to obtain digital images in some fluoroscopic equipment. The electrical signal from the video camera attached to the output phosphor may be digitized. Alternatively, the TV camera may be replaced by a digital device such as a charge-coupled-device (CCD) camera or other digital detector. However the digital image is acquired, the use of digital technology offers the possibility of some methods of dose reduction. One method makes use of the fact that a brief high-intensity pulse of radiation may create an entire image of the output phosphor. The lines composing the image are progressively scanned (i.e., the image on the camera, namely the TV lines, is scanned or painted in a natural sequence, left to right followed by right to left and so on from top to bottom) to provide the picture that appears on a monitor during a brief time period (one sixtieth of a second). The x-ray beam is turned off while the image is being scanned, thereby decreasing patient dose, and then pulsed back on for the next image. These systems are known as "pulsed progressive" systems and are commonly used to lower patient dose.

Use of Last-Image-Hold Feature for Dose Reduction

Another dose reduction technique that is particularly effective in digital fluoroscopy systems is "last image hold." In last image hold, an image is stored from the last time that the foot switch was depressed. In a digital system, this image could be composed of several frames of information that have been added together to reduce the effect of quantum noise that would be particularly apparent in a single frame.

HIGH-LEVEL-CONTROL INTERVENTIONAL PROCEDURES

Justification for Use of High-Level-Control Interventional Procedures

Interventional procedures are invasive procedures performed by a physician with the aid of fluoroscopic imaging. The interventional physician, usually a radiologist or cardiologist, inserts catheters into vessels or directly into patient tissues for the purpose of drainage, biopsy, or alteration of vascular occlusions or malformations. For these procedures, **high-level-control fluoroscopy (HLCF)** is often employed. HLCF is an operating mode for state-of-the-art fluoroscopic equipment in which exposure rates are substantially higher than those normally allowed in routine procedures. The higher exposure rate allows visualization of smaller and lower contrast objects that do not usually appear during standard fluoroscopy. HLCF, therefore, is used for interventional procedures in which visualization of fine catheters or not easily seen structures is crucial. An audible signal constantly reminds personnel that the HLC mode is engaged.

Public Health Advisory about the Dangers of Overexposure of Patients and Exposure Rate Limits

Some fluoroscopically guided therapeutic interventional procedures have the potential for substantial patient exposure. On September 30, 1974, the Food and Drug Administration (FDA) issued a public health advisory to alert health care workers to the dangers of overexposure of patients through the use of high-level fluoroscopy. The FDA X-Ray Equipment Standards, enacted in 1994, limited the tabletop exposure rate of fluoroscopic equipment for routine procedures to 10 R per minute unless an HLC mode was present, in which case routine fluoroscopy was limited to 5 R per minute when the system was not in HLC mode and unlimited when it was in HLC mode.[17] The authors of the standards felt that the high-level capability was necessary for certain vital situations involving therapeutic interventional procedures in which the potential risks to the patient of increased radiation exposure would be subordinate to a successful medical outcome of an

From the U.S. Food and Drug Administration: *Public health advisory: avoidance of serious x-ray-induced skin injuries to patients during fluoroscopically guided procedures*, Rockville, Md, September 30, 1994, FDA.

> ### BOX 8-8
> #### Procedures Involving Extended Fluoroscopic Time
>
> Percutaneous transluminal angioplasty
> Radiofrequency cardiac catheter ablation
> Vascular embolization
> Stent and filter placement
> Thrombolytic and fibrinolytic procedures
> Percutaneous transhepatic cholangiography
> Endoscopic retrograde cholangiopancreatography
> Transjugular intrahepatic portosystemic shunt
> Percutaneous nephrostomy
> Biliary drainage
> Urinary or biliary stone removal

intervention. The HLC mode, although allowing unlimited exposure, required continuous, positive-pressure manual operation (e.g., continuously depressing a foot switch) and a continuous audible signal to remind personnel that the high-level fluoroscopic mode was in use. In this mode, patient exposure rates have been estimated to range from 20 to 120 R per minute. When the rule was enacted, total patient exposure was limited by the heat-loading capabilities of the x-ray tube. The thinking was that the tube would reach its heat limit before any detectable nonstochastic radiation injury could occur. By the early 1990s, advances in x-ray tube technology and the development of vascular interventional procedures that require long fluoroscopy times (Box 8-8) had created a situation in which serious skin reactions had been reported in some patients. Radiogenic skin injuries such as erythema (diffuse reddening) or desquamation (sloughing off of skin cells) are deterministic effects in which the severity of the disorder increases with radiation dose. As the data in Table 8-2 show, a half hour of total beam-on time at one location on a patient's skin is sufficient to produce erythema. The effect does not appear for approximately 10 days. Because manifestation of skin injury is delayed, a radiologist would not usually be the first

TABLE 8-2

Radiation-Induced Skin Injuries

Effect	Typical Threshold Absorbed Dose (Gy)*	Hours of Fluoroscopic "On Time" to Reach Threshold[†]		Time to Onset of Effect[‡]
		Usual Fluoroscopic Dose Rate of 0.02 Gy/Min (2 Rads/Min)	High-Level Dose Rate of 0.2 Gy/Min (20 Rads/Min)	
Early transient erythema	2	1.7	0.17	Hours
Temporary epilation	3	2.5	0.25	3 wk
Main erythema	6	5.0	0.50	10 days
Permanent epilation	7	5.8	0.58	3 wk
Dry desquamation	10	8.3	0.83	4 wk
Dermal atrophy	11	9.2	0.92	0.14 wk
Telangiectasis	12	10.0	1.00	0.52 wk
Moist desquamation	15	12.5	1.25	4 wk
Late erythema	15	12.5	1.25	6-10 wk
Dermal necrosis	18	15.0	1.50	0.10 wk
Secondary ulceration	20	16.7	1.67	0.6 wk

Modified from Wagner LK, Eifel PJ, Geise RA: *J Vasc Interv Radiol* 5:71, 1994.
*The unit for absorbed dose is the gray (Gy) in the International System of units. One Gy is equivalent to 100 rads in the traditional system of radiation units.
[†]Time required to deliver the typical threshold dose at the specified dose rate.
[‡]Time after single irradiation to observation of effect.

person to observe the onset of the symptoms. Therefore, patient monitoring, radiation dosimetry, and accurate record keeping are important for the future medical management of adverse reactions. The FDA has recommended that a notation be placed in the patient's record if skin dose is received in the range of 1 to 2 gray (Gy) (100 to 200 rads). The location of the area of the patient's skin that received the absorbed dose should also be noted using a diagram, annotated photograph, or narrative description.

Use of Fluoroscopic Equipment by Nonradiologist Physicians

Because of increasing use of C-arm fluoroscopes and fluoroscopes on stationary equipment with HLC mode by nonradiologist physicians performing interventional procedures and other potentially lengthy cases, and the fact that such procedures are capable of subjecting the patient and the equipment operator and other personnel near the fluoroscopic equipment to substantial doses of ionizing radiation, there is need for ongoing education and training of these physicians and equipment operators in the safe use of such fluoroscopic equipment. Some of the reasons for high radiation exposures during interventional procedures include the fluoroscopic tube being operated for longer periods of time in continuous and not pulsed mode, failure to use the protective curtain or floating shields on the stationary fluoroscopic equipment's image intensifier as a means of protection, and extensive use of cine as a recording medium. Monitoring and documenting procedural fluoroscopic time are essential. The responsibility for monitoring and documentation generally belongs to the radiographer assisting with the procedure. Also, if due to the intensity of a particular situation, a physician loses track of how long a procedure is taking and how much radiation is being delivered to a localized area of the patient's body, it becomes the radiographer's ethical responsibility to call this to the physician's attention in the interest of safety of all concerned. In the event of a critical situation in which there is excessive fluoroscopic operation time, the radiographer should notify an appropriate supervisor who should then follow the imaging facility's established protocol.

The National Cancer Institute and the Society of Interventional Radiology have conjointly designed some guidelines to assist physicians in developing strategies that will enable them to fulfill their interventional clinical objectives while controlling patient radiation dose and minimizing exposure to occupationally exposed personnel and any other assisting personnel. These strategies are listed in Box 8-9.

AMOUNT OF RADIATION RECEIVED BY PATIENTS UNDERGOING DIAGNOSTIC IMAGING PROCEDURES

Concern about Risk of Exposure from Diagnostic Imaging Procedures

Because increased numbers of people in the United States are undergoing diagnostic imaging procedures

---

BOX 8-9

Strategies to Manage Radiation Dose to Patients, Operators, and Staff during Interventional Fluoroscopy

Immediate	Long-Term
Optimize Dose to Patient	
Use proper radiologic technique:	Include medical physicist in decisions:
• Maximize distance between x-ray tube and patient	• Machine selection and maintenance
• Minimize distance between patient and image receptor	Incorporate dose-reduction technologies and dose-measurement devices in equipment
• Limit use of electronic magnification	
Control fluoroscopic time:	
• Limit use to necessary evaluation of moving structures	Establish a facility quality improvement program that includes an appropriate x-ray equipment quality assurance program, overseen by a medical physicist, which includes equipment evaluation/inspection at appropriate intervals
• Employ last-image-hold to review findings	
Control images:	
• Limit acquisition to essential diagnostic and documentation purposes	
Reduce dose:	
• Reduce field size (collimate) and minimize field overlap	
• Use pulsed fluoroscopy and low frame rate	
Minimize Dose to Operators and Staff	
Keep hands out of the beam	Improve ergonomics of operations and staff:
Use movable shields	• Train operators and staff in ergonomically good positioning when using fluoroscopy equipment; periodically assess their practice
Maintain awareness of body position relative to the x-ray beam:	• Identify and provide the ergonomically best personal protective gear for operators and staff
• Horizontal x-ray beam—operator and staff should stand on the side of the image receptor	• Urge manufacturers to develop ergonomically improved personal protective gear
• Vertical x-ray beam—the image receptor should be above the table	• Recommend research to improve ergonomics for personal protective gear
Wear adequate protection	
• Protective well-fitted lead apron	
• Leaded glasses	

From the National Cancer Institute, Division of Cancer Epidemiology and Genetics, Radiation Epidemiology Branch: *Interventional fluoroscopy: reducing radiation risks for patients and staff*, NIH Publication No. 05-5286, Rockville, Md, March 2005, National Institutes of Health.

each year, concern about the risk of exposure (the possibility of inducing a radiogenic cancer or genetic defect after irradiation) from these procedures is growing. Imaging personnel must reduce the risk to patients whenever possible by employing radiation control practices that produce good images with lower radiation exposure.

Ways to Specify the Amount of Radiation Received by a Patient from a Diagnostic Imaging Procedure

In general, the amount of radiation received by a patient from diagnostic imaging procedures may be specified in four ways: (1) entrance skin exposure, (2) skin dose, (3) gonadal dose, and (4) bone marrow dose. Although each type of specification has significance in estimating the risk to the patient, entrance skin exposure is the most frequently reported because it is the simplest to determine.

Entrance Skin Exposure (ESE)

Conversion of Entrance Skin Exposure to Patient Skin Dose

Entrance skin exposure (ESE) may be converted to *patient skin dose* by using well-documented multiplicative factors. As later discussed, ESE measurements are relatively easy to obtain. When actual patient measurements are not available, reasonably accurate ESE estimates can still be made, which is why ESE is so widely used in assessing the amount of radiation received by a patient.

Measuring Skin Dose Directly

Thermoluminescent dosimeters (TLDs) are the sensing devices most often used to measure skin dose directly. (The characteristics, components, and function of the TLD are described in Chapter 10.) A small, relatively thin pack of TLDs is secured to the patient's skin in the middle of the clinical area of interest and exposed during a radiographic procedure. Because lithium fluoride (LiF), the sensing material in the TLD, responds in a manner similar to human tissue when exposed to ionizing radiation, an accurate determination of surface dose can be made. (See Table 1-5 for a list of permissible skin entrance exposures for

various radiographic examinations.) In fluoroscopy, the amount of radiation that a patient receives is usually estimated by measuring the radiation exposure rate at the tabletop and multiplying this by the fluoro time.

Skin Dose

Skin dose in general represents the absorbed dose to the most superficial layers of the skin. This region is called the *epidermis*. It is composed of five layers: (1) the horny, or outer, layer; (2) translucent, or clear, layer; (3) granular layer; (4) prickle cell layer; and (5) germinal, or basal, cell layer. The thickness of the epidermis varies from one anatomic area to another. It is greater in areas such as the palms of the hands and soles of the feet. The primary function of the epidermis is to protect underlying tissues and structures.

Gonadal Dose

Difference in Gonadal Dose Received by Human Males and Females

Because genetic effects may result from exposure to ionizing radiation, protection of the reproductive organs is of particular concern in diagnostic radiology. (See Table 1-8 for a list of typical gonadal doses from various radiographic examinations.) For several examinations identified in the table, differences exist between the dosage received by human males and females. Protection of the ovaries by overlying tissue accounts for these differences. In diagnostic radiology, the relatively low **gonadal dose** for a single human is considered insignificant. However, when the low gonadal dose is applied to the entire population, the dose becomes far more significant.

Genetically Significant Dose (GSD)

The concept of **genetically significant dose (GSD)** is used to assess the impact of gonadal dose. GSD is the equivalent dose (EqD) to the reproductive organs that, if received by every human, would be expected to bring about an identical gross genetic injury to the total population, as does the sum of the actual doses received by exposed individual members of the population. In other words, if a maximum of 500 people inhabited the earth and each person received an equivalent dose of

0.005 Sv (0.5 rem) gonadal radiation, the gross genetic effect would be identical to the effect occurring when 50 individual inhabitants each receive 0.05 Sv (5 rem) of gonadal radiation and the other 450 inhabitants do not receive an equivalent dose. In simple terms the GSD concept suggests that the consequences of substantial absorbed doses of gonadal radiation become significantly less when averaged over an entire population rather than applied to just a few of its members.

Genetically Significant Dose Considerations

The GSD takes into consideration the fact that some people receive radiation to their reproductive organs during a given year, whereas others do not. Also, it accounts for the fact that radiation exposure in members of the population who cannot bear children (e.g., those who are beyond reproductive years) has no genetic impact. Hence, the GSD is the average annual gonadal equivalent dose to members of the population who are of childbearing age. It includes the number of children who may be expected to be conceived by members of the exposed population in a given year. According to the U.S. Public Health Service, the estimated GSD for the population of the United States is about 0.20 millisievert (mSv) (20 millirem [mrem]).

Bone Marrow Dose

In human beings, bone marrow is of great importance because it contains large numbers of stem, or precursor, blood cells that could be depleted or destroyed by substantial exposure to ionizing radiation. The **bone marrow dose** is a dose of radiation delivered to that organ. Since radiation dose to bone marrow may be responsible for radiation-induced leukemia, the dose to this organ becomes very significant.[5] Bone marrow dose may also be referred to as the *mean marrow dose*. It can be defined as "the average radiation dose to the entire active bone marrow."[5] For example, if in the course of performing a specific radiographic procedure, 25% of the active bone marrow were in the useful beam and received an average absorbed dose of 0.8 mGy (80 mrads), the mean marrow dose is 0.2 mGy (20 mrads). The radiation dose absorbed by an organ such as bone marrow cannot be measured accurately by a direct method; it can only be esti-

mated. In diagnostic radiology the bone marrow dose provides an estimate of patient absorbed dose even though hematologic effects are generally negligible for doses associated with this discipline.

Table 1-7 provides typical bone marrow doses for various radiographic examinations performed on human adults. The levels indicated in Table 1-7 are usually less for children because the active bone marrow is more evenly spread out, and significantly lower technical radiographic exposure factors are used. Although each dose listed in Table 1-7 results from fragmentary exposure of the human body, it is averaged over the whole body.

THE PREGNANT PATIENT

Determining the Possibility of Pregnancy

Whenever a female of childbearing age is to undergo an x-ray examination, it is essential that the radiographer carefully question the patient regarding any possibility of pregnancy. Part of this questioning involves asking the patient for the date of her last menstrual period (LMP). If the patient is to receive substantial pelvic irradiation and there is some doubt about her pregnancy status, then, providing there are no overriding medical concerns, it is strongly recommended that the result of a pregnancy test be obtained before irradiating the pelvis. For all female patients of childbearing age, utilizing a gonadal shield when the uterus and ovaries are within the field of view is advisable as long as the presence of the shield would not disrupt the interpretation of the image. A shield is also recommended if the ovaries and uterus are less than 5 cm from any edge of the field.

Irradiation of an Unknown Pregnancy

Even with all of these precautionary steps, it is likely that a radiographer will see many occasions when a patient who was absolutely certain that she could not be pregnant would later find that she was so at the time of her x-ray examination. This discovery usually is communicated to the imaging department by the patient's obstetrician and is accompanied by a request for the amount of radiation dose that the patient's embryo-fetus received from the x-ray study. In the following discussion, we attempt to illustrate in a simplified manner how the radiography team can appropriately respond to such queries by presenting several case examples.

The first step in the process is to list the particulars of the x-ray examination in as much detail as possible. A useful form can be developed to assist in this process (Fig. 8-34). The information that is needed to develop this form is listed in Box 8-10.

Procedure to Follow and Responsibility for Absorbed Equivalent Dose Determination to the Patient's Embryo-Fetus

When these details have been collected and listed on an appropriate summary form, they must be conveyed to the radiation safety officer or to the medical physicist providing x-ray quality assurance services. It is then that person's task to determine the absorbed equivalent dose to the patient's embryo-fetus. The

Facility: _____

Imaging Department

**REQUEST FOR PATIENT RADIATION DOSE
PATIENT X-RAY EXAM RECORD**

Patient's name: _____   X-ray study #: _____
Date of birth: _____   Exam date: _____
Date of last menstrual period: _____
Referring physician: _____
Physician requesting radiation dose: _____
Radiologist: _____   Radiographer: _____
Examination: _____   X-ray room unit: _____

RADIOGRAPHIC

Projection	Patient thickness	Film	kVp	mAs	SID	Number of films	Gonadal shield

FLUOROSCOPIC

Anatomic location	kVp (mean)	mA (mean)	Fluoro time	Exam description

SPOT FILMS

Anatomic location	kVp	mA	Time (msec)	Number of spots	Special details

FIG. 8-34. Request for patient radiation dose form.

calculation process incorporates actual measurements of radiation output on the involved x-ray unit or units with the examination data list supplied by the radiographer. It also uses published absorbed dose data tables. What eventually is obtained and presented by the medical physicist, radiologist, or radiation safety officer to the patient's physician is a calculated estimate of the approximate equivalent dose to the embryo-fetus as a result of the x-ray examination.

Sample Cases to Estimate Approximate Equivalent Dose to the Embryo-Fetus

Several typical cases (somewhat simplified) are presented to illustrate one of the methods that might be used to obtain this calculated estimate. It is not the purpose here to give an advanced presentation but rather to offer a basic method that makes use of fundamental principles and shows the importance of the radiographer's input in the process. The most significant principle is the correction to the measured radiation output at a given kVp as a result of the patient's thickness and the distance from the image receptor to the tabletop. The radiation output is specified in milliroentgens per milliampere-second (mR/mAs). Although the SI unit of exposure is the coulomb/kilogram, x-ray tube output is usually measured in milliroentgens per milliampere-second because the ionization chambers used to perform the measurements are still calibrated in roentgens. Therefore, in this section the traditional unit of exposure is used. The product of radiation output at the patient's radiation entrance surface and the milliampere-second used for the x-ray projection considered yields the ESE for that view. It is this value that we seek to obtain for each x-ray exposure given to the patient. The most common measurement of milliroentgens per milliampere-second is at a distance of 40 inches from the x-ray tube target. For a patient with thickness T in centimeters and a typical distance of 2 inches from film to tabletop, the radiation output at the patient's entrance surface is given in Equation 8-1:

Equation 8-1

$$(mR/mAs)_s = (mR/mAs)_{40''} \times \{40''/[SID - (T/2.54) - 2'']\}^2$$

Then to obtain the ESE for a given x-ray projection, use Equation 8-2:

Equation 8-2

$$ESE = (mR/mAs)_s \times mAs \text{ for the projection}$$

After the ESE has been found for each x-ray exposure, it is necessary to obtain conversion factors that will yield a value for the uterine absorbed dose attributable to each exposure. In 1977 the National Council on Radiation Protection and Measurements (NCRP) published Report No. 54, "Medical Radiation Exposure of Pregnant and Potentially Pregnant Women." Table 4 in this report has been a very useful resource for helping establish the uterine absorbed dose. Although other useful and more recent data tables exist, this table has been reproduced here as Table 8-3 to illustrate a simple method for fetal dose estimation. To use the table, it is necessary to know for each x-ray view the ESE, the anatomic location, the beam quality (HVL), and the image receptor size.

TABLE 8-3

Embryo (Uterine) Doses for Selected X-Ray Projections (mrad/R)*,†

Anatomy or Study	Projection	SID (inches)	Image Receptor Size (inches)‡	Beam Quality (HVL mm Al)					
				1.5	2.0	2.5	3.0	3.5	4.0
Pelvis, lumbopelvic	AP	40	17 × 14	142	212	283	353	421	486
	LAT	40	14 × 17	13	25	39	56	75	97
Abdominal§	AP	40	14 × 17	133	199	265	330	392	451
	PA	40	14 × 17	56	90	130	174	222	273
	LAT	40	14 × 17	13	23	37	53	71	91
Lumbar spine	AP	40	14 × 17	128	189	250	309	366	419
	LAT	40	14 × 17	9	17	27	39	53	69
Hip	AP (1)	40	10 × 12	105	153	200	244	285	324
	AP (2)	40	17 × 14	136	203	269	333	395	454
Full spine (chiropractic)	AP	40	14 × 36	154	231	308	384	457	527
Urethrogram	AP	40	10 × 12	135	200	265	327	386	441
Upper GI	AP	40	14 × 17	9.5	16	25	34	45	56
Femur (one side)	AP	40	7 × 17	1.6	3.0	4.8	6.9	9.4	12
Cholecystography	PA	40	10 × 12	0.7	1.5	2.6	4.1	6.0	8.3
Chest	AP	72	14 × 17	0.3	0.7	1.3	2.0	3.1	4.3
	PA	72	14 × 17	0.3	0.6	1.2	2.0	3.0	4.5
	LAT	72	14 × 17	0.1	0.3	0.5	0.8	1.2	1.8
Ribs, barium swallow	AP	40	14 × 17	0.1	0.3	0.5	0.9	1.4	2.0
	PA	40	14 × 17	0.1	0.3	0.5	0.9	1.5	2.2
	LAT	40	14 × 17	0.03	0.08	0.2	0.3	0.4	0.6
Thoracic spine	AP	40	14 × 17	0.2	0.4	0.8	1.4	4.1	3.0
	LAT	40	14 × 17	0.04	0.1	0.2	0.4	0.5	0.8
Skull, cervical spine, scapula, shoulder, humerus	—	40	—	<0.01	<0.01	<0.01	<0.01	<0.01	<0.01

Data from National Council on Radiation Protection and Measurements: *Medical radiation exposure of pregnant and potentially pregnant women*, Report No. 54, Washington, DC, 1977, NCRP.

AP, Anteroposterior; *GI*, gastrointestinal; *LAT*, lateral; *PA*, posteroanterior.

*Average dose to the uterus (mrad) for 1 roentgen entrance skin exposure (free-in-air).

†From Rosenstein (1976).

‡Field size is collimated to the image receptor.

§Includes retrograde pyelogram; kidney, ureter, and bladder (KUB); barium enema, lumbosacral spine, intravenous pyelogram (IVP); renal arteriogram.

Sample Cases to Obtain an Approximate Estimate of the Fetal Equivalent Dose

Now we shall consider several typical x-ray examinations and obtain an approximate estimate of the fetal equivalent dose resulting from each study. Three separate cases (A, B, and C) are presented as examples.

CASE A: OBSTRUCTION SERIES

X-ray projection details:
PA chest radiograph

(1) 110 kVp, 14 mAs, 72″ SID, 14″ × 17″ film,

25-cm patient thickness

Erect AP abdomen

(1) 70 kVp, 60 mAs, 40″ SID, 14″ × 17″ film,

20-cm patient thickness

Supine abdomen

(1) 70 kVp, 60 mAs, 40″ SID, 14″ × 17″ film,

20-cm patient thickness

The first step is to obtain the value of mR/mAs for each projection. To determine this value, a reference value $(mR/mAs)_{40''}$ is needed for the x-ray unit involved and the kVp used. To comply with state rules and regulations, a medical physicist measures these values yearly for each x-ray tube. If the measured reference mR/mAs values for the three projections are 9.35, 3.79, and 3.79, respectively, then substituting these numbers into Equation 8-1 along with the corresponding SIDs and patient thicknesses yields $(mR/mAs)_s$ PA chest = 4.13, $(mR/mAs)_s$, erect AP abdomen = 6.7, and supine abdomen = 6.7, respectively. From Equation 8-2 the ESE value is then given by

ESE PA chest: 4.13 × 14 = 58 mR = 0.058 R

ESE erect AP abdomen: 6.7 × 60 = 402 mR = 0.402 R

ESE supine abdomen: 6.7 × 60 = 402 mR = 0.402 R

For the chest field, HVL is approximately 4 mm Al, while for the abdominal fields we shall use 2 mm Al. Then from Table 8-3 the uterine dose conversion factors are 4.5 millirads (mrads)/R, 199 mrads/R, and 199 mrads/R. Multiplying these values by the ESE for each view gives a fetal dose estimate (FDE) for each, namely:

PA chest FDE = 0.058 × 4.5 = 0.3 mrad

Erect AP abdomen FDE = 0.402 × 199 = 80 mrad

Supine abdomen FDE = 0.402 × 199 = 80 mrad

The total FDE is therefore 160 mrads. For diagnostic x-rays, 1 mrad is the same as 1 mrem, and consequently the calculated approximate equivalent dose to the patient's embryo-fetus from her obstruction series is 160 mrem (1.6 mSv).

For reference purposes this value of equivalent dose to the embryo-fetus is substantially less than the 500 mrem (5 mSv) recommended by the NCRP as a maximum equivalent dose to the embryo-fetus during the 9-month gestation period.

CASE B: CHEST AND THORACIC SPINE STUDY

X-ray projection details:
PA chest radiograph:

(1) 120 kVp, 10 mAs, 72″ SID, 14″ × 17″ film,

28-cm patient thickness

Lateral chest radiograph:

(1) 120 kVp, 30 mAs, 72″ SID, 14″ × 17″ film,

36-cm patient thickness

AP thoracic spine:

(1) 80 kVp, 50 mAs, 40″ SID, 7″ × 17″ film,

28-cm patient thickness

Lateral thoracic spine:

(1) 90 kVp, 150 mAs, 40″ SID, 7″ × 17″ film,

36-cm patient thickness

CALCULATION

MEASURED	FROM EQUATION 8-1
PA chest $(mR/mAs)_{40''}$ = 9.5	$(mR/mAs)_s$ = 4.9
Lateral chest $(mR/mAs)_{40''}$ = 9.5	$(mR/mAs)_s$ = 5.6
AP T-spine $(mR/mAs)_{40''}$ = 5.5	$(mR/mAs)_s$ = 12.1
Lateral T-spine $(mR/mAs)_{40''}$ = 7.6	$(mR/mAs)_s$ = 21.4

FROM EQUATION 8-2

ESE (PA chest) = 49 mR = 0.049 R
ESE (lateral chest) = 168 mR = 0.168 R
ESE (AP T-spine) = 0.605 R
ESE (lateral T-spine) = 3.21 R

The HVLs used for each view are 4.5 mm Al, 4.5 mm Al, 2.5 mm Al, and 3 mm Al, respectively. Then from Table 8-3 we obtain the uterine dose rates associated with each projection:

PA chest	4.5 mrads/R
Lateral chest	1.8 mrad/R
AP T-spine	0.8 mrad/R
Lateral T-spine	0.4 mrad/R

The approximate fetal equivalent dose for each projection is as follows:

PA chest	$4.5 \times 0.049 = 0.22$ mrem
Lateral chest	$1.8 \times 0.168 = 0.30$ mrem
AP T-spine	$0.8 \times 0.605 = 0.48$ mrem
Lateral T-spine	$0.4 \times 3.21 = 1.28$ mrem

This amounts to a total estimated equivalent dose to the embryo-fetus of 2.3 mrem (23 microsievert). This value is negligible compared with the NCRP maximum equivalent dose value.

CASE C: MODIFIED UPPER GI EXAM

X-ray projection details:
    Fluoroscopy: 115 kVp, 4.5 mA (mean values), 3.5 minutes
    Spot films (4): 110 kVp, 200 mA, 20 msec (mean values)

CALCULATION DETAILS From measured data on the involved fluoroscopic unit, the entrance exposure rate to the patient is about 1.25 R per milliampere-minute. Therefore, the ESE for the delivered fluoroscopic radiation is obtained from the product:

$$1.25 \text{ R/mA-min.} \times 4.5 \text{ mA} \times 3.5 \text{ min.} = 19.7 \text{ R}$$

From measured spot film radiation output, for the technique factors used in this study, the x-ray output at the patient's entrance surface is 50 mR/mAs.* Therefore, the total ESE for the four spot films is given by

$$4 \times 50 \text{ mR/mAs} \times 200 \text{ mA} \times .020 \text{ seconds} = 800 \text{ mR} = 0.8 \text{ R}$$

Using HVL values of 4.0 and 3.5 mm Al, respectively, the uterine dose rates obtained from Table 8-3 are as follows:
    Averaged fluoroscopic exposures: 56 mrads/R
    Spot films: 45 mrads/R
    The estimated approximate equivalent dose to the embryo-fetus from this modified upper gastrointestinal (UGI) study is then

---

*For the spot films the entrance surface of the patient is only about 18 inches from the x-ray tube target, and that is why the value of mR/mAs can be so high.

$$56 \times 19.7 + 45 \times 0.8 = 1.14 \text{ rem (11.4 mSv)}$$

For this modified UGI study on a heavy patient, we have obtained a fetal equivalent dose estimate that is more than twice the NCRP recommended maximum fetal equivalent dose of 0.5 rem (5 mSv). This result, however, is far below the range between 10 and 20 rem (100 to 200 mSv) at which therapeutic abortion has historically been considered. If the embryo-fetus were in its most sensitive stage (i.e., early first trimester), then possibly some genetic studies might be undertaken. Otherwise, in most situations, increased follow-up would be the course of action.

OTHER DIAGNOSTIC EXAMS AND IMAGING MODALITIES

Patient Dose in Mammography

Mammography is used to detect breast cancer that is not palpable in physical examinations (Fig. 8-35, A and B). Experts agree that yearly mammographic screening of women 50 years of age and older leads to earlier detection of breast cancer. Earlier treatment saves lives and reduces suffering. The value of mammography in younger women is somewhat controversial. The controversy has little to do with radiation risk (induction of breast cancer by radiation). Although it is still mentioned occasionally in the popular press, cancer researchers generally agree that radiation risk resulting from the small doses associated with mammography is negligible in all women.[18-20] Federal regulations for FDA certification of screening mammography facilities state that the mean dose to the glandular tissue of a 4.5-cm compressed breast using a screen-film mammography system should not exceed 3 mGy (300 mrads) per view.[21] Studies have shown that well-calibrated mammographic systems are capable of providing excellent imaging performance with an average glandular dose of not more than 2 mGy (200 mrads).[22] The age recommendation for screening is controversial because mammography is less accurate in the detection of breast cancer in younger women and likely to result in many false-positive readings, leading to

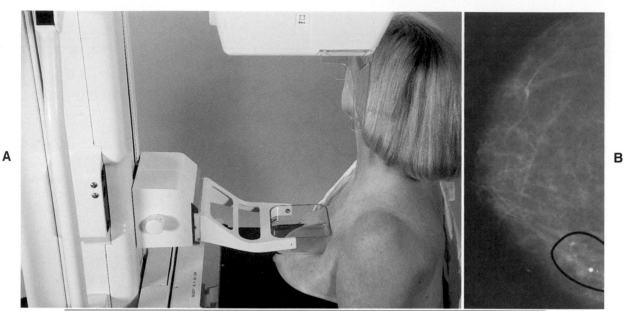

FIG. 8-35. A, Mammography of the breast using the craniocaudal projection. **B,** Mammography can be used to detect breast cancer. (**A** From Ballinger PW, Frank ED: *Merrill's atlas of radiographic positions and radiologic procedures,* ed 10, vol 2, St Louis, 2003, Mosby.)

unnecessary biopsies in that population. The increased density of the breast of younger women tends to reduce radiographic contrast, and therefore mammography may be less sensitive in the average younger woman than in the average older woman. Nevertheless, earlier detection of more aggressive cancers is assumed to save lives in general. Consequently, the efficacy of screening mammography in women under 50 is a subject that has generated a great deal of interest.

Mammography Screening

As of this writing, the authors support the recommendations of the American College of Radiology, the American Cancer Society, and the American Medical Association. These groups advocate annual mammography screening or mammography screening at least every other year for women between the ages of 40 and 49. Before the onset of menopause, a baseline mammogram is also highly recommended for comparison with mammograms taken at a later age. The interested reader should contact these organizations for their latest policy statements on this subject.

Dose Reduction in Mammography

Dose reduction in mammography can be achieved by limiting the number of projections taken. Axillary projections should be done only upon request of the radiologist. If mammography is performed as a routine screening procedure, it is prudent to perform only craniocaudal and mediolateral projections of each breast with adequate compression to uniformly demonstrate breast tissue from the nipple to the most posterior portion.

Digital Mammography

A description of digital radiography was provided earlier in this chapter. In the latest (and most expensive) systems that are used for breast imaging, digital radiography has replaced film-based mammography to provide optimal quality images.

Patient Dose in Computed Tomography

Radiation Exposure

Computed tomography (CT) is defined as the "process by which a computer-reconstructed transverse (or axial) image of a patient is created by an x-ray tube and detector assembly rotating 360 degrees about a specified area of the body."[23] CT may also be referred to as *computed axial tomography (CAT)*. Although a discussion of CT equipment, function, and procedure is not within the scope of this text, patient dose resulting from exposure to ionizing radiation is relevant because CT is a frequently employed diagnostic x-ray imaging modality that is considered to be a relatively high radiation exposure examination. Currently this is of even more concern because of the increasing use of multislice spiral (helical) CT scanners employing small slice thickness. With higher radiation exposure to the patient, there is an increased associated cancer risk. For this reason, physicians ordering such procedures must weigh the benefits of the procedure for the patient in terms of medical information gained and determine if these benefits outweigh the risk involved.

Concerns Related to Patient Dose: Skin Dose and Dose Distribution

Two concerns relate to patient dose in CT scanning. One concern is the *skin* dose, and the other is the *dose distribution* during the scanning procedure. When compared with any routine radiographic projection of an adult cranium or a single AP projection of the abdomen, the entrance exposure received by the patient after a succession of adjacent scans is greater than the entrance exposure from an individual x-ray projection. However, when a patient undergoes an ordinary but complicated x-ray examination, many radiographs involving different projections are obtained. If the doses from this extensive radiographic series are added together, the sum is comparable to the dose from a CT examination. Still another consideration exists. CT examinations generally expose a smaller mass of tissue than that exposed during an ordinary x-ray series. This is because the CT x-ray beam is more tightly collimated than the conventional radiographic beam. The entrance exposure from a CT examination also may be compared with the entrance exposure received during a routine fluoroscopic examination. In this instance, the entrance exposure received during a CT examination is generally considerably less than that received during a routine fluoroscopic procedure.

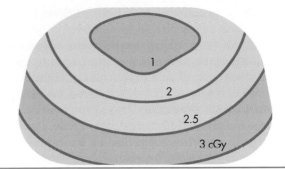

FIG. 8-36. Typical distribution of the doses deposited in a single-slice CT examination. For multiple contiguous slices, the doses may be twice these values.

The dose distribution resulting from a CT scan is not the same as the dose distribution occurring in routine radiologic procedures (Fig. 8-36). Because CT scanners use an x-ray beam that is tightly collimated, the amount of scatter radiation generated is lower than the scatter produced by the less tightly collimated radiographic beam. Also because of this, the mass of human tissue exposed to radiation falls off rapidly outside the plane of concern during the production of any given scan. Although in single slice scanners only one cross-sectional tomographic plane (slice) is exposed and imaged at a time (in the latest generation of scanners multiple slices are acquired simultaneously), some overlap of the margins of the x-ray beam occurs when each single tomographic section is made. Also, when as usual a series of adjacent slices are obtained, some radiation scatters from the slice being made into the adjacent slices (*interslice scatter*). Both of these contribute to dose increase and are the reasons that a succession of adjacent tomographic sections (slices) imparts a higher absorbed dose than would a single tomographic section.

Approximate Doses for Head and Body CT Imaging

Depending on the type of CT imaging system and the examination technique, Bushong identifies typical average CT dose range from 30 to 50 mGy (3000 to 5000 mrads) during head imaging and 40 to 60 mGy (4000 to 6000 mrads) during body imaging.[5] Actual doses delivered during any CT scanning procedure depend on the type of scanner being used and the radiation technical exposure factors selected. The tight collimation of the CT beam makes possible its accurate placement relative to the area of anatomy to be studied, which permits CT technologists to avoid exposing selected radiosensitive organs (e.g., the eyes).

Direct Patient Shielding

Direct patient shielding is not typically used in CT. Because of the rotational nature of the exposure, a shield is no more effective than the collimators that already exist on the device. Because the beam is so tightly collimated to the slice thickness, exposure to anatomy outside the field of view is usually only caused by internal scatter. Generally, in CT, anatomy does not appear in the primary x-ray beam unless it is part of the intended field of view.

Spiral/Helical CT

Spiral CT presents a greater challenge for assessing patient dose than does conventional CT. It is defined as a "data acquisition method that combines a continuous gantry rotation with a continuous table movement to form a spiral path of scan data."[23] It is also called *helical CT*.

When spiral scan pitch ratio (pitch), which is the relationship between the movement or advance of the patient couch (also known as table increment "I") and the x-ray beam collimator dimension (let us call it "Z" so that pitch = I/Z) is about 1, spiral CT patient dose is comparable with that produced by conventional CT. However, when the pitch is higher (e.g., 2:1), patient dose is reduced in comparison with conventional CT because less of the patient is exposed during the scan. The reverse also is true; patient dose increases at a lower pitch.

Other Factors That Influence Patient Dose

Patient dose also may be influenced by other factors. Changes in noise level (the random variation in pixel brightness seen when an image is made of too few photons, i.e., if the mA is made too low in a CT scan), pixel (individual picture element) size, and slice thickness all affect patient dose. The use of smaller pixel sizes for better resolution, the selection of thinner slices, and the increase of tube mA all increase the patient's absorbed dose. These relationships are summarized as follows.

Summary of Relationships Equation:

$$D = K\left(\frac{SNR^2}{e^3h}\right)$$

where *SNR* is the "signal-to-noise" ratio (i.e., the comparison of the average CT number in a region with the statistical variation of CT number in that region), *e* is the size of the smallest resolvable object, and *h* is the slice thickness. *K* is simply a constant of proportionality that depends on the special properties or characteristics of each scanner. The value of this constant is determined by measurement. The signal-to-noise ratio is an indicator of the "smoothness" of the image and is related to the ability to detect low-contrast objects (e.g., a liver tumor within liver tissues). The equation shows that the dose is proportional to the square of the SNR and therefore attempting to increase the SNR (by increasing the tube mA) results in a noticeably higher patient dose. Dose also increases if CT technologists attempt to resolve smaller objects by setting thinner slice widths without sacrificing any SNR.

Goal of CT Imaging from a Radiation Protection Point of View

From a radiation protection point of view, the goal of CT imaging should be to obtain the best possible image while delivering a reasonable dose of ionizing radiation to the patient (optimize the dose to the patient). In the absence of specially designed scan protocols, the fulfillment of this responsibility lies with the technologist performing the examination.

PEDIATRIC CONSIDERATIONS

Vulnerability of Children to Radiation Exposure

With regard to the potential for biologic damage from exposure to ionizing radiation, children are much more vulnerable to both the late somatic effects and genetic effects of radiation than are adults. Hence, children require special consideration when undergoing diagnostic x-ray studies. Appropriate radiation protection methods must be used for each procedure.

Some of these methods are described in the following sections. Because children have a greater life expectancy, they may easily survive long enough to develop a leukemia induced by radiation or develop a radiogenic malignancy such as lung or thyroid cancer. In fact, according to studies published by Beebe and others in 1978, the risk of a radiation-induced leukemia in children after a substantial dose of ionizing radiation is about two times that of adults.[24] For low doses such as those generally encountered in diagnostic radiology, data are still inconclusive (see Chapter 6). With this consideration in mind, radiographers must take every precaution to minimize exposure to all pediatric patients.

Children Require Smaller Radiation Doses Than Adults Do

In general, smaller doses of ionizing radiation are sufficient to obtain useful images in pediatric imaging procedures than are necessary for adult imaging procedures. For example, an entrance exposure below 5 mR results from an AP projection of an infant's chest,[25] whereas the same projection or a PA projection of an adult's chest yields an entrance exposure ranging from 10 to 25 mR (see Table 1-5).

Patient Motion and Motion Reduction Methods

Patient motion is frequently a problem in diagnostic pediatric radiography. Because of the limited ability of children to understand the radiologic procedure and, in most cases, their limited ability to cooperate, children are less likely to remain still during a radiographic or fluoroscopic exposure. To solve or at least minimize this problem, the radiographer must employ very short exposure times by selecting a high mA station and also using effective immobilization techniques. For some examinations, such as chest radiography, special pediatric immobilization devices are available to hold the pediatric patient securely and safely in the required position, thus providing adequate immobilization (see Fig. 8-3). The use of such techniques along with the use of appropriate radiographic or fluoroscopic technical exposure factors and correct image processing methods greatly reduces or eliminates the need for repeat examinations that will increase patient dose.

Gaining Cooperation during the Procedure

The presence of technologists who have experience working with children is helpful. Rooms specially earmarked for pediatric studies also are beneficial. Such rooms contain not only the appropriate restraint devices but also suitable entertainment and distracting devices such as cartoon posters and puppets. The examination progresses most efficiently with the best hope for patient cooperation when the child feels less intimidated.

Gonadal Shielding and Gonadal Dose

The radiographer should be familiar with particular difficulties related to gonadal shielding in pediatric studies. First, if the gonadal tissue is more than 2 cm from the edge of the field of view (assuming good collimation), the use of a gonadal shield does not significantly affect the gonadal dose because in that case the dose is caused mainly by internal scatter. In small girls, the variation in anatomic location of the ovaries requires shielding of the iliac wings as well as the sacral area when shielding is needed.[25] Effective shielding may not be possible for some studies because it obscures the anatomy of interest.

Collimation

Collimation is especially important in pediatric studies. The automatic collimation system reduces the radiation field size to the dimensions of the image receptor, but because many pediatric patients are significantly smaller than the image receptor, further manual adjustment of collimation is sometimes necessary. As in any other radiographic study, reducing the field size to the anatomy of interest not only reduces patient exposure but also increases recorded image quality by decreasing scatter. Projection orientation also is important. Female patients who may be imaged in either PA or AP projection will receive significantly lower doses to the breast tissues in a PA projection.[26]

Patient Protection Adult and Child: Similarities and Necessary Changes

Essentially, the same patient protection methods used to reduce the radiation exposure for adults may be employed to reduce the radiation exposure for pediatric patients. In general, the techniques discussed in this chapter may be applied to meet the needs of infants or children. It should also be strongly noted that CT technical exposure factors normally used for adults are not appropriate for young children. The scan kVp can be lowered as well as the mAs per obtained slice. Unfortunately, many facilities have in the past routinely used the same factors for both adults and small children and continue to do so today because of an unwillingness to develop new scanning protocols because of the conflicting demands of pediatric protocols. Because of the overall vulnerability of children to ionizing radiation, it is imperative that facilities and imaging personnel make every conscious effort to develop and use protocols that are in the best interest of the children entrusted to their care.

PROTECTING THE PREGNANT OR POTENTIALLY PREGNANT PATIENT

Position of the American College of Radiology (ACR) on Abdominal Radiologic Exams of Female Patients

Because much evidence suggests that the developing embryo-fetus is especially radiation sensitive, special care is taken in radiography to prevent unnecessary exposure of the abdominal area of pregnant females. Unfortunately, many women are not aware that they are pregnant during the earliest stage of pregnancy, which means that exposure of the abdominal area of potentially pregnant (i.e., fertile) women is a concern. In 1970 the International Commission on Radiation Protection (ICRP) proposed a 10-day rule.[27] Based on the low degree of probability that a woman would be pregnant during the first 10 days after the onset of menstruation, this rule suggests that abdominal x-ray examinations of fertile women be postponed until sometime during the first 10 days after the onset of the next menstrual cycle if the results of the examination are not important in connection with an immediate

illness. However, such scheduling is difficult in many imaging departments, where sustained contact among the radiologist, the referring physician, and the patient is unlikely. Because most fertile women are not pregnant at any given time, the 10-day rule may unnecessarily postpone examinations for the majority of female patients. For this reason, the 10-day rule is now obsolete. The official position of the American College of Radiology (ACR), the major professional organization of radiologists in the United States, is as follows: "Abdominal radiological exams that have been requested after full consideration of the clinical status of a patient, including the possibility of pregnancy, need not be postponed or selectively scheduled."[28]

Elective Examinations

When the referring physician does not consider radiologic procedures urgent, they may be regarded as elective examinations and can be booked at an appropriate time to meet patient needs and safety. In NCRP Report No. 102, a recommendation was made to facilitate scheduling of elective examinations.[29,30] This recommendation states that elective abdominal examinations of women of childbearing years should be performed during the first few days following the onset of menses to minimize the possible irradiation of an embryo (Box 8-11).

Inadvertent Irradiation of a Pregnancy

In the event that a pregnant patient is inadvertently irradiated, a radiologic physicist should perform the

---

BOX 8-11

Recommendation from NCRP No. 102 to Facilitate Scheduling of Elective Procedures

Ideally, an elective abdominal examination of a woman of childbearing age should be performed during the first few days following the onset of menses to minimize the possibility of irradiating an embryo. In practice, the timeliness of medical needs should be the primary consideration in deciding the timing of the examination.

From National Council of Radiation Protection and Measurements (NCRP). Medical x-ray, electron beam, and gamma-ray protection up to 50 MeV (equipment, design, performance, and use). Report No. 102, Bethesda, Md, 1989, NCRP.

BOX 8-12

Position of the NCRP Concerning Risk and Fetal Exposure Regarding Termination of Pregnancy[30]

This risk is considered to be negligible at 5 rad or less when compared to other risks of pregnancy, and the risk of malformations is significantly increased above control levels only at doses above 15 rad. Therefore, the exposure of the fetus to radiation arising from diagnostic procedures would rarely be cause, by itself, for terminating a pregnancy. If there are reasons other than possible radiation effects to consider a therapeutic abortion, the attending physician should discuss those reasons with the patient so that it is clear that the radiation exposure is not being used as an excuse for terminating the pregnancy.

From National Council on Radiation Protection and Measurements (NCRP): Medical exposure of pregnant and potentially pregnant women, Report No. 54, Washington, D.C., 1977, NCRP.

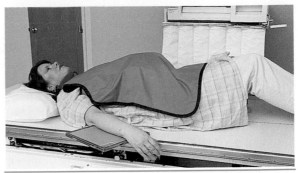

FIG. 8-37. To protect a developing embryo-fetus from unnecessary radiation exposure, place a lead apron over the female patient's lower abdomen and pelvic region when they do not have to be included in the area to be irradiated.

calculations necessary to determine fetal exposure. This may include taking measurements using phantoms to simulate the patient and using ion chambers to record exposure. The following question sometimes arises: Should a therapeutic abortion be performed to prevent the birth of an infant because of radiation exposure during pregnancy? Studies of groups such as the atomic bomb survivors of Hiroshima have shown that damage to the newborn is unlikely for doses below 20 rads. Because most medical procedures result in fetal exposures of less than 1 rad, the risk of abnormality is small. The position of the National Council on Radiation Protection and Measurements is stated in Box 8-12.[30]

Irradiating a Pregnant Patient

If the physician feels it is in the best interest of a pregnant or potentially pregnant patient to undergo a radiologic examination, the examination should be performed without delay. Under such circumstances, special efforts should be made to minimize the dose of radiation the patient receives to her lower abdomen and pelvic region. This can be accomplished by selecting technical exposure factors that are appropriate for the examination (i.e., by using the smallest exposure

that will generate a diagnostically useful radiograph) and by precisely collimating the radiographic beam to include only the anatomic area of interest. When the patient's lower abdomen and pelvic region do not have to be included in the area to be irradiated, they should be protected with a lead apron or other suitable protective contact shield so that a developing embryo-fetus does not receive unnecessary radiation exposure (Fig. 8-37).

SUMMARY

➤ Effective communication with the patient is the first step in holistic patient care.
  ■ Imaging procedures should be explained in simple terms.
  ■ Patients must have an opportunity to ask questions and receive truthful answers within ethical limits.
➤ Adequate immobilization of the patient is necessary to eliminate voluntary motion.
  ■ Restraining devices are available to immobilize either the whole body or the individual body part to be radiographed.
  ■ Involuntary motion can be compensated for by shortening exposure time with an appropriate increase in mA and by using very-high-speed image receptors.
➤ X-ray beam limitation devices must be used to confine the useful beam before it enters the anatomic area of clinical interest.

■ Aperture diaphragms, cones, and extension cylinders and the light-localizing variable-aperture rectangular collimator are the beam limitation devices used.

■ The patient's skin surface should always be at least 15 cm below the collimator to minimize exposure to the epidermis.

■ Good coincidence between the x-ray beam and the light-localizing beam of the collimator is necessary; both alignment and width dimensions of the two beams must correspond to within 2% of the SID.

■ According to the regulatory standard presently in effect, 2% of the SID is required with PBL devices.

➤ Exposure to the patient's skin may be reduced through proper filtration of the radiographic beam.

■ Inherent filtration amounting to 0.5-mm aluminum equivalent is required.

■ Together the inherent and added filtration constitute the total filtration. Stationary x-ray units operating above 70 kVp are required to have a total filtration of 2.5-mm aluminum equivalent.

■ The HVL of the beam is measured to determine whether an x-ray beam is adequately filtered.

➤ Protective shielding may be used to reduce or eliminate radiation exposure to radiosensitive body organs and tissues.

■ The reproductive organs should be protected from exposure to the useful beam when they are in or within approximately 5 cm of a properly collimated beam, unless this would compromise the diagnostic value of the study.

■ Correctly placed, appropriate gonadal shielding can greatly reduce the exposure received by both sexes (50% reduction for females, 90% to 95% reduction for males).

➤ The clear lead shadow shield and a PA projection can significantly reduce the dose to the breast of a young patient undergoing a scoliosis examination.

➤ Compensating filters are used in radiography to provide uniform imaging of body parts when considerable variation in thickness or tissue composition exists.

➤ Appropriate technical exposure factors for each examination must be selected.

■ Techniques chosen should ensure a diagnostic image of optimal quality with minimum patient dose.

■ Standardized technique charts should be available for each x-ray unit to help provide a uniform selection of technical exposure factors. High kVp and lower mAs should be chosen whenever possible to reduce the amount of radiation received by the patient, yet maintain acceptable radiographic contrast.

➤ Although the use of radiographic grids increases patient dose in radiography, their use for examination of thicker body parts is a fair compromise because they remove scattered radiation emanating from the patient that would otherwise degrade the recorded image.

■ An air gap technique can be used as an alternative to the use of a grid.

➤ Repeat radiographic exposures must be minimized to prevent the patient's skin and gonads from receiving a double dose of radiation.

➤ To limit the effects of inverse square falloff of radiation intensity with distance during a mobile radiographic examination, an SSD of at least 12 inches (30 cm) must be used.

➤ With digital radiography, the latent image formed by x-ray photons on a radiation detector is actually an electronic latent image. It is called a *digital image* because it is produced by computer representation of anatomical information. The image receptor is divided into small detector elements that make up the picture elements, or pixels, of the digital image. The pixels collectively represent the information contained in a volume of tissue. Radiographers must select correct technical exposure factors the first time to avoid overexposing patients when digital images are obtained.

➤ Computed radiography results when the invisible, or latent, image generated in conventional radiography is produced in a digital format using computer technology. The digital image can be displayed on a monitor for viewing, and it can be printed on a laser film when hard copy is needed.

➤ Fluoroscopic procedures produce the greatest patient radiation exposure rate in diagnostic radiology.

■ Minimize patient exposure time whenever possible.

- Limit the size of the fluoroscopic field to include only the area of anatomy that is of clinical interest.
- Employ the practice of intermittent, or pulsed, fluoroscopy to reduce the overall length of exposure.
- Select the correct technical exposure factors to help minimize the amount of radiation received by a patient.
- Ensure that the x-ray source-to-skin distance (SSD) is no less than 15 inches (38 cm) for stationary (fixed) fluoroscopes and no less than 12 inches (30 cm) for mobile fluoroscopes.

➤ During C-arm fluoroscopic procedures, the patient-image intensifier distance should be as short as possible.

➤ Cinefluorography can result in the highest patient doses of all diagnostic procedures.
- Reduce patient dose by using intermittent activation of the fluoroscope to locate the catheter, limiting the time of the cine run, and using the last-hold feature to view the most recent image.

➤ HLC fluoroscopy is used for interventional procedures.
- The operating mode uses exposure rates that are substantially higher than those allowed for routine fluoroscopic procedures.
- If skin dose is received in the range of 1 to 2 Gy (100 to 200 rads), the FDA requires that a notation be placed in the patient's record.

➤ The amount of radiation received by a patient from diagnostic radiologic procedures may be specified as ESE, skin dose, gonadal dose, or bone marrow dose.
- ESE is the easiest to obtain and most widely used.
- The estimated GSD for the population of the United States is about 0.20 mSv (20 mrem).

➤ Nonpalpable breast cancer may be detected through mammography.
- Federal regulations state that the mean dose to the glandular tissue of a 4.5-cm compressed breast using a screen-film mammography system should not exceed 3 mGy (300 mrads) per view.

➤ CT scanning is considered a relatively high radiation exposure diagnostic procedure because of increasing use of multislice spiral (helical) CT scanners employing small slice thickness.

- Skin dose and dose distribution are two concerns.
- In spiral CT, patient dose is comparable with that of conventional CT when pitch ratio is about 1; patient dose is reduced when pitch is higher and increased when pitch is lower.

➤ Children are much more vulnerable than adults to both the late somatic and genetic effects of ionizing radiation.
- Use a PA projection to protect breasts of female patients.
- In small girls, shielding of the ovaries requires shielding of the iliac wings as well as the sacral area when shielding is needed.
- Adequate collimation of the radiographic beam to include only the area of clinical interest is essential.

➤ A developing embryo-fetus is especially sensitive to exposure from ionizing radiation.
- Use the smallest technical exposure factors that will generate a diagnostically useful radiographic image, carefully collimate the beam to include only the anatomic area of interest, and cover the lower abdomen and pelvic region with a suitable contact shield if they do not need to be included in the examination.
- A radiologic physicist should determine fetal dose if a pregnant patient is inadvertently irradiated.

References

1. Torres LS: *Basic medical techniques and patient care for radiologic technologists,* ed 5, p. 20, Philadelphia, 1997, Lippincott Williams & Wilkins.
2. Edwards C, Statkiewicz-Sherer MA, Ritenour ER: *Radiation protection for dental radiographers,* Denver, 1984, Multi-Media.
3. National Council on Radiation Protection and Measurements (NCRP): *Medical x-ray, electron beam and gamma ray protection for energies up to 50 MeV: equipment design, performance, and use,* Report No. 102, Bethesda, Md, 1989, NCRP.
4. Frank ED: Technical aspects of mammography: In Carlton RR, Adler AM: *Principles of radiographic imaging: an art and a science,* ed 3, Albany, 2001, Delmar.
5. Bushong SC: *Radiologic science for technologists: physics, biology and protection,* ed 8, p. 589, St Louis, 2004, Mosby.

6. Gray J et al: *Quality control in diagnostic imaging*, Baltimore, 1983, University Park Press.

7. Hendee WR, Chaney EL, Rossi RP: *Radiologic physics equipment and quality control*, Chicago, 1977, Year Book.

8. McKinney W: *Radiographic processing and quality control*, Philadelphia, 1988, JB Lippincott.

9. Eastman Kodak Company, Rochester, New York, Available at http://Kodak.com/global/en/health/productsByType/medFilmSys/film/gen/hyperg.jhtml.

10. FDA Publication No. 86-8265, Pre-surgical chest x-ray screening examinations, Washington, DC, Superintendent of Documents, US Government Printing Office.

11. Roberts TD: *The effect of computers in imaging and radiation safety*. Available at http://XrayCredits.com. Accessed September 3, 2004.

12. Seeram E: Digital image processing, *RadiolTechnol*, 75:6, 2004.

13. Cullinan AM, Cullinan JE: *Producing quality radiographs*, ed 2, Philadelphia, 1994, JB Lippincott.

14. Ballinger PW, Frank ED: *Merrill's atlas of radiographic positions and radiologic procedures*, ed 10, vol 1, St Louis, 2003, Mosby.

15. Carlton RR, Adler AM: *Principles of radiographic imaging: an art and a science*, ed 3, Albany, 2001, Delmar.

16. National Council on Radiation Protection and Measurements (NCRP): *Medical x-ray, electron beam and gamma-ray protection for energies up to 50 MeV (equipment design, performance and use)*, Report No. 102, Bethesda, Md, 1989, NCRP.

17. Office of the Federal Register: *Federal Register* August 15, 1972 (37 FR 16461), Washington, DC, 1972, US Government Printing Office.

18. Huda W, Sourkes AM, Bews JA et al: Radiation doses due to breast imaging in Manitoba: 1978-1988, *Radiology* 177:812, 1990.

19. Ritenour ER, Hendee WR: Screening mammography: a risk vs risk decision, *Invest Radiol* 24:17, 1989.

20. Taubes G: The breast-screening brawl, *Science* 275:1056, 1997.

21. Office of the Federal Register: *Federal Register* 42CFR494 (d). 251, 53525, Washington, DC, US Government Printing Office.

22. Yaffe M, Mawdslwy GE: Equipment requirements and quality control for mammography, in specification, acceptance testing and quality control of diagnostic x-ray imaging equipment. In Siebert JA, Barnes GT, Gould RG, editors: *American Association of Physicists in Medicine, medical physics monograph No. 20*, College Park, Md, 1994, American Association of Physicists in Medicine.

23. Ballinger PW, Frank ED: *Merrill's atlas of radiographic positions and radiologic procedures*, ed 10, vol 3, p. 352-353, St Louis, 2003, Mosby.

24. Beebe GW, Kato H, Land DE: Studies of the mortality of A-bomb survivors. 6. Mortality and radiation dose, 1950-1974, *Radiat Res* 75:138, 1978.

25. National Council on Radiation Protection and Measurements (NCRP): *Radiation protection in pediatric radiology*, Report No. 68, Washington, DC, 1981, NCRP.

26. Bontrager KL: *Textbook of positioning and related anatomy*, ed 4, St Louis, 1997, Mosby.

27. International Commission on Radiation Protection: *Protection of the patient in x-ray diagnosis*, Publication No. 16, Oxford, England, 1970, Pergamon Press.

28. Reynold FB: Prepared remarks for the October 20, 1976, American College of Radiology press conference.

29. National Council on Radiation Protection and Measurements (NCRP): *Medical x-ray, electron beam and gamma-ray protection up to 50 MeV (equipment design, performance and use)*, Report No. 102, Bethesda, Md, 1989, NCRP.

30. National Council on Radiation Protection and Measurements (NCRP): *Medical exposure of pregnant and potentially pregnant women*, Report No. 54, Washington, DC, 1977, NCRP.

GENERAL DISCUSSION QUESTIONS

1. How does the patient benefit from effective communication with the radiographer during an imaging procedure?

2. What can the radiographer do to eliminate the problem of voluntary patient motion and how can involuntary motion be compensated for during radiography?

3. How do aperture diaphragms, cones and cylinders, and collimators reduce the amount of scattered radiation being produced during a radiographic examination?

4. How does filtration of the radiographic beam reduce exposure to the patient's skin and superficial tissues?

5. When should half-value layer of a diagnostic x-ray tube be measured?

6. When should gonadal shielding not be used during a radiographic examination?

7. How can the dose to the breast of a young female patient be reduced when performing a radiographic examination for scoliosis?

8. Why does the use of carbon fiber in a radiographic film-cassette lower patient dose?

9. Why is the use of a radiographic grid a fair compromise, if the use of it increases patient dose?

10. What can a radiographer do to avoid overexposing the patient when using a computed radiographic system?

11. What effect does the use of intermittent, or pulsed, fluoroscopy have on patient dose?

12. Why is there concern over the use of mobile C-arm fluoroscopes during surgical, vascular, interventional, or other potentially lengthy procedures?

13. What dose reduction techniques can radiologists or cardiologists implement to reduce exposure during cinefluorographic procedures?

14. What strategies can physicians use during interventional fluoroscopic procedures to control patient radiation dose and minimize exposure to occupationally exposed personnel and any other assisting personnel?

15. What is the position of the American College of Radiology (ACR) regarding abdominal radiologic examinations of pregnant or potentially pregnant patients?

REVIEW QUESTIONS

1. **The radiographic beam should be collimated so that it is which of the following?**
   A. Slightly larger than the image receptor
   B. No larger than the image receptor
   C. Twice as large as the image receptor
   D. Four times as large as the image receptor

2. **Both alignment and length and width dimensions of the radiographic and light beams must correspond to within:**
   A. 1% of the SID
   B. 2% of the SID
   C. 5% of the SID
   D. 10% of the SID

3. **What is the function of a filter in diagnostic radiology?**
   A. To permit only alpha rays to reach the patient's skin
   B. To permit only beta particles to interact with the atoms of the patient's body
   C. To decrease the x-radiation dose to the patient's skin and superficial tissue
   D. To remove gamma radiation from the useful beam

4. **HVL may be defined as the thickness of a designated absorber required to do which of the following?**
   A. Increase the intensity of the primary beam by 50% of its initial value
   B. Increase the intensity of the primary beam by 25% of its initial value
   C. Decrease the intensity of the primary beam by 50% of its initial value
   D. Decrease the intensity of the primary beam by 25% of its initial value

5. **A woman who is 3 months pregnant has been in a motor vehicle accident. The emergency room physician suspects there is injury to her cervical spine and thus feels justified in ordering an x-ray to aid in determining the extent of the patient's injury. Because the patient is pregnant, the radiographer should:**
   1. **Select the smallest technical exposure factors that will produce a diagnostically useful radiograph**
   2. **Adequately and precisely collimate the radiographic beam to include only the anatomic area of interest**
   3. **Shield the patient's lower abdomen and pelvic region with a suitable protective contact shield**
   A. 1 only
   B. 2 only
   C. 3 only
   D. 1, 2, and 3

6. **Pediatric patients require special consideration and appropriate radiation protection procedures because they are more vulnerable to which of the following?**
   A. Both the late somatic effects and genetic effects of radiation
   B. Only the late somatic effects of radiation
   C. Only the genetic effects of radiation
   D. Only the early somatic effects of radiation

7. **The use of the PA projection during a juvenile scoliosis radiographic examination results in which of the following?**
   A. Higher entrance exposure dose to the anterior body surface, thereby significantly increasing the dose to the breast
   B. Lower entrance exposure dose to the anterior body surface, thereby significantly reducing the dose to the breast
   C. Poorer quality radiographs that necessitate a repeat examination
   D. Radiographs that do not adequately demonstrate spinal curvature

8. **Federal regulations in the United States for Food and Drug Administration Certification of screening mammography facilities state that the mean dose to the glandular tissue of a 4.5-cm compressed breast using a screen-film mammography system should *not* exceed which of the following?**
   A. 1 mGy (100 rads) per view
   B. 3 mGy (300 rads) per view
   C. 5 mGy (500 rads) per view
   D. 7 mGy (700 rads) per view

9. **To *decrease* patient exposure during fluoroscopic procedures, the fluoroscopist can:**
   1. Limit the size of the fluoroscopic field to include only the area of anatomy that is of clinical interest
   2. Employ the practice of intermittent, or pulsed, fluoroscopy to reduce the overall length of exposure
   3. Choose to use a conventional fluoroscope instead of an image intensification fluoroscope

   A. 1 and 2 only
   B. 1 and 3 only
   C. 2 and 3 only
   D. 1, 2, and 3

10. **If a maximum of 500 people were inhabiting the earth and each person received an equivalent dose (EqD) of 0.005 Sv (0.5 rem) gonadal radiation, the gross genetic effect would be _____ the effect occurring when 50 individual inhabitants each receive 0.05 Sv (5 rem) of gonadal radiation and no equivalent dose is received by other inhabitants.**
   A. Greatly different than
   B. Slightly different than
   C. Almost the same as
   D. Identical to

9 Protection of Imaging Personnel During Diagnostic X-Ray Procedures

KEY TERMS

Bucky slot shielding device
control-booth barrier
controlled area
cumulative effective dose
   (CumEfD) limit
diagnostic-type protective tube
   housing
distance

genetically significant dose
   (GSD)
inverse square law (ISL)
leakage radiation
occupancy factor (T)
occupational risk
primary protective barrier
primary radiation

scatter radiation
secondary protective barrier
shielding
time
uncontrolled area
use factor (U)
workload (W)

OBJECTIVES

After completing this chapter, the reader will be able to perform the following:

- State the annual occupational effective dose limit for whole body exposure of diagnostic imaging personnel during routine operations and explain the significance of the ALARA concept for these individuals.
- Explain the reason that occupational exposure of diagnostic imaging personnel must be limited and state the most important reason for allowing a larger equivalent dose for radiation workers than for the population as a whole.
- Identify the type of x-radiation that poses the greatest occupational hazard in diagnostic radiology and explain the various ways this hazard can be reduced or eliminated.
- Explain the way various methods and techniques that reduce patient exposure during a diagnostic examination also reduce exposure for the radiographer and other diagnostic personnel.
- Discuss the responsibilities of the employer for protecting declared pregnant diagnostic imaging personnel from radiation exposure.
- List and explain the three basic principles of radiation protection that can be used for personnel exposure reduction.
- State and explain the inverse square law by solving mathematical problems applying its concept.
- Explain the purpose of a diagnostic-type protective tube housing, differentiate between a primary and a secondary protective barrier, and list examples of each.
- Describe the construction of protective structural shielding, and list the factors that govern the selection of appropriate construction materials.
- List and describe the protective garments that may be worn to reduce whole- or partial-body exposure, and discuss the circumstances in which such garments are worn.
- Explain the various methods and devices that may be used to reduce exposure for personnel during routine fluoroscopic examinations and during interventional procedures that use high-level-control fluoroscopy.
- Explain the various methods and devices that may be used to reduce the radiographer's exposure during a mobile radiographic examination.
- Explain the variation in dose rate caused by scatter radiation near the entrance and exit surfaces of the patient during C-arm fluoroscopy.
- Describe methods used to provide patient restraint during a diagnostic x-ray procedure and identify individuals who might use them.
- List the three categories of radiation sources that may be generated in an x-ray room; list the considerations on which the design of radiation-absorbent barriers should be based; and explain the importance of each.
- Differentiate between a controlled area and an uncontrolled area.
- Discuss new approaches to shielding design.

While fulfilling professional responsibilities associated with diagnostic imaging, radiographers may be exposed to secondary radiation (scatter or leakage). Some x-ray procedures increase the radiographer's risk of exposure (Box 9-1). When participating in any procedure that may result in occupational exposure, the radiographer must employ appropriate methods of protection against ionizing radiation. This chapter presents an overview of methods that may be used to reduce exposure for imaging professionals during diagnostic x-ray procedures.

ANNUAL LIMIT FOR OCCUPATIONALLY EXPOSED PERSONNEL

Effective Dose Limits

Federal government standards, enforcing a recommendation of the National Council on Radiation Protection and Measurements (NCRP) (previously discussed in Chapter 7), permit diagnostic imaging personnel to receive an "annual occupational effective dose (EfD) of 50 millisievert (mSv) (5 rem)"[1] for whole-body exposure during routine operations. This effective dose does not include personal medical and natural background exposure. To ensure that the lifetime risk of occupationally exposed persons remains acceptable, an additional recommendation indicates that the *lifetime effective dose* in mSv should not exceed 10 times the occupationally exposed person's age in years. Hence a **cumulative effective dose (CumEfD) limit** has been established for the whole body that limits a radiation worker's lifetime effective dose to his or her age in years times 10 mSv (years × 1 rem).

Annual Occupational and Nonoccupational Effective Dose Limits

The annual occupational effective dose limit of 50 mSv (5 rem) is an upper boundary limit. It is greater than the annual effective dose limit allowed for individual members of the general population not occupationally exposed. That limit is 1 mSv (0.1 rem) for continuous or frequent exposures from artificial sources other than medical irradiation and natural background radiation[1] and 5 mSv (0.5 rem) for infrequent annual exposure.[1] The 1 mSv (0.1 rem) annual effective dose limit set for members of the general public is designed to limit that exposure "to reasonable levels of risk comparable with risks from other common sources—i.e., about 10^{-4} to 10^{-6} annually"[1] (10^{-4} to 10^{-6} means an excess cancer risk of one chance in 10,000 to one chance in 1 million per year). The 5 mSv (0.5 rem) maximal annual effective dose limit recommendation "is made because annual exposures in excess of the 1 mSv recommendation, usually to a small group of people, need not be regarded as especially hazardous, provided it does not occur often to the same groups and that the average exposure to individuals in these groups does not exceed an average annual effective dose of about 1 mSv."[1] Both these limits "will keep the annual equivalent dose to those organs and tissues that are considered in the effective dose system below levels of concern for deterministic effects."[1]

Allowance for a Larger Equivalent Dose for Radiation Workers

Valid reasons exist for allowance of a larger equivalent dose (EqD) (the product of the average absorbed dose [D] in a tissue or organ in the human body and its associated radiation weighting factor [W_R] chosen for the type and energy of the radiation in question [see Chapter 3 for additional information]) for radiation workers. Among the most important of these reasons is that the workforce in radiation-related jobs is small

---

BOX 9-1

Imaging Procedures That Increase the Radiographer's Risk of Exposure

- General fluoroscopy
- Interventional procedures that employ high-level-control fluoroscopy (HLCF)
- Mobile examinations
- General radiographic procedures
- C-arm fluoroscopy

when compared with the population as a whole. Thus, the amount of radiation received by this workforce can be larger than the amount received by the general public without altering the **genetically significant dose (GSD),** the average annual gonadal equivalent dose to members of the population who are of child-bearing age (see Chapter 8). This means that the extra amount of radiation absorbed by the radiation work-force does not significantly increase the total number of deleterious mutations in the United States. Although the radiographer and other diagnostic imaging personnel are allowed to absorb more radia-tion, the equivalent dose received must be minimized whenever possible. This reduces the potential for somatic and genetic damage.

ALARA CONCEPT

In addition to the effective dose limiting system, another radiation protection principle exists—the ALARA concept. As defined in Chapter 7, this concept holds that occupational exposure of the radiographer and other occupationally exposed persons should be kept "as low as reasonably achiev-able," with consideration of economic and social factors. This implies that actual effective and equiva-lent dose values should be kept well below their allow-able maximal limits. The best way for radiologists and radiographers to do this is to conscientiously employ appropriate radiation-control procedures such as, for example, adequate collimation of the radiographic beam (Fig. 9-1). Because continual use of such radia-tion protection-awareness procedures ensures a high degree of safety from most radiation exposures, radiog-raphy is not considered a hazardous profession. The **occupational risk** (i.e., the possibility of developing a radiogenic cancer or the induction of a genetic defect as a consequence of the radiation exposure received) for monitored diagnostic imaging personnel may be compared with the occupational risk for persons employed in other industries generally considered rea-sonably safe such as government and trade. These jobs have a risk of fatal accidents generally estimated to be about $1 \times 10^{-4} \, y^{-1}$.[1] The annual risk for radiation workers is unlikely to exceed this rate.

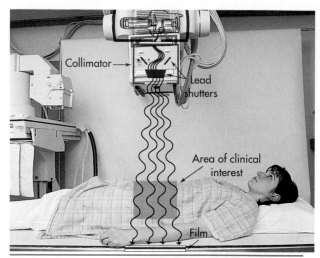

FIG. 9-1. Radiographic beam collimation (restricting the x-ray beam to the area of clinical interest) limits the production of scattered radiation. This radiation-control procedure helps keep the radiographer's occupational exposure as low as rea-sonably achievable (ALARA).

DOSE REDUCTION METHODS AND TECHNIQUES

Avoiding Repeat Examinations

Methods and techniques that reduce patient exposure also reduce exposure for the radiographer. For example, when using screen-film systems, repeat examinations should be avoided whenever possible to eliminate additional occupational exposure. Other such consid-erations are identified in this chapter.

The Patient as a Source of Scattered Radiation

During a diagnostic examination, the patient becomes a source of scattered radiation as a consequence of the Compton interaction process (see Chapter 2). At a 90-degree angle to the primary x-ray beam, at a distance of 1 m (3.3 feet), the scattered x-ray intensity is gen-erally approximately 1/1000 of the intensity of the primary x-ray beam.

Scattered Radiation—Occupational Hazard

Because scattered radiation poses the greatest occupational hazard in diagnostic radiology, the use of any device or appropriate technique that lessens the amount of scattered radiation significantly reduces occupational exposure of diagnostic imaging personnel. Beam limitation devices such as the positive beam limitation (PBL)–equipped light-localizing variable-aperture rectangular collimator restrict the size of the radiographic beam so that its margins do not extend beyond the image receptor. This reduction in beam size results in a decrease in the number of x-ray photons available to undergo Compton scatter. Because scatter is reduced, the radiographer's occupational exposure is reduced.

Filtration of the Diagnostic X-Ray Beam

When a radiographic beam is properly filtered, nonuseful low-energy photons are removed from the primary beam. Without proper filtration, a relatively high percentage of the normally excluded low-energy photons interact with the tissues of the patient's body. A portion of these photons undergo Compton scatter. The radiographer's equivalent dose could therefore increase as a result of exposure to this excess scattered radiation. Most of these low-energy photons, however, are absorbed in the patient, increasing the patient's absorbed dose and contributing nothing to the radiographic image. Thus filtration primarily benefits the patient.

Protective Apparel

Protective lead aprons (Fig. 9-2, A) and shielded barriers (Fig. 9-2, B) function as gonadal shields for diagnostic imaging personnel. These devices protect them from secondary (scatter and leakage) radiation.

Technical Exposure Factors

Technical exposure factors control the quantity of scattered radiation produced, although this effect is not very great. Higher peak kilovoltage techniques increase the mean energy of the photons composing the radiographic beam and also require lower photon

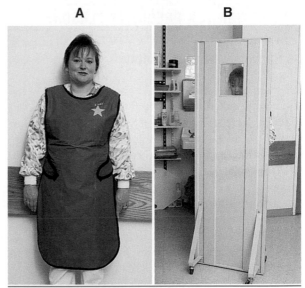

A   B

FIG. 9-2. **A,** A lead apron protects occupationally exposed personnel from scattered radiation. **B,** A lead mobile x-ray barrier of 0.5- or 1.0-mm lead equivalent provides protection from scattered radiation. It may be used during special procedures, in the operating room, and in cardiac units.

beam intensity (i.e., lower milliamperage). As the average energy of the beam increases, the percentage of radiation that is forward-scattered increases. Therefore less side-scattered radiation is available to reach the imaging personnel, and their equivalent dose is reduced.

Use of High-Speed Image Receptor Systems

When high-speed image receptor systems are used, smaller radiographic exposure (less milliamperage) is required, which results in fewer x-ray photons being available to produce Compton scatter. Because of this reduction in Compton scatter, personnel exposure is decreased.

Correct Radiographic Film Processing Techniques

Finally, the use of correct radiographic film processing techniques leads to a decrease in the number of repeat examinations required, with a resultant reduction in exposure to the radiographer.

PROTECTION FOR PREGNANT PERSONNEL

Imaging Department Protocol

Pregnant diagnostic imaging department staff members should be able to continue performing their duties without interruption of employment if they follow established radiation safety practices. Most health care facilities have policies for protecting pregnant personnel from radiation. Under these policies, an imaging professional who becomes pregnant first informs her supervisor. After this voluntary "declaration" has been made, the health care facility officially recognizes the pregnancy. The facility, through its radiation safety officer, provides essential counseling and furnishes an appropriate additional monitor. This device is to be worn at waist level during all radiation procedures. When a protective lead apron is worn, the additional monitor should be worn at waist level beneath the garment. The purpose of this additional monitor is to ensure that the monthly equivalent dose to the embryo-fetus does not exceed 0.5 mSv (0.05 rem). This equivalent dose limit excludes both medical and natural background radiation. It is designed to significantly restrict the total lifetime risk of leukemia and other malignancies in persons exposed in utero.

Acknowledgment of Counseling and Understanding of Radiation Safety Measures

After receiving radiation safety counseling, the pregnant radiologic technologist must read and sign a form acknowledging that she has received counseling and understands the ways to implement appropriate measures to ensure the safety of the embryo-fetus. For additionally monitored pregnant personnel, monitoring badge companies provide a separate monthly report that tracks the exposure of the worker and the embryo-fetus. A copy of this report is sent to the health care facility's radiation safety officer.

Protective Apparel

Protective maternity apparel should be available for pregnant radiologists and radiographers. Maternity protective aprons consist of 0.5-mm lead equivalent over their entire length and width, and also have an extra 1-mm lead equivalent protective panel that runs transversely across the width of the apron to provide added safety for the embryo-fetus.

Wraparound protective aprons of 0.5-mm lead equivalent can also be used during pregnancy. The size of the apron must be appropriate for the pregnant worker to ensure safety and provide reasonable comfort.

Work Schedule Alteration

In accordance with ALARA guidelines, work schedules are designed to evenly distribute radiation exposure risk to all employees. If a declared pregnant radiographer is reassigned to a lower radiation exposure risk area, other unknowing potentially pregnant radiographers can be subject to increased risk. Therefore, the declared pregnant radiographer does not necessarily need to be reassigned to a lower radiation exposure as a direct consequence of a declared pregnancy. However, it is imperative that the equivalent dose to the embryo-fetus from occupational exposure of the mother does not exceed the NCRP recommended monthly equivalent dose limit of 0.5 mSv (0.05 rem) or a limit of 5.0 mSv (0.50 rem) during the entire pregnancy (see Chapter 7, pp. 157 and 159).

BASIC PRINCIPLES OF RADIATION PROTECTION FOR PERSONNEL EXPOSURE REDUCTION

The three basic principles of radiation protection are *time, distance, and shielding.* Occupational radiation exposure of imaging personnel can be minimized by the use of these cardinal principles. Shortening the length of time spent in a room where x-radiation is being produced, standing at the greatest distance possible from an energized x-ray beam, and interposing a radiation-absorbent shielding material between the radiation worker and the source of radiation will reduce occupational exposure.

Time

The amount of radiation a worker receives is directly proportional to the length of **time** that the individual is exposed to ionizing radiation. As the length of exposure time increases, the radiation dose received increases in direct proportion. The reverse is also true. As the length of exposure time decreases, the radiation dose decreases in direct proportion. During fluoroscopy, reduced exposure time will decrease both patient and personnel exposure. For this reason, most fluoroscopic x-ray units are equipped with 5-minute timers to alert the radiologist or other authorized equipment operator that a specific period of time has elapsed. To minimize radiation exposure and utilize the cardinal principle of time effectively for this purpose, a radiographer should only be present in a fluoroscopic room when needed to perform relevant patient care and to fulfill respective duties associated with the procedure. When the presence of the radiographer is not required in the fluoroscopic room, the radiographer should remain behind a protective barrier.

Distance

Distance is the most effective means of protection from ionizing radiation. Imaging personnel receive significantly less radiation exposure by standing farther away from a source of radiation because there will be a significant decrease in the radiation level.

Application of the Inverse Square Law

The **inverse square law (ISL)** expresses the relationship between distance and intensity (quantity) of radiation and governs the dose received. The law is stated as follows: "The intensity of radiation is inversely proportional to the square of the distance from the source." To be more precise, as the distance between the radiation source and a measurement point increases, the quantity of radiation measured at the more distant position decreases by the square of the ratio of the original distance from the source to that of the new distance from the source (Fig. 9-3). This decrease in radiation intensity physically occurs because the area, which the same flux of x-rays at the original location now covers at the new location, has increased by the square of the relative distance change. For example, when the distance from the x-ray target, a point source of radiation, is doubled, the radiation at the new location spans an area four times larger than the original area. However, because the same amount

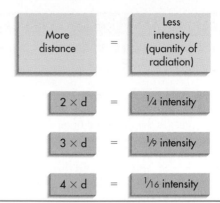

FIG. 9-3. As the distance between the source of radiation and any given measurement point increases, radiation intensity (quantity) measured at that point decreases by the square of the relative change in distance between the new location and the old.

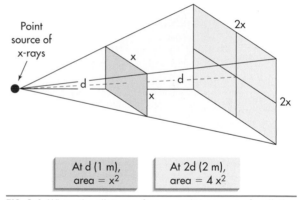

FIG. 9-4. When the distance from a point source of radiation is doubled, the radiation at the new location spans an area four times larger than the original area. However, the intensity at the new distance is only one fourth the original intensity.

of radiation exists to cover this larger area, the intensity at the new distance consequently decreases by a factor of four (Fig. 9-4).

The ISL may be stated as a formula, shown in the equation in Box 9-2. A mathematical example is also provided. The ISL for radiation should be utilized, whenever possible, to reduce the radiographer's exposure from sources of x-radiation. (This law also may be applied to sources of gamma and neutron radiation.)

BOX 9-2

Inverse Square Law Formula and Example

$$\frac{I_1}{I_2} = \frac{(d_2)^2}{(d_1)^2}$$

where I_1 expresses the exposure (intensity) at the original distance, I_2 expresses the exposure (intensity) at the new distance, d_1 expresses the original distance from the source of radiation, and d_2 expresses the new distance from the source of radiation.

EXAMPLE: If a radiographer stands 1 m away from an x-ray tube and is subject to an exposure rate of 2 mR per hour, what will the exposure rate be if the same radiographer moves to a position located 2 m from the x-ray tube?

ANSWER:

$$\frac{I_1}{I_2} = \frac{(d_2)^2}{(d_1)^2}$$

$$\frac{2}{I_2} = \frac{(2)^2}{(1)^2}$$

$$\frac{2}{I_2} = \frac{4}{1}(cross - multiply)$$

$$4I_2 = 2$$

$$I_2 = 0.5\,mR/hr$$

The ISL also implies that if a radiographer moves closer to a source of radiation, the radiation exposure to the radiographer *dramatically* increases. For example, according to the ISL, if the radiographer stands 2 feet away from an x-ray source instead of 6 feet, the radiographer's radiation exposure increases by a factor of $(6/2)^2 = 9$.

Shielding

When it is not possible to use the cardinal principles of time or distance to minimize occupational radiation exposure, protective lead-equivalent **shielding** of appropriate thickness may be used to provide protection from radiation. The most common materials used for structural protective barriers are lead and concrete. Accessory protective devices such as aprons, gloves, and thyroid shields are made of lead-impregnated

vinyl. This apparel provides protection from ionizing radiation when it is not possible to remain behind a stationary (fixed) or mobile protective barrier. The effectiveness of shielding materials (i.e., their ability to attenuate radiation) depends on their atomic number, density, and thickness.

Protective Structural Shielding

Structural barriers such as walls and doors in an x-ray room provide radiation shielding for both imaging department personnel and the general public. This protection is necessary to ensure that occupational and nonoccupational annual effective dose limits are not exceeded. Lead sheets of appropriate thickness placed in the walls of the radiographic or fluoroscopic room are generally used to provide proper shielding. A qualified medical physicist will determine the exact protection requirements for a particular imaging facility. Radiographers should understand the concept of shielding but are not responsible for determining barrier thickness.

Primary Protective Barrier The purpose of a **primary protective barrier** is to prevent direct, or unscattered, radiation from reaching personnel or members of the general public on the other side of the barrier. The primary beam is made up of the x-ray photons that follow straight-line paths between all sets of collimator shutters. Primary protective barriers are located perpendicular to the undeflected line of travel of the x-ray beam (Fig. 9-5). If the peak energy of the beam is 130 kVp, the primary protective barrier in a typical installation consists of 1/16-inch lead and extends 7 feet (2.1 m) upward from the floor of the x-ray room when the x-ray tube is 5 to 7 feet from the wall in question.

Secondary Protective Barrier Secondary radiation consists of radiation that has been deflected from the primary beam. Leakage from the tube housing (photons that pass through the housing because the lead shielding around the tube for practical reasons cannot be made perfect) and scatter (primarily from the patient) make up the secondary radiation. A **secondary protective barrier** protects against secondary radiation (leakage and scatter radiation). Any wall or barrier that is never struck by the primary x-ray beam is classified as a secondary barrier (see Fig. 9-5). This does not mean that secondary radiation cannot hit primary barriers as well. A secondary barrier should overlap the primary protective barrier by about

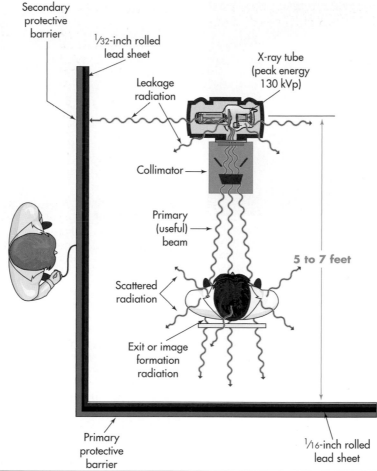

FIG. 9-5. Protective barriers are lined with lead to protect personnel and the general public from radiation. The primary protective barrier is located perpendicular to the undeflected line of travel of the x-ray beam. The walls that are not in the direct line of travel of the primary beam are called *secondary protective barriers,* because they are designed to shield against secondary (leakage and scattered) radiation.

1/2 inch. In a typical installation, the secondary barrier consists of 1/32-inch lead.

Control-booth barrier X-ray rooms housing stationary (fixed) radiographic equipment contain a **control-booth barrier** for the protection of the radiographer. This barrier must extend 7 feet (2.1 m) upward from the floor and must be permanently secured to it. Diagnostic x-rays should scatter a minimum of two times before reaching any area behind this barrier. Because this booth intercepts leakage and scattered radiation only, it may be

regarded as a secondary protective barrier. To ensure maximal protection during radiographic exposures, personnel must remain completely behind the barrier. The radiographer may observe the patient through the lead glass window in the booth (Fig. 9-6). This window typically consists of 1.5-mm lead equivalent. With the appropriate lead equivalent in the barrier, exposure of the radiographer shall not exceed a maximum allowance of 1 mSv (100 mrem) per week; in actual practice in a well-designed facility, exposure should not exceed 0.02 mSv (2 mrem) per week. For further

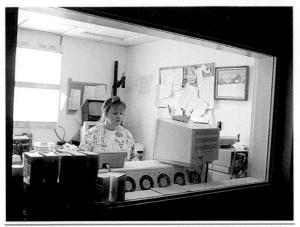

FIG. 9-6. While making a radiographic exposure with a stationary radiographic unit, the radiographer must remain completely within the control-booth barrier (behind the fixed protective barrier) for safety. The radiographer may observe the patient through the lead glass observation window in the control booth.

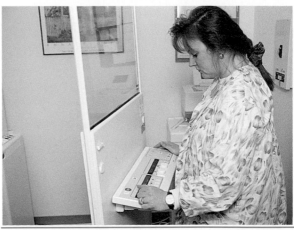

FIG. 9-7. A clear lead-plastic secondary protective barrier impregnated with approximately 30% lead lends a modern appearance to the facility.

protection, the exposure cord must be short enough so that the exposure switch can be operated only when the radiographer is completely behind the control-booth barrier.

Clear lead-plastic secondary protective barrier Clear lead-plastic material impregnated with approximately 30% lead by weight may be fashioned into an effective secondary protective barrier, such as for the control booth (Fig. 9-7). This creates a modern appearance for the facility and permits a panoramic view allowing diagnostic imaging personnel to observe the patient more completely. These modular x-ray barriers are shatter-resistant, can extend 7 feet upward from the floor, and are available in lead equivalency from 0.3 to 2 mm.

Clear lead-plastic overhead protective barrier Clear lead-plastic protective barriers also can be used as overhead x-ray barriers (Fig. 9-8) to provide an open view during special procedures and cardiac catheterization. This shielding typically offers 0.5-mm lead equivalency protection.

Accessory Protective Devices

As stated earlier in this chapter, accessory protective shielding includes aprons, gloves, and thyroid shields made of lead-impregnated vinyl.

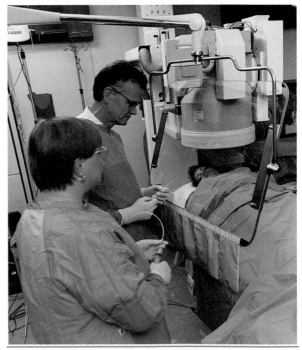

FIG. 9-8. A clear lead-plastic overhead protective barrier used during special procedures and cardiac catheterization. (Courtesy Fluke Biomedical.)

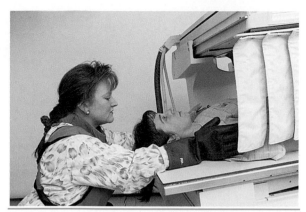

FIG. 9-9. A lead apron, gloves, and thyroid shield protect the radiographer from scattered radiation.

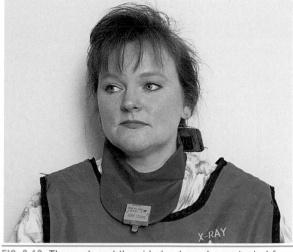

FIG. 9-10. The neck and thyroid gland can be protected from radiation exposure through the use of a 0.5-mm lead-equivalent protective shield.

Lead Aprons and Gloves Wraparound protective lead aprons and leaded gloves, if the radiographer's hands will be near the x-ray beam (Fig. 9-9), should be used whenever the radiographer cannot remain behind a protective lead barrier during an exposure. If the peak energy of the x-ray beam is 100 kVp, a protective lead apron must be equivalent to at least a 0.25-mm thickness of lead. A lead apron of 0.5- or 1-mm lead equivalent affords much greater protection. All three of these thicknesses are available for protective apparel. However, 0.5-mm lead equivalent is the most widely used and recommended thickness in diagnostic imaging.

Neck and Thyroid Shield A neck and thyroid shield (Fig. 9-10) can guard the thyroid area of occupationally exposed people during general fluoroscopy and x-ray special procedures. It should be a minimum of 0.5-mm lead equivalent.

Protective Eyeglasses Scatter Radiation to the lens of the eyes of diagnostic imaging personnel can be substantially reduced by wearing protective eyeglasses (Fig. 9-11) with optically clear lenses that contain a minimal lead equivalent protection of 0.35 mm. Side shields on the glasses are also available for procedures that require turning of the head. A wraparound frame containing optically clear lenses with a 0.5-mm lead equivalency is also available.

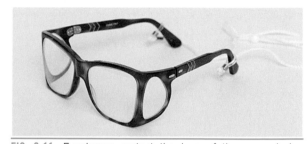

FIG. 9-11. Eyeglasses protect the lens of the eyes during general fluoroscopy and special procedures. (Shown are glasses with wrap-around frames; other styles are also available.)

DIAGNOSTIC-TYPE PROTECTIVE TUBE HOUSING

Requirement

A lead-lined metal **diagnostic-type protective tube housing** (Fig. 9-12) is required to protect both the radiographer and patient from off-focus, or leakage, radiation by restricting the emission of x-rays to the area of the useful, or primary, beam (those x-rays emitted through the x-ray tube window or port).

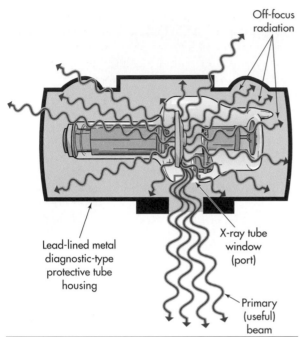

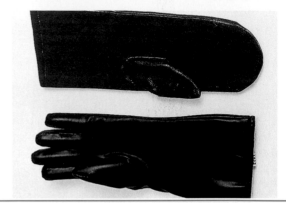

FIG. 9-13. Lead gloves.

FIG. 9-12. A lead-lined metal diagnostic-type protective tube housing protects the radiographer and the patient from off-focus, or leakage, radiation by restricting x-ray emission to the area of the primary (useful) beam.

X-Ray Tube Housing Construction

The housing enclosing the x-ray tube must be constructed so that leakage radiation measured at a distance of 1 m (3.3 feet) from the x-ray source does not exceed 100 mR/hour (2.58×10^{-5} C/kg)/hour when the tube is operated at its highest voltage at the highest current that allows continuous operation. Although the x-ray tube housing is designed to protect the operator from the hazard of electric shock, the radiographer must be careful when handling this piece of equipment and its adjoining part, the collimator. When manipulating the tube housing for a radiographic examination, the radiographer should avoid handling or severely bending the high- tension cables that connect to the positive and negative terminals of the x-ray tube. No one should touch the tube housing or high-tension cables while a radiographic exposure is in progress.

PROTECTION DURING FLUOROSCOPIC PROCEDURES

Personnel Protection

To ensure protection from scattered radiation emanating from the patient during a fluoroscopic examination, the radiographer should stand as far away from the patient as is practical and should move closer to the patient only when assistance is required. A protective apron of at least 0.5-mm lead equivalent must be worn during all fluoroscopic procedures. Protective lead gloves of at least 0.25-mm lead equivalent (Fig. 9-13) should be worn whenever the hands must be placed near the fluoroscopic field. Imaging personnel assisting during a fluoroscopic examination also should wear thyroid shields of 0.5-mm lead equivalent if they are standing in close proximity to the patient being examined (Fig. 9-14). If immediate presence assisting a radiologist during a fluoroscopic examination is not required near the x-ray table, the radiographer should either stand behind the radiologist who is also wearing protective apparel, or stand behind the control-booth barrier until his or her services are required. To protect personnel who must move around the x-ray room during a fluoroscopic examination, a wraparound protective apron is recommended.

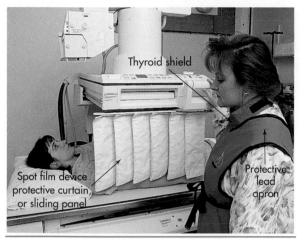

FIG. 9-14. Scattered radiation produced during a fluoroscopic examination can be absorbed by a spot-film device protective curtain, or sliding panel, with a minimum of 0.25-mm lead equivalent placed between the fluoroscopist and the patient.

Dose Reduction Techniques

Many of the methods and devices that reduce the radiographer's exposure when operating stationary (fixed) radiographic equipment also reduce the dose received by the radiographer and the radiologist during a fluoroscopic procedure. These methods and devices include adequate beam collimation, filtration, gonadal shielding, control of technical exposure factors, high-speed image receptor systems, correct radiographic film processing, adequate structural shielding, appropriate source-to-skin distance, use of a cumulative timing device, and housing of the x-ray tube in a diagnostic-type protective encasement. Some additional requirements are included in the federal government specifications for the use of fluoroscopic equipment to ensure adequate protection for both the radiographer and radiologist.

Remote Control Fluoroscopic Systems

In Chapter 8, possible arrangements of image intensified fluoroscopic imaging systems were described (see page 194). Of the fluoroscopic equipment arrange-ments discussed in Chapter 8, the remote control unit provides imaging personnel the best radiation protection opportunity. This system permits the radiologist and assisting radiographer to remain outside of the fluoroscopic room at a control console located behind a protective barrier until needed. This increases imaging personnel safety because distance is used as a means of increased protection. With remote equipment, the radiologist and assisting radiographer can view the patient directly through clear protective shielding and will enter the x-ray room only when absolutely necessary to provide essential patient care or perform procedural functions.

Spot Film Device Protective Curtain

A spot film device protective curtain, or sliding panel, with a minimum of 0.25-mm lead equivalent should normally be positioned between the fluoroscopist and the patient to intercept scattered radiation above the tabletop (see Fig. 9-14).

Bucky Slot Shielding Device

A Bucky slot shielding device (Fig. 9-15) of at least 0.25-mm lead equivalent must automatically cover the Bucky slot opening in the side of the x-ray table during a standard fluoroscopic examination when the Bucky tray is positioned at the foot end of the table. This shielding device protects the radiologist and radiographer at gonadal level. Without this device and the spot film protective curtain in place, the exposure rate to the fluoroscopist would exceed 100 mR per hour at a distance of 2 feet from the side of the x-ray table.

Rotational Scheduling of Personnel

Diagnostic imaging personnel receive the highest occupational exposure during fluoroscopy, mobile radiography, and special procedures. Scheduling personnel to spend less time in these higher-radiation tasks can decrease this exposure. Radiographers may be assigned to clinical areas in a rotational pattern. This type of scheduling uses the cardinal principle of time as a means of additional radiation protection.

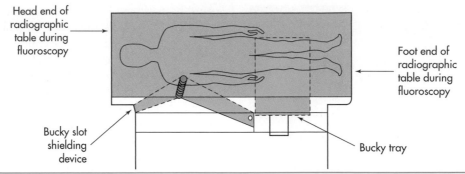

FIG. 9-15. To provide protection at gonadal level for the fluoroscopist, the Bucky slot shielding device should be at least 0.25-mm lead equivalent.

PROTECTION DURING MOBILE RADIOGRAPHIC EXAMINATIONS

Use of Protective Garments

Mobile radiographic equipment creates special radiation protection considerations for the radiographer. Suitable protective garments should be worn by the radiographer whenever structural or mobile protective shielding is unavailable. A protective apron should be assigned to each mobile unit so that it is immediately available for the radiographer.

Distance as a Means of Protection

Some mobile units are equipped with a remote control exposure device. This permits the radiographer to leave the immediate vicinity and uses distance as an effective means of protection from radiation. For the vast majority of mobile units that are non-remote-controlled, the cord leading to the exposure switch must be long enough to permit the radiographer to stand at least 2 m (approximately 6 feet) from the patient, the x-ray tube, and the useful beam. This permits the radiographer to take advantage of the inverse square effect of exposure reduction with distance.

Where the Radiographer Should Stand During a Mobile Radiographic Procedure

The radiographer should attempt to stand at right angles (90 degrees) to the x-ray beam scattering object

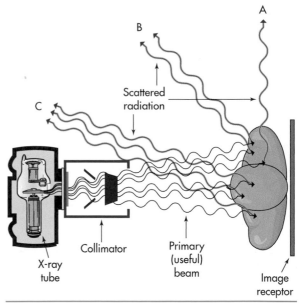

FIG. 9-16. When the protective factors of distance and shielding have been accounted for, the radiographer will receive the least amount of scattered radiation by standing at a right angle (90 degrees) to the scattering object (the patient) (in position *A*). The most scattered radiation would be received at point *C* because of backscatter coming from the patient. (Intensity or quantity of x-ray exposure at any given point is indicated in this picture by the number of scattered x-rays reaching that point.)

(the patient) line; when the protection factors of distance and shielding have been accounted for, this is the place at which the least amount of scattered radiation is received (Fig. 9-16). However, because distance and shielding have much more influence on the reduction of exposure to the technologist, these factors should be addressed first.

PROTECTION DURING C-ARM FLUOROSCOPY

Personnel Exposure from Scattered Radiation

Safety procedures are particularly important when mobile fluoroscopy (C-arm) systems are used. Because patterns of exposure direction are less predictable and the equipment is frequently operated by physicians whose training and experience in radiation safety may not match those of an experienced radiologist, the radiographer should exercise special vigilance. For C-arm devices with similar fields of view, the dose rate to personnel located within a meter of the patient is comparable to that of routine fluoroscopy—approximately several milligray (mGy) per hour. Exposure of personnel is caused by scatter from the patient. During operating room procedures in which cross-table exposures are used (Fig. 9-17), an understanding of the patterns of x-ray scatter is particularly useful. The exposure rate caused by scatter near the entrance surface of the patient (the x-ray tube side) exceeds the exposure rate caused by scatter near the exit surface of the patient (the image intensifier side). The difference in the amount of scatter, typically a factor of 2 or 3, is caused by the higher radiation intensity at the entrance surface of the patient. Thus the location of the lower potential scatter dose is on the side of the patient away from the x-ray tube (i.e., the image intensifier side). Obviously, the radiographer should never encounter the actual useful beam.

Need for Protective Apparel for All Personnel and Monitoring of Imaging Personnel

The C-arm fluoroscope can be manipulated into almost any position and remain in an energized state for long periods of time to accommodate, for example, an orthopedic surgeon performing an open reduction of a fractured hip in the operating room or a vascular surgeon performing an interventional procedure. When radiographers and other medical personnel participate in procedures that require this unit to be energized for long periods of time, they are subject to

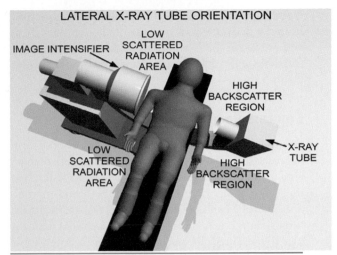

FIG. 9-17. Cross-table exposure using a C-arm fluoroscope. The exposure rate caused by scatter near the entrance surface of the patient (the x-ray tube side) exceeds the exposure rate caused by scatter near the exit surface of the patient (the image intensifier side). The location of lower potential scatter dose is on the side of the patient away from the x-ray tube (i.e., the image intensifier side). (Courtesy Mark Rzeszotarski.)

increased radiation exposure. Also, the physical configuration of a C-arm fluoroscopic unit limits the methods that can be used to achieve protection from scattered radiation. For this reason, personnel that routinely operate a C-arm fluoroscope or those who are in the immediate area of the unit when it is energized must wear a lead apron. This garment should be 0.5-mm lead equivalent to ensure adequate protection. A neck and thyroid shield of 0.5-mm lead equivalent should also be worn. Appropriate monitoring of imaging personnel (see Chapter 10) who are normally involved in C-arm fluoroscopic procedures is mandatory.

Positioning of the C-Arm Fluoroscope

As discussed in Chapter 8 (see pp. 198 and 200), the positioning of a C-arm fluoroscope with the x-ray tube over the table and the image intensifier underneath the table results in higher exposure of the patient and increased scatter radiation. As scatter increases, radiation exposure of all personnel in the immediate vicinity of the C-arm also increases. Therefore, just from the perspective of increased radiation safety, it is best to reverse the C-arm to place the x-ray tube under the table and the image intensifier over the table (see Fig. 8-33).

Exposure Reduction for Personnel

Personnel radiation exposure is reduced when C-arm fluoroscope beam-on time is minimized. When some type of image storage device (e.g., last-image-hold) is used in conjunction with the unit, beam-on time decreases and exposure reduction increases. If the image intensifier is positioned as close to the patient as possible, the required fluoroscopic x-ray beam intensity is minimized. This equipment-patient arrangement also permits the image intensifier to function more effectively as a scatter barrier between the patient and the person operating the C-arm fluoroscope.

PROTECTION DURING HIGH-LEVEL-CONTROL INTERVENTIONAL PROCEDURES

Increased Importance of Radiation Safety Techniques

All the standard precautions and procedures for the reduction of dose to personnel are applicable during interventional procedures. These radiation safety techniques take on an increased importance in interventional procedures because of the extended length of some of these procedures (see Table 8-2), the large number of digital and cineradiographic images that are taken, and in certain studies the frequent use of the high-level-control (high-dose) mode of operation, in which the exposure rate may significantly exceed the rate used in routine fluoroscopy.

Knowledge of Dose Reduction Techniques Required by the Radiographer

Although the duration of the procedure and the number of the exposures taken are under the control of the radiologist or other interventional physician, the radiographer should be knowledgeable in the application of dose reduction techniques. The radiog-

rapher should verify that dose-reducing features are available and in good working order. These include the presence of high-quality low-dose fluoroscopy mode, pulsed beam operation, collimation, optimal beam filtration, removable grids, variable optical aperture, "roadmapping," time-interval differences, and "last-image-hold" mode.

In last-image-hold mode, the last exposure remains on the viewing monitor so that the operator does not need to expose again simply to review the position of a catheter in relation to landmarks when no new information is needed. If possible, the beam entry side could be changed during the procedure to reduce total dose to any one area of skin.

High-level-control is to be used sparingly and only when increased visualization is necessary during a critical maneuver such as embolization or deployment of devices such as stents.[2] Records should be kept so that the cumulative fluoroscopic exposure time may be determined (as opposed to an unspecified number of resets of the 5-minute timer).

How the Radiologist or Other Interventional Physician Can Reduce Radiation Exposure

The radiologist or other interventional physician can reduce radiation exposure by shortening the duration of the procedure, thereby decreasing fluoroscopic beam-on time; taking fewer digital and cineradiographic images; reducing the use of continuous as contrasted to pulsed mode of operation; keeping the protective curtain, if present, on the image intensifier or scatter shield in place during a procedure; and regularly using the last-image-hold feature to view the most recent fluoroscopic image. These good safety practices will substantially decrease exposure of all participating personnel and of the patient as well.

Extremity Monitoring

Because the hands and forearms of physicians performing interventional procedures can be subject to large radiation exposures if the safety protocol is not carefully followed—and sometimes this may not be possible—it is imperative that extremities be monitored. Physicians need to be aware of the recommended dose limits that have been established for extremities. The National Council of Radiation Protection and Measurements currently recommends an annual equivalent dose limit to localized areas of the skin and hands of 500 mSv (50 rem) (see Table 7-3). To avoid remotely approaching this limit and consequently increasing the possibility of adverse effects, protective gloves should be worn whenever possible by any physician whose hands will of necessity often be close to the fluoroscopic beam.

PATIENT RESTRAINT

Radiographers should *never* stand in the primary (useful) beam to restrain a patient during a radiographic exposure (Fig. 9-18, A). When patient restraint is necessary, mechanical restraining devices may be used to immobilize the patient whenever possible. If mechanical means of restraint are not feasible, nonoccupationally exposed persons wearing appropriate protective apparel are to perform this function. These individuals should be positioned so that their lead-protected torsos are not struck by the primary, or direct, beam (Fig. 9-18, B). Holding patients can be necessary when they are unable to support themselves. For example, a weak elderly patient may be unable to stand alone and raise his arms above his head for a lateral chest x-ray. In this situation, a nonoccupationally exposed person (relative or friend) may hold the patient in position during the exposure. A mechanical restraining device is often used to hold an infant in the upright position for chest radiographs. If such a device is not available, the child must be physically held (usually by a parent) during the exposure. The radiographer should take care that these exposed individuals do not stand in the useful beam while holding the patient during the exposure. Pregnant women are *never* to be permitted to assist in holding a patient during an exposure.

DOORS TO X-RAY ROOMS

Radiographic and fluoroscopic exposures should be made only when doors are closed. This practice affords a substantial degree of protection for persons in areas adjacent to the room door because in most facilities

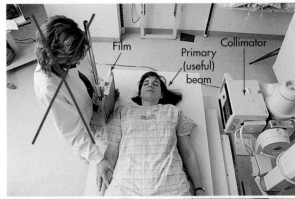

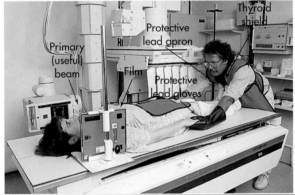

FIG. 9-18. A, The radiographer should never stand in the primary (useful) beam to restrain the patient. **B,** A nonoccupationally exposed person restraining a patient during a radiographic exposure should wear a lead apron, gloves, and thyroid shield and stand outside the primary beam.

room doors have attenuation for diagnostic energy x-rays equivalent to that provided by 1/32-inch of lead.

DIAGNOSTIC X-RAY SUITE PROTECTION DESIGN

Requirement for Radiation-Absorbent Barriers

To reduce the equivalent dose to radiographers, nonoccupationally exposed personnel, and the general public to levels deemed statistically safe by both federal and international bodies, every room in which a diagnostic x-ray unit is housed must be equipped with radiation-absorbent barriers. The design of these barriers is based on considerations listed in Box 9-3.

BOX 9-3

Radiation-Absorbent Barrier Design Considerations

- The mean energy of the x-rays that will strike the barrier
- Whether the barrier is of a primary or secondary nature
- The distance from the x-ray source to a position of occupancy 1 foot from the barrier
- The workload of the unit
- The use factor of the unit
- The occupancy factor behind the barrier
- The intrinsic shielding (e.g., tube housing attenuation) of the x-ray unit
- Whether the area beyond the barrier is "controlled" or "uncontrolled"

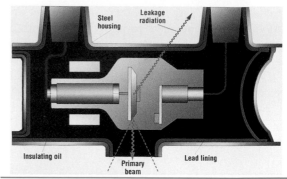

FIG. 9-19. Primary radiation emerges directly from the collimator and spreads throughout the room.

Reason for Overshielding

The shielding designer must take all the factors identified in Box 9-3 into account to meet necessary radiation protection standards. In addition, the designer should plan conservatively to satisfy future regulatory limits that may be more stringent. This and the ALARA principle (mentioned earlier in this chapter) are two reasons why many diagnostic x-ray facilities are overshielded. Spending some extra money up front for additional shielding is far easier and much less expensive than adding it after the suite has been completed.

Radiation Shielding Categories

Three categories of radiation sources can be generated in an x-ray room. They are classified as follows:
1. Primary radiation
2. Scatter radiation
3. Leakage radiation

The latter two categories are collectively known as *secondary radiation*.

Primary Radiation

Primary radiation emerges directly from the x-ray tube collimator (Fig. 9-19) and moves without deflection toward a wall, door, viewing window, and so on.

Because of this tendency, primary radiation also is known as *direct radiation*. Energy from direct radiation has not been degraded by scatter, and substantial proportions of the initial beam may not have been attenuated. Therefore a wall in the path of direct radiation requires the most radiation protection shielding to ensure the safety of personnel and the public. In a typical x-ray suite, the most common primary radiation barrier is that behind the wall Bucky unit.

Scatter Radiation

Scatter radiation results whenever a diagnostic x-ray beam passes through matter. Compton interactions between the x-ray photons and the electrons of the atoms within the attenuating object deflect x-ray photons from their initial trajectories. As a result, photons emerge from the object in all directions (Fig. 9-20). Scattered radiation is greatly reduced in intensity relative to the incident beam. It also is somewhat weakened in energy and consequently in penetrating power. The amount of shielding required to protect against scatter radiation is therefore almost always much less than that for primary radiation. In general, the patient is the major source of scatter radiation.

Leakage Radiation

Leakage radiation is radiation generated in the x-ray tube that does not exit from the collimator opening but rather penetrates through the protective tube-housing and, to some degree, through the sides of the collimator (see Figs. 9-19 and 9-20). Leakage radiation is therefore always present in some amount. When

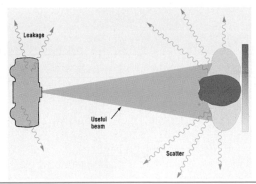

FIG. 9-20. Scatter radiation emerges from the patient and spreads in all directions.

shielding is planned for a secondary barrier, the potential contributions from leakage radiation must be added to those from the scatter radiation reaching that barrier.

Calculation Considerations

Workload

Because a diagnostic x-ray unit does not produce radiation 24 hours per day, 7 days per week, a parameter must be used to reflect the unit's radiation-on time in the determination of barrier shielding requirements. The quantity that best describes the weekly radiation use of a diagnostic x-ray unit is called its **workload (W).** The workload is essentially the radiation output weighted time during the week that the unit is actually delivering radiation. Workloads are specified either in units of milliampere-seconds (mA) per week or milliampere-minutes (mA-min) per week. The following example illustrates this concept.

EXAMPLE: A radiographic x-ray suite is in operation 5 days per week. The average number of patients per day is 20, and the average number of films per patient is 3. The average technical exposure factors are 90 kVp, 300 mA, 0.1 sec. Find the weekly workload.

$$W = (300\,mA \times 0.1\,sec) \times (5\,days/wk) \times$$
$$(20\,patients/day) \times (3\,films/patient)$$
$$= 9000\,mA/wk$$
$$= 150\,mA\text{-}min/wk$$

Note that the kVp is not used in the workload calculation. It is, however, an important parameter in the calculation of barrier-shielding thickness.

Inverse Square Law

Just as the intensity of light fades with separation from its source, the strength of an x-ray beam is weakened as the distance from its source increases. The ISL, introduced earlier in this chapter, is the mathematical relation describing this property and is a fundamental component of radiation protection. As such, the ISL plays a major role in the design of radiation safety barriers. An illustration of its use for this purpose is shown here.

EXAMPLE: At a distance of 1 m from an x-ray tube target, the exposure rate measured by a radiation survey meter was 500 milliroentgens (mR) per hour. What would that instrument read if it were moved back an extra 2 m? As already seen, ISL is mathematically given by the following proportion:

$$\frac{I_1}{I_2} = \frac{(d_2)^2}{(d_1)^2}$$

If the given data are substituted into the above relation and cross-multiplied, the following result is obtained:

$$(3)^2 I_2 = 500(1)^2$$

$$I_2 = 500/9$$
$$= 55.6\,mR/hr$$

This result demonstrates an enormous reduction in radiation intensity. Its direct consequence is a greatly reduced barrier-shielding thickness requirement.

Use Factor (U)

If radiation, whether primary or secondary, is never directed at a particular wall or structure, then ordinary or existing construction is sufficient. Most structures in a diagnostic x-ray suite, however, are struck by radiation to some degree for some fraction of the weekly beam-on time. The **use factor (U)** is a quantity that was introduced to select this fractional contact time.

For primary radiation, the use factor represents the portion of beam-on time during the week that the

TABLE 9-1

Use Factors Recommended by the ICRP

Use Factor	Primary Barrier
Full use (U = 1)	Floors of radiation rooms except dental installations, doors, walls, and ceilings of radiation rooms exposed routinely to the primary beam
Partial use (U = 1/4)	Doors and walls of radiation rooms not exposed routinely to the primary beam; also, floors of dental installations
Occasional use (U = 1/16)	Ceilings of radiation rooms not exposed routinely to the primary beam; because of the low use factor, shielding requirements for a ceiling are usually determined by secondary rather than primary beam considerations

From International Commission on Radiological Protection (ICRP): *Report of Committee III on protection against x-rays up to energies of 3 MeV and beta and gamma rays from sealed sources*, ICRP Publication No. 3, New York, 1960, Pergamon Press.

x-ray beam is directed at a primary barrier. Consider a typical radiographic suite with a wall Bucky unit. If 50% of the x-ray examinations involve this device, the wall behind the Bucky unit has a U (primary) = 1/2.

Because scatter and leakage radiation emerge in all directions in the x-ray room, every wall, door, viewing window, and other surface will always be struck by some quantity of radiation. Therefore U (secondary) = 1 for all radiation-accessible structures.

Table 9-1 presents the most current recommended use factor values. The use factor also may be referred to as the *beam direction factor*.

Occupancy Factor (T)

Radiation barriers are installed to protect personnel and the general public from radiation that otherwise would reach them uninhibited. If no one will ever be present beyond an existing wall in a particular area while the x-ray unit is being operated, the addition of supplementary shielding to that wall is unnecessary. The opposite situation is an area in which someone is always present. When planning radiation protection shielding for a diagnostic x-ray suite, the designer must consider not only zero and full occupancy cases but also the more common partial occupancy situation. The **occupancy factor (T)** is used to modify the shielding requirement for a particular barrier by taking into account the fraction of the workweek that the space beyond the barrier is occupied. Table 9-2 lists the latest recommended values for T.

Controlled and Uncontrolled Areas

If a region adjacent to a wall of an x-ray room is used only by occupationally exposed personnel (e.g., radiographers), that location is designated as a **controlled area.** Conversely, a nearby hall or corridor that is frequented by the general public is classified as an **uncontrolled area.** For the latter, the weekly maximum permitted equivalent dose (MPED) is equal to 20 microsievert (μSv), or 2 mrem; for controlled areas, it is a relatively much larger amount, 1000 μSv (100 mrem). The main reason for this disparity lies in the fact that the occupationally exposed population is only a tiny fraction of the overall population. Therefore, the potential for detrimental radiobiologic effects to the general public as a whole as a result of the higher MPED to occupationally exposed personnel is statistically negligible. Thus, whether the area beyond a structure is designated as controlled or uncontrolled is significant in determining the amount of radiation shielding to be added to that structure. The following sections discuss the use of these concepts in the determination of radiation shielding requirements.

Calculating Barrier Shielding Requirements

For each wall, door, and other barrier in an x-ray room that is to provide protection against radiation, the product of W × U × T must be determined. The workload is generally fixed by the overall use of the x-ray unit, whereas the use and occupancy factors are

TABLE 9-2

Suggested Occupancy Factors*†

Location	Occupancy Factor (T)
Administrative or clerical offices; laboratories, pharmacies, and other work areas fully occupied by an individual; receptionist areas, attended waiting rooms, children's indoor play areas, adjacent x-ray rooms, film reading areas, nurses' stations, x-ray control rooms	1
Rooms used for patient examinations and treatments	1/2
Corridors, patient rooms, employee lounges, and staff rest rooms	1/5
Corridor doors‡	1/8
Public toilets, unattended vending areas, storage rooms, outdoor areas with seating, unattended waiting rooms, patient holding areas	1/20
Outdoor areas with only transient pedestrians or vehicular traffic, unattended parking lots, vehicular drop off areas (unattended), attics, stairways, unattended elevators, janitors' closets	1/40

*For use as a guide in planning shielding where other occupancy data are not available.

†When using a low occupancy factor for a room immediately adjacent to an x-ray room, care should be taken to also consider the areas further removed from the x-ray room. These areas may have significantly higher occupancy factors than the adjacent room and may therefore be more important in shielding design despite the larger distances involved.

‡The occupancy factor for the area just outside a corridor door can often be reasonably assumed to be lower than the occupancy factor for the corridor.

Modified from National Council on Radiation Protection and Measurements (NCRP): *Structural shielding design for medical x-ray imaging facilities*, Report No. 147, Table 4.1, p 31, Bethesda, MD, 2004, NCRP.

usually different among various barriers. The protection planner also must know whether the barrier is a primary or secondary one and whether the area beyond the barrier is controlled or uncontrolled.

Prior to the recent publication of NCRP Report No. 147,[3] the most common method used to determine shielding requirements for diagnostic installations was to employ the precalculated tables located in Appendix C of NCRP Report No. 49.[4] Table 9-3 is a reproduction of one of these tables. The data within this table are utilized to illustrate in a simple manner how virtually all of the present-day existing shielding for diagnostic installations has been calculated.

Primary Barrier Calculation

The primary radiation intensity for a selected kVp at the barrier location can be determined by making exposure measurements on the x-ray unit. This information may then be used to determine the amount of shielding necessary to attenuate the radiation to permissible levels. The values shown in Table 9-3 are based on such output measurements averaged over many typical x-ray units. The following example

demonstrates determination of the primary barrier shielding requirement in a controlled area for an average-usage radiographic room.

EXAMPLE: Average kVp = 100

$$U = \frac{1}{2}$$

$$T = 1$$

$$W = 15,000 \ mAs/wk = 250 \ mA\text{-}min/wk$$

Distance from x-ray source to occupied area = 3 m

SOLUTION:

$$W \times U \times T = (250)(1/2)(1) = 125 \times mA\text{-}min/wk$$

From Table 9-3, a shielding requirement of 0.65-mm lead or approximately 1/32-inch lead is obtained.

Secondary Barrier Calculation

Secondary barriers intercept both scatter and leakage radiation. No additional shielding against secondary radiation is needed for areas already protected against

TABLE 9-3

Minimal Shielding Requirements for Radiographic Installations

WUT* in mA-Min

A100 kV[†]	125 kV[†]	150 kV[†]	Distance in Meters from Source to Occupied Area										
1000	400	200	1.5	2.1	3.0	4.2	6.1	8.4	12.2				
500	200	100		1.5	2.1	3.0	4.2	6.1	8.4	12.2			
250	100	50			1.5	2.1	3.0	4.2	6.1	8.4	12.2		
125	50	25				1.5	2.1	3.0	4.2	6.1	8.4	12.2	
62.5	25	12.5					1.5	2.1	3.0	4.2	6.1	8.4	12.2

Type of Area	Material	Primary Protective Barrier Thickness[‡]										
Controlled	Lead, mm	1.95	1.65	1.4	1.15	0.9	0.65	0.45	0.3	0.2	0.1	0.1
Noncontrolled	Lead, mm	2.9	2.6	2.3	2.05	1.75	1.5	1.2	0.95	0.75	0.55	0.35
Controlled	Concrete, cm[§]	18	15.5	13.5	11.5	9.5	7	5.5	4	2.5	1.5	0.5
Noncontrolled	Concrete, cm[§]	25	23	20.5	18.5	16.5	14	12	10	8		

Type of Area	Material	Secondary Protective Barrier Thickness[‡]										
Controlled	Lead, mm	0.55	0.45	0.35	0.3	0	0	0	0	0	0	0
Noncontrolled	Lead, mm	1.3	1.05	0.75	0.65	0.45	0.35	0.3	0.05	0	0	0
Controlled	Concrete, cm[‡]	5	3.5	2.5	2	0	0	0	0	0	0	0
Noncontrolled	Concrete, cm[‡]	11.5	9.5	7.5	5.5	4	3	2	0.5	0	0	0

From National Council on Radiation Protection and Measurements (NCRP): *Structural shielding design and evaluation for medical use of x-rays and gamma rays with energies up to 10 meV*, Report No. 49, Appendix C, p 66, Washington DC, 1976, NCRP.
*W, weekly workload in mA-min; U, use factor; T, occupancy factor.
[†]Peak pulsating x-ray tube potential.
[‡]Barrier thickness based on 150 kV.
[§]Thickness based on concrete density of 2.35 g/cm^3 (147 lb/ft^3).

primary radiation. Because scatter and leakage radiation emerge in all directions, the use factor for these is always one.

Scatter Radiation The intensity and energy of the scatter radiation at the location of a barrier are unknown. Therefore the following is assumed to determine barrier shielding requirements:

1. The energy of the scatter radiation is equal to the primary radiation.
2. The intensity of radiation scattered at 90 degrees at a distance of 1 m from its source is reduced by a factor of 1000 relative to the primary radiation for a field size of 400 cm^2 (about 8 inches × 8 inches). The greater the x-ray field dimension at the source of the scatter radiation (usually the patient), the

larger the amount of generated scatter radiation. The ISL plays an important role in shielding determination, but in the case of scatter radiation the distance is measured from the center of the patient rather than from the x-ray tube target. The following exercise demonstrates the way to determine a lead shielding requirement in a controlled area against scatter radiation.

EXAMPLE: Find the amount of lead shielding needed to protect a controlled area against scatter radiation for full occupancy if the area is at a distance of 2.1 m from the center of the patient. The weekly workload = 1000 mA-min and the mean kVp = 100.

SOLUTION:

$$U = 1$$

$$T = 1$$

$$W = 1000$$

$$W \times U \times T = 100\ \text{mA-min/wk}$$

From Table 9-3 a shielding requirement of 0.45-mm lead is obtained, which is less than 1/32 inch (1/32 inch = 0.79 mm). In practice, 1/32-inch lead shielding would be recommended.

Leakage Radiation Leakage radiation does not emerge directly from the collimator opening but rather penetrates through the x-ray tube housing walls or through the sides of the collimator when the x-ray beam is "on." Leakage radiation is therefore an additional radiation output that shielding designers must consider. Regulatory standards mandate that the maximum permissible leakage exposure rate at 1 m from the target of a diagnostic x-ray tube in all directions cannot exceed 100 mR/hour when the tube is being operated continuously at its maximal permitted kVp and mA combination.

Leakage radiation is always present when the x-ray tube is on, even if the collimator jaws are tightly closed. Because of the attenuation that occurs when leakage radiation penetrates the tube housing walls, it is essentially a monoenergetic beam; thus, the concept of half-value layer (HVL) may be used at barriers to reduce leakage radiation levels to permissible values. A long-standing rule of thumb regarding leakage radiation is stated as follows.

If the barrier shielding requirements for scatter and leakage differ by more than 3 HVLs, install the larger shielding value; however if the difference is less than 3 HVLs, add 1 HVL to the larger shielding requirement and ignore the smaller shielding requirement.

EXAMPLE: Suppose that shielding must be added to a wall that is subject only to secondary radiation to protect a controlled area. Given the following information, find the total thickness of lead needed.

HVL for scatter and leakage radiation: Each = 0.24-mm lead

Shielding requirement for scatter radiation alone = 0.95-mm lead

Shielding requirement for leakage radiation alone = 0.4-mm lead

SOLUTION: The difference in barrier shielding requirements for scatter and leakage = 0.55-mm lead, which is less than 3 HVL, which = 3 × 0.24-mm lead, or 0.72-mm lead. Therefore, using the rule of thumb that the total shielding requirement is 0.95 mm + 1 HVL, a total thickness of 0.95 + 0.24 = 1.19 mm lead must be installed.

New Approaches to Shielding

At the time of this writing, virtually all installed shielding was designed according to the NCRP Report No. 49, which is more than 20 years old. The examples given in this chapter follow those guidelines. Some of the techniques described in this report were based on very conservative estimates and graphic data for shielding that may now be handled by computer modeling. Following a very long and exhausting effort, NCRP Report 49 has been rewritten and is now superseded by the material presented in NCRP Report No. 147. Table 9-2 of this edition in fact is reproduced from NCRP 147. The methods described in NCRP 147 will be followed from now on. Despite the trend toward decreasing the maximum dose limits and consequently the appropriate design limits for installations, experts do not expect that retrofitting of additional shielding will be necessary in existing installations. The techniques in NCRP 49 were sufficiently conservative (in terms of overshielding) to accommodate the lower dose limits. New approaches will ensure that installations are designed in accordance with current limits.

Among the new approaches to shielding design detailed in NCRP 147, a more rigorous analysis of workload incorporates the range of kVps actually used. Also, the true role of leakage radiation in state-of-the-art equipment is now modeled explicitly, along with scatter. The current rule of adding an HVL, if leakage and scatter barrier requirements are similar, has been abandoned in favor of exact calculations. Use factors now reflect a true percentage of the time that the beam is directed at various barriers. Some existing shielding that was generally ignored in older design calculations, such as the patient table, Bucky, and cassette holder, are included in the new designs. Finally, the suggested occupancy factors have been reevaluated to approximate more closely the percentage of the time that

TABLE 9-4

Brief Summary of NCRP 147 New Shielding Guidelines*

Item	New Approach
Workload	More realistic use of contemporary survey data
Leakage and scatter	Explicit barrier calculations
Use factor	Adjusted for beam direction data reflecting actual usage patterns
Occupancy factor	Realistic assumptions of occupancy of low-occupancy areas (e.g., stairwells)

*Based on National Council on Radiation Protection and Measurements (NCRP): *Structural shielding design for medical imaging facilities*, Report No. 147, Bethesda, Md., 2004, NCRP.

workers are expected to be present (See Table 9-2). Under NCRP 49 a minimal occupancy factor of at least $1/16$ was assumed. Under the revised guidelines, occupancy factors for areas such as closets and stairways may be placed as low as $1/40$. Some of the changes in the revision of NCRP 49 are listed in Table 9-4.

SUMMARY

➤ An annual occupational effective dose of 50 mSv (5 rem) for whole-body exposure during routine operations and an annual effective dose of 1 mSv (0.1 rem) for individuals of the general population have been established.
➤ A CumEfD limits a radiation worker's whole-body lifetime effective dose to his/her age times 10 mSv (years × 1 rem).
➤ Radiation workers can receive a larger equivalent dose than the general public without altering the GSD.
➤ Occupational exposure must be kept ALARA.
➤ The following methods of reducing scatter radiation also reduce the occupational hazard for the radiographer:
  ■ Use of beam-limitation devices, higher kVp and lower mA techniques, appropriate beam filtration, and adequate protective shielding.

■ Correct use of protective apparel (lead aprons, gloves, thyroid shields).
■ Reduction of repeat examinations.
➤ The basic principles of time, distance, and shielding can be used to minimize occupational radiation exposure.
➤ Pregnant radiographers can wear an additional monitoring device at waist level to ensure that monthly equivalent dose does not exceed 0.5 mSv (0.05 rem).
➤ Primary and secondary protective barriers must be designed to ensure annual effective dose limits are not exceeded.
➤ To protect the radiographer and patient from leakage radiation, lead-lined metal diagnostic-type protective tube housing must be used.
➤ The following are required to protect the radiographer during routine fluoroscopy:
  ■ The radiographer, in addition to wearing appropriate protective apparel, should stand as far away from the patient as is practical and move closer to the patient only when assistance is required.
  ■ A spot-film device protective curtain and Bucky slot shielding device must be used.
  ■ The x-ray beam must be adequately collimated, and high-speed image receptor systems and a cumulative timing device should be used.
➤ The following are required to protect the radiographer during mobile radiographic exams:
  ■ The radiographer must wear protective garments.
  ■ The radiographer should stand at least 6 feet from the patient, x-ray tube, and useful beam.
  ■ The radiographer should stand at a right angle to the x-ray beam-scattering object (the patient) line.
➤ Limited exposure time and dose reduction features are required to protect the radiographer during high-level-control fluoroscopy.
➤ Distance is the most effective means of protection from ionizing radiation.
➤ If the peak energy of the x-ray beam is 100 kVp, a lead apron of at least 0.25-mm lead-equivalent thickness should be worn if the radiographer cannot remain behind a protective barrier. A lead apron

of 0.5- or 1-mm lead-equivalent thickness affords much greater protection.

■ Lead gloves, a thyroid shield, and protective glasses are sometimes required.

➤ Radiographers should never stand in the primary beam to hold a patient during a radiographic exposure.

➤ When designing diagnostic x-ray suites, equivalent dose to radiation workers, nonoccupationally exposed personnel, and the general public must be taken into consideration.

■ Facilities must be equipped with radiation-absorbent barriers.

■ Occupancy factor, workload, and use factor must be considered when determining thickness requirements for a protective barrier. Whether an area beyond a structure is designated as a controlled or uncontrolled area is significant in determining the amount of radiation shielding to be added to that structure.

References

1. National Council on Radiation Protection and Measurements (NCRP): *Limitation of exposure to ionizing radiation*, Report No. 116, Bethesda, Md, 1993, NCRP.
2. Marx MV: *Interventional procedures: risks to patients and personnel, in radiation risk*, Reston, Va, 1996, American College of Radiology, Commission on Physics and Radiation Safety.
3. National Council on Radiation Protection and Measurements (NCRP): *Structural shielding design for medical x-ray imaging facilities*, Report No. 147, Bethesda, Md, 2004, NCRP.
4. National Council on Radiation Protection and Measurements (NCRP): *Structural shielding design and evaluation for medical use of x-rays and gamma rays with energies up to 10 meV*, Report No. 49, Washington DC, 1976, NCRP.

GENERAL DISCUSSION QUESTIONS

1. Why has a cumulative effective dose limit for the whole body been established for radiation workers?
2. Why can radiation workers receive a larger equivalent dose than members of the general population?
3. What can a radiographer do during a radiographic procedure to reduce scattered radiation from a patient?
4. When an additional radiation monitor is worn by a pregnant radiographer to monitor equivalent dose to the embryo-fetus, where should the monitor be placed if a protective lead apron is worn?
5. Why is it *not* necessary to reassign a declared pregnant radiographer to a lower radiation exposure risk area?
6. Why is the control-booth barrier considered a secondary protective barrier?
7. Where should a radiographer, whose immediate presence is *not* required during a fluoroscopic procedure, stand in an x-ray room until his or her services are required?
8. How can the use of a remote-control exposure device on a mobile radiographic unit reduce exposure for the radiographer?
9. Why is it best to position the image intensifier of a C-arm fluoroscope close to the patient during any x-radiation procedure?
10. How can the radiologist reduce radiation exposure for himself or herself and for assisting personnel during a high-level-control interventional procedure?
11. What documentation of radiation exposure should be kept by the assisting radiographer during a high-level-control interventional procedure?
12. When should the radiographer stand in the primary beam to restrain a patient during a radiographic exposure?
13. What factors must the shielding designer take into account to meet necessary radiation protection standards?
14. What quantity *best* describes the weekly radiation usage of a diagnostic x-ray unit?
15. What mathematical relationship plays a major role in the design of radiation safety barriers?

REVIEW QUESTIONS

1. **When performing a mobile radiographic examination, if the protection factors of distance and shielding are equal, the radiographer should stand at a _____ to the scattering object (the patient) line.**
   A. 30-degree angle
   B. 45-degree angle
   C. 75-degree angle
   D. 90-degree angle

2. **Diagnostic imaging personnel may receive an annual occupational effective dose of _____ for whole-body exposure during routine operations.**
   A. 1 mSv (0.1 rem)
   B. 5 mSv (0.5 rem)
   C. 25 mSv (2.5 rem)
   D. 50 mSv (5 rem)

3. **At a 90-degree angle to the primary x-ray beam, at a distance of 1 m (3.3 feet), the scattered radiation is what fraction of the intensity of the primary beam?**
   A. 1/10
   B. 1/100
   C. 1/1000
   D. 1/10,000

4. **If a radiographer stands 6 m away from an x-ray tube and receives an exposure rate of 4 mR per hour, what will the exposure rate be if the same radiographer moves to stand at a position located 12 m from the x-ray tube?**
   A. 1 mR per hour
   B. 2 mR per hour
   C. 3 mR per hour
   D. 4 mR per hour

5. **A diagnostic-type protective tube housing must be constructed so that leakage radiation measured at a distance of 1 m from the x-ray source does *not* exceed _____ when the tube is operated at its highest voltage at the highest current that allows continuous operation.**
   A. 500 mR per hour (2.58×10^{-5} C/kg/hr)
   B. 300 mR per hour (2.58×10^{-5} C/kg/hr)
   C. 100 mR per hour (2.58×10^{-5} C/kg/hr)
   D. 50 mR per hour (2.58×10^{-5} C/kg/hr)

6. **If the Bucky slot shielding device and spot-film device protective curtain, or sliding panel, were *not* in the correct position during a routine fluoroscopic examination, what would the fluoroscopist do?**
   A. Exceed an exposure rate of 100 mR per hour at a distance of 2 feet from the side of the x-ray table
   B. Not exceed an exposure rate of 100 mR per hour at a distance of 2 feet from the side of the x-ray table
   C. Exceed an exposure rate of 250 mR per hour at a distance of 2 feet from the side of the x-ray table
   D. Exceed an exposure rate of 500 mR per hour at a distance of 2 feet from the side of the x-ray table

7. **Units of either mAs/wk or mA-min/wk are used to determine the _____ for a specific x-ray room.**
   A. Distance factor
   B. Occupancy factor
   C. Use factor
   D. Workload

8. **A Bucky slot shielding device of at least _____ must automatically cover the Bucky slot opening in the side of the x-ray table during a fluoroscopic examination when the Bucky tray is positioned at the foot end of the table.**
   A. 0.25-mm aluminum equivalent
   B. 0.25-mm lead equivalent
   C. 0.5-mm aluminum equivalent
   D. 0.5-mm lead equivalent

9. **For mobile radiographic units, which are not equipped with remote control exposure devices, the cord leading to the exposure switch must be long enough to permit the radiographer to stand *at least* _____ from the patient, the x-ray tube, and the useful beam to reduce occupational exposure.**
   A. 1 m
   B. 2 m
   C. 3 m
   D. 5 m

10. **Of the following factors, which is considered when determining thickness requirements for protective barriers?**
    1. Occupancy factor (T)
    2. Workload (W)
    3. Use factor (U)
    A. 1 only
    B. 2 only
    C. 3 only
    D. 1, 2, and 3

KEY TERMS

characteristic curve
control badge
densitometer
extremity dosimeter
film badges
Geiger-Müller (GM) detector
ionization chamber–type survey
 meter (cutie pie)

optical density
optically stimulated
 luminescence (OSL) dosimeter
personnel dosimeter
personnel dosimetry
personnel monitoring report
pocket ionization chamber
 (pocket dosimeter)

proportional counter
radiation-dosimetry film
radiation survey instruments
thermoluminescent dosimeter
 (TLD)
TLD analyzer

OBJECTIVES

After completing this chapter, the reader will be able to perform the following:

- State the reason why a radiation worker should wear a personnel dosimeter and explain the function and characteristics of such devices.
- Identify the appropriate location on the body where the personnel dosimeter(s) should be worn during the following procedures or conditions: (1) routine radiographic procedures, (2) fluoroscopic procedures, (3) special radiographic procedures, (4) pregnancy.
- Describe the various components of the film badge, optically stimulated luminescence (OSL) dosimeter, pocket ionization chamber, and thermoluminescent dosimeter (TLD) and explain the use of each of these devices as personnel monitors.
- Explain the function of radiation survey instruments.

Continued

OBJECTIVES—*cont'd*

- List three gas-filled radiation survey instruments.
- Explain the requirements for radiation survey instruments.
- Explain the purpose of the following instruments: (1) ionization chamber–type survey meter (cutie pie), (2) proportional counter, (3) Geiger-Müller (GM) detector.
- Identify the radiation survey instrument that can be used to calibrate radiographic and fluoroscopic x-ray equipment.

Some means of monitoring personnel exposure must be employed to ensure that occupational radiation exposure levels are kept well below the annual effective dose (EfD) limit. The radiographer and other occupationally exposed persons must be aware of the various personnel and area radiation exposure monitoring devices and their functions. This chapter provides an overview of personnel and area monitoring.

PERSONNEL MONITORING

Requirement for Personnel Monitoring

Personnel dosimetry—monitoring of radiation exposure to any person occupationally exposed regularly to ionizing radiation is recommended. Exposure monitoring of personnel is *required* whenever radiation workers are likely to risk receiving 10% or more of the annual occupational effective dose limit of 50 mSv (5 rem) in any single year. In keeping with the ALARA (as low as reasonably achievable) concept, most health care facilities issue dosimetry devices when personnel might receive about 1% of the annual occupational effective dose limit in any month, or approximately 0.5 mSv (50 mrem). Exposure monitoring is accomplished through the wearing of personnel dosimeters.

Purpose of Personnel Dosimeter

The **personnel dosimeter** provides an indication of the working habits and working conditions of diagnostic imaging personnel. It determines occupational exposure by detecting and measuring the quantity of ionizing radiation to which the dosimeter has been exposed over a period of time. This instrument, however, does not protect the wearer from exposure.

Placement of Personnel Dosimeter

During Routine Radiographic Procedures

A personnel monitoring device records only the exposure received in the area where it is worn. During routine radiographic procedures, when a protective apron is not being used, the primary personnel dosimeter should be attached to the clothing on the front of the body at collar level to approximate the location of maximal radiation dose to the thyroid and head and neck (Fig. 10-1). Consistency of location in wearing the dosimeter is the responsibility of the individual wearing the device. A list of the types of personnel monitors available to diagnostic imaging personnel is found in Box 10-1. Discussion of each of the personnel monitoring devices follows.

When a Protective Apron Is Worn

Fluoroscopy and special radiographic procedures produce the highest occupational radiation exposure

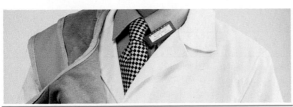

FIG. 10-1. To approximate the maximum radiation dose to the thyroid and the head and neck during routine radiographic procedures, the primary personnel monitor should be attached to the clothing on the front of the body at collar level.

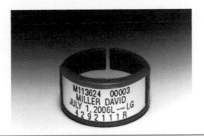

FIG. 10-2. Extremity dosimeter (thermoluminescent dosimeter [TLD] ring badge) can be used to monitor the equivalent dose to the hands. (Courtesy Landauer, Inc., Glenwood, Ill.)

BOX 10-1

Personnel Monitoring Devices Currently Available

1. Film badge
2. Extremity dosimeter (TLD ring badge)
3. Optically stimulated luminescence (OSL) dosimeter
4. Pocket ionization chamber (pocket dosimeter)
5. Thermoluminescent dosimeter (TLD)

---

for diagnostic imaging personnel. When a protective lead apron is used during such procedures, the dosimeter should be worn outside the apron at collar level on the anterior surface of the body (see Fig. 9-10) because the unprotected head, neck, and lenses of the eye receive 10 to 20 times more exposure than the protected body trunk. When the dosimeter is located at collar level, it also provides a reading of the approximate equivalent dose to the thyroid gland and eyes of the occupationally exposed person. If the lead apron's shielding integrity is not compromised, a dosimeter reading that is within acceptable limits outside of the apron ensures a minimal reading under the apron.

As a Second Monitor When a Protective Apron Is Worn

During special radiographic procedures, some health care facilities may prefer to have diagnostic imaging personnel wear two separate monitoring devices. The first, or primary, dosimeter is to be worn outside the protective apparel at collar level to monitor the approximate equivalent dose to the thyroid gland and eyes; the second dosimeter should be worn beneath a wraparound-style lead apron at waist level to monitor the approximate equivalent dose to the lower body trunk.

As a Monitor for the Embryo-Fetus

In addition to a primary dosimeter worn at collar level, pregnant diagnostic imaging personnel should be issued a second monitoring device to record the radiation dose to the abdomen during gestation. This monitor will provide an estimate of the equivalent dose to the embryo-fetus.

Extremity Dosimeter

It is recommended that an **extremity dosimeter,** or TLD ring badge (Fig. 10-2), be worn by an imaging professional as a second monitor when performing radiographic procedures that require the hands to be near the primary x-ray beam. This monitor measures the approximate equivalent dose to the hands of the wearer of the dosimeter. The badge cover contains information such as the account number, participant's name and number, wear date, indication of hand (right or left), size, and reference number of the TLD ring dosimeter. All of this is laser-etched to ensure permanent identification, which allows the extremity dosimeter to be worn during scrub procedures without fear of damaging the identification. The reusable TLD element of the dosimeter is encapsulated within the engraved cover.

TABLE 10-1

Occupational Exposure Values for a Typical Year

Category	Number of Workers (Thousands)		Average Annual Effective Dose (mSv)		Collective Effective Dose (Person-Sv)*
	All	Exposed	All	Exposed	
Medicine	584	277	0.7	1.5	416
Industry	350	156	1.2	2.4	380
Nuclear power	151	91	3.6	5.6	550
Flight crews/flight attendants	97	97	1.7	1.7	165
Other[†]					789
				Total	**2300**

Compiled from data found in NCRP Report No. 101, Tables 4.1 to 4.3, pp. 65-70.

*See Chapter 3, page 60.

[†]Includes workers in the U.S. government (Dept. of Energy, U.S. Public Health Service), uranium mining, well logging, miscellaneous workers, visitors to facilities, etc.

Record of Radiation Exposure

A record of exposure should be part of the employment record of all radiation workers. Table 10-1 gives occupational exposure values (gathered from personnel dosimeter readings) for a typical year. The values represent the average annual effective dose to the whole body.

PERSONNEL DOSIMETERS

Characteristics

A personnel dosimeter must be lightweight and easy to carry. It should be made of materials durable enough to tolerate *normal* daily use. The dosimeter must be able to detect and record both small and large exposures in a consistent and reliable manner. Outside influences such as very warm weather, humidity, and ordinary mechanical shock should not affect performance of the instrument. Because many employees in a health care facility may be required to wear radiation monitors, they should be reasonably inexpensive to purchase and maintain. This permits health care facilities to monitor large numbers of radiation workers in a cost-effective manner.

Types

Four types of personnel dosimeters are used to measure individual exposure of the body to ionizing radiation: film badges, optically stimulated luminescent (OSL) dosimeters, pocket ionization chambers, and thermoluminescent dosimeters (TLDs). Extremity dosimeters (TLD ring badges), previously discussed, are used for monitoring of the hands only.

Film Badges

Film badges (Fig. 10-3) are still used and are an economical type of personnel monitoring device. In general, they record whole-body radiation exposure accumulated at a low rate over a long period of time.

The film badge is composed of three parts: a durable, lightweight plastic film holder; an assortment of metal filters; and a film packet. The film holder should be made of a plastic material of a low atomic number to filter low-energy x-radiation, gamma radiation, and beta radiation. Inside the plastic holder are metal filters of aluminum or copper that are secured in a permanent position. These filters allow the measurement of the approximate energy of the radiation reaching the dosimeter. Penetrating radiations cast a faint shadow of the filters on the processed dosimetry film, whereas soft radiations cast a more pronounced image

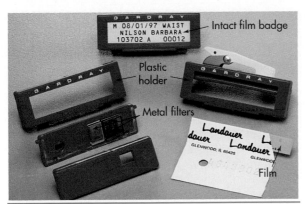

FIG. 10-3. Disassembled film badge, demonstrating badge components: plastic holder, metal filters, and film packet. (Courtesy Landauer, Inc., Glenwood, Ill.)

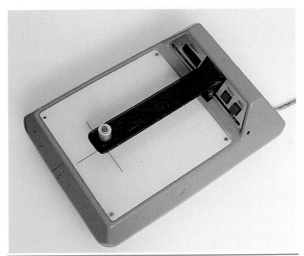

FIG. 10-4. The densitometer, an instrument that measures occupational exposure by comparing optical densities of exposed film badge (dosimetry) films.

of the filters. The density of the *image cast by the filters* permits estimation of the energy of the radiation. From these data the radiation dose can be evaluated as deep (penetrating) or shallow (nonpenetrating). In addition, the direction from which the radiation reached the film (from front to back or from back to front) can be estimated from the appearance of the filter shadows imaged on the processed dosimetry film. The filter images may also be used to determine whether the exposure was the result of excessive amounts of scattered radiation or a single exposure from a primary beam. Excessive exposure to scatter, such as that produced by poor working habits (e.g., radiographer standing too close to a patient during an exposure) or poor facility design, results in a relatively fuzzy image of the filters because the film badge was irradiated from many different angles. A single exposure from a primary beam, such as that which would result if a radiographer inadvertently left the film badge on a table during an exposure (the badge may have fallen off while the radiographer was positioning the patient and gone unnoticed), results in a sharply defined image.

Radiation-Dosimetry Film Inside the Film Badge The **radiation-dosimetry film** contained in the radiographic film packet is similar to dental film. This film is sensitive to doses ranging from as low as 0.1 mSv (10 mrem) to as high as 5000 mSv (500 rem). Doses less than 0.1 mSv (10 mrem) are not usually detected and will be reported as minimal (M) on a personnel monitoring report. The outside of the film packet

forms a light-free envelope for the dosimetry film. Inside the envelope, a sheet of lead foil backs the film to absorb scatter radiation coming from behind the dosimeter. Radiation interacting with the film in the badge causes the film to darken once it is developed. After processing, the density, or degree of blackening, of the image of the filters recorded on the dosimeter film is proportional to the amount of radiation received and the energy of the radiation. An instrument called a **densitometer** (Fig. 10-4) is used to measure this density. It measures **optical density**, the intensity of light transmitted through a given area of the dosimetry film, and compares it with the intensity of light incident on the anterior side of the film. The amount of radiation to which the film was exposed is determined by locating the exposure value of a control film of a similar optical density on a **characteristic curve**. For example, in the characteristic curve shown in Fig. 10-5, if the optical density of the dosimeter film is determined to be 0.5, the film badge has received slightly more than 0.1 mSv (10 rem).

Function of Control Badge The monitoring company that supplies a health care facility with film badges provides a **control badge** with each batch of badges. This control badge serves as a basis of comparison with the remaining film badges after they have

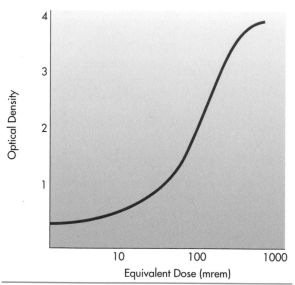

FIG. 10-5. Typical characteristic curve.

been returned to the monitoring company for processing. Because the control badge is supposed to be kept in a radiation-free area within an imaging facility, its optical density reading should be zero. After processing, if a control badge reading above zero is indicated, then the batch of badges may have been exposed to radiation while in transit to or from the health care facility. To ensure that false readings are not recorded, the control badge reading is reported to the health care facility. This reading, if different from zero, must be subtracted from each of the remaining film badges in the batch to ensure accuracy in exposure reporting.

Personnel Monitoring Reports Results from personnel monitoring programs must be recorded accurately and maintained for review to meet state and federal regulations. To comply with such requirements, health care facilities frequently use established dosimetry services. These monitoring services process film badges and other types of personnel dosimeters such as the OSL dosimeter (described subsequently) and supply a written **personnel monitoring report** (Fig. 10-6, A) for the health care facility. This report lists the deep, eye, and shallow occupational exposure of each person in the facility as measured by the exposed monitors. Information on the report is arranged in a series of columns. These columns include the information listed in Box 10-2.

BOX 10-2

Information Found on a Personnel Monitoring Report

1. Personal data: participant's identification number, name, birth date, and sex
2. Type of dosimeter: *P* represents Luxel optically stimulated luminescence (OSL) dosimeter* for x-ray, beta, and gamma radiation; *J* represents Luxel OSL dosimeter for x-ray, beta, gamma, and fast neutron radiation; *U* represents a finger badge used to monitor x-radiation and gamma and beta radiation; *G* represents a film badge reading
3. Radiation quality (e.g., x-rays, beta particle, neutron, combined radiation exposure)
4. Equivalent dose data, including current deep, eye, and shallow recorded dose equivalents (millirems) for the time indicated on the report (e.g., from the first day of a given month to the last day of that month)
5. Cumulative equivalent doses for deep, eye, and shallow radiation exposures for the calendar quarter (3 months), the year to date, and lifetime radiation
6. Inception date (month and year) that the monitoring company began keeping dosimeter records for a given dosimeter for an individual listed on the account who is wearing a monitoring device

*Luxel OSL dosimeter is manufactured by Landauer, Inc., Glenwood, Ill.

The cumulative columns shown in Fig. 10-6, A provide a continuous audit of actual absorbed radiation equivalent dose. These totals can be compared with allowable values established by regulatory agencies. Whenever the letter M appears under the current monitoring period or in the cumulative columns, it signifies that an equivalent dose below the minimum measurable radiation quantity was recorded during that time. The minimal reporting levels vary according to the dosimeter type and radiation quality as follows:

X-ray, gamma:	1 mrem
Beta:	10 mrem
Neutron:	20 mrem fast, 10 mrem thermal
Fetal:	1 mrem
Rings:	30 mrem

LANDAUER®

Landauer, Inc. 2 Science Road Glenwood, Illinois 60425-1586
Telephone: (708) 755-7000 Facsimile: (708) 755-7016
www.landauerinc.com

SAMPLE ORGANIZATION
RADIATION SAFETY OFFICER
1000 HIGH TECH AVENUE
GLENWOOD, IL 60425

RADIATION DOSIMETRY REPORT

ACCOUNT NO.	SERIES CODE	ANALYTICAL WORK ORDER	REPORT DATE	DOSIMETER RECEIVED	REPORT TIME IN WORK DAYS	PAGE NO.
103702	RAD	9920800151	06/11/04	06/07/04	4	1

FOR MONITORING PERIOD:

PARTICIPANT NUMBER	ID NUMBER	NAME	BIRTH DATE	SEX	DOSIMETER	USE	RADIATION QUALITY	DOSE EQ. FOR PERIODS (05/01/04-05/31/04) DEEP DDE	EYE LDE	SHALLOW SDE	QUARTERLY ACCUM. (QTR 2) DEEP DDE	EYE LDE	SHALLOW SDE	YEAR TO DATE (2004) DEEP DDE	EYE LDE	SHALLOW SDE	LIFETIME DEEP DDE	EYE LDE	SHALLOW SDE	RECORDS FOR YEAR	INCEPTION DATE (MM/YY)
0000H	CONTROL				Ja	CNTRL	PN	M	M	M											
	CONTROL				Pa	CNTRL	P	M	M	M											
	CONTROL				U	CNTRL	NF			M											
00191	ADDISON, JOHN	336235619	08/31/1968	M	Ja	WHBODY		90	90	90	90	90	90	100	100	100	200	200	200	5	07/97
								60	60	60	60	60	60	70	70	70	170	170	170		07/97
								30	30	30	30	30	30	30	30	30	30	30	30		07/97
00192	JORGENSON, MIKE	471740095	10/04/1968	M	Pa	WHBODY		M	M	M	M	M	M	M	M	M	M	M	M	5	07/97
					U	RFINGR		M		M			M			70			100		07/97
00193	THOMAS, LEE	384846378	11/22/1964	M	Pa	WHBODY		ABSENT			M	M	M	M	M	M		M	M	5	07/97
					U	RFINGR		ABSENT					M			M			M		07/97
00196	WALKER, JANE	587336640	06/09/1960	F	Pa	WHBODY		3	3	3	12	11	11	12	11	11	22	21	21	5	11/97
00197	EDWARD, CHRIS	489635774	02/14/1966	M	Pa	WHBODY		M	M	M	M	M	M	M	M	M	M	M	M	5	01/98
00198	ZERR, ROBERT	982446591	07/15/1945	M	Pa	WHBODY NOTE		40 CALCULATED	40	40	160	160	160	200	200	200	240	240	240	5	07/98
00199	ADAMS, JANE	335148621	08/25/1951	F	Pa	WHBODY		M	M	M	M	M	M	9	10	12	9	10	12	5	07/98
00200	MEYER, STEVE	416395887	03/21/1947	M	Pa	COLLAR	PL	105	105	105	6	162	165	11	327	334	51	1247	1284	5	08/98
					Pa	WAIST / ASSIGN / NOTE		M / 4 / 105	M / 105	M / 105 / 140			400			690			2180		08/98
					U	RFINGR		ASSIGNED DOSE BASED ON EDE 1 CALCULATION													08/98
00202	HARRIS, KATHY	352235619	06/15/1972	F	Pa	WHBODY		M	M	M	M	M	M	M	M	M	M	M	M	4	02/99
					U	RFINGR		M	M	M			M			M			30		02/99

M: MINIMAL REPORTING SERVICE OF 1 MREM
ELECTRONIC MEDIA TO FOLLOW THIS REPORT

QUALITY CONTROL RELEASE: VS

20 - PR   6774 - RFT130 - RPT130 - N1

- 02013

NVLAP LAB CODE 100518-0**

FIG. 10-6. **A,** Personnel monitoring report must include the items of information shown here. (Courtesy Landauer, Inc., Glenwood, Ill.) *Continued*

OCCUPATIONAL DOSE RECORD FOR A MONITORING PERIOD

This form is for use in place of certain reports required by NRC licensees, OSHA and state regulations. It reflects data provided to or by your account and contains information for NRC Form 5 and other equivalent forms.

Prepared by

LANDAUER®

Landauer, Inc.   2 Science Road   Glenwood, Illinois 60425-1586
Telephone: (708) 755-7000   Facsimile: (708) 755-7016

ACCOUNT NUMBER	SERIES CODE	PARTICIPANT NUMBER
103702	A	00010

1. NAME (LAST, FIRST, MIDDLE INITIAL)	2. IDENTIFICATION NUMBER	3. ID TYPE	4. SEX	5. DATE OF BIRTH
ROTH P	564-38-2390	SSN	X MALE ☐ FEMALE	06/18/56

6. MONITORING PERIOD	7. LICENSEE NAME	8. LICENSE NUMBER(S)
01/01/03 - 12/31/03	SAMPLE	

9A: X RECORD   ☐ ESTIMATE
9B: X ROUTINE   ☐ PSE

INTAKES

10A. RADIONUCLIDE	10B. CLASS	10C. MODE	10D. INTAKE IN µCi

DOSES (in rem)

DEEP DOSE EQUIVALENT (DDE)	11.	0.410
EYE DOSE EQUIVALENT TO THE LENS OF THE EYE (LDE)	12.	0.410
SHALLOW DOSE EQUIVALENT, WHOLE BODY (SDE, WB)	13.	0.410
SHALLOW DOSE EQUIVALENT, MAX EXTREMITY (SDE, ME)	14.	ND
COMMITTED EFFECTIVE DOSE EQUIVALENT (CEDE)	15.	
COMMITTED DOSE EQUIVALENT, MAXIMALLY EXPOSED ORGAN (CDE)	16.	
TOTAL EFFECTIVE DOSE EQUIVALENT (BLOCKS 11 + 15) (TEDE)	17.	0.410
TOTAL ORGAN DOSE EQUIVALENT, MAX ORGAN (BLOCKS 11 + 16) (TODE)	18.	0.410

19. COMMENTS

PERMANENT TO DATE (IN REM)

DDE   : 5.060
LDE   : 5.390
SDE, WB : 5.160
SDE, ME : 4.960
TEDE   : 5.060

20. SIGNATURE - LICENSEE	DATE SIGNED	21. DATE PREPARED
		03/24/04

- FORM 5 A NI L 1 17 M INCEPTION DATE: 01/01/87

FIG. 10-6, cont'd B, Report showing a summary of occupational exposure. (Courtesy Landauer, Inc., Glenwood, Ill.)

Change in Employment by Radiation Worker

When changing employment, the radiation worker must convey the data pertinent to accumulated permanent equivalent dose to the new employer so that this information can be placed on file. Fig. 10-6, *B* is an example of an appropriate summary of an occupational exposure report. A copy of such a report should be given to the radiation worker on termination of employment.

Main Advantage of the Film Badge The main advantage of the film badge is that the radiographic film itself, which is maintained by the monitoring company, constitutes a permanent legal record of personnel exposure. In health care facilities that have a well-structured radiation safety program, personnel monitoring reports are received and reviewed by the radiation safety officer (RSO). Film badge readings that exceed a trigger level set by the health care facility are investigated to ascertain the cause of that reading. Such a process should be an integral component of the facility's radiation safety programs. This practice is compatible with the ALARA policy (i.e., keeping radiation exposures to personnel *as low as reasonably achievable*).

Other Advantages of the Film Badge The film badge has other benefits. This monitoring device is reasonably economical, costing only a few dollars per unit per month. It can be used to monitor x-radiation, gamma radiation, and all but very-low-energy beta radiation in a reliable manner. Moreover, the film badge can discriminate between the types of radiation and the energies of each of these radiations. Another advantage is its mechanical integrity. For example, the dosimeter will not be damaged if the badge is accidentally dropped.

Objectionable Characteristics of the Film Badge The film badge does have some objectionable characteristics. Temperature and humidity extremes can cause fogging of the dosimetry film over long periods of time. This effect increases with the length of time that the badge is worn and can result in a substantially inaccurate high exposure reading. Film badge dosimetry film must be shipped to the monitoring company for processing and exposure determination. Because this task takes time, a radiation worker's exposure cannot be determined on the day of occurrence. Manufacturers usually recommend 1 month as the period of time that a film badge should be worn for personnel monitoring before being read. However, for those groups of workers who will be monitored even though their likelihood and history of any significant radiation exposure are low and nonexistent, a quarterly badge monitoring is available.

Film Badge Dosimeter Sensitivity Other types of personnel dosimeters are more sensitive to ionizing radiation and are therefore more effective monitors in some situations. The film badge dosimeter is most sensitive to photons having an energy level of 50 keV; for values above and below this energy range, dosimetry film sensitivity decreases.

Optically Stimulated Luminescence (OSL) Dosimeter

The **optically stimulated luminescence (OSL) dosimeter** (Fig. 10-7) for personnel monitoring provides the best features of traditional film and thermoluminescent dosimeters while eliminating some of the disadvantages. The OSL dosimeter shown in Fig. 10-7 contains an aluminum oxide (Al_2O_3) detector (thin layer). When the dosimeter is "read out," OSL occurs when the dosimeter is struck by laser light at selected frequencies. When such laser light is incident upon the sensing material, it becomes luminescent in proportion to the amount of radiation exposure received. The OSL technology is actually similar to the way in which a luminous dial watch displays information.[1]

Although the OSL dosimeter can be worn for up to 1 year, it is common practice to wear it for a period of two months. Like traditional film badge monitors, OSL dosimeters must be shipped to the monitoring company for reading and exposure determination. Because this task takes time, occupational exposure cannot be determined on the day of occurrence.

Energy Discrimination As can be seen in Fig. 10-7, three different filters are incorporated into the detector packet of the OSL dosimeter. The filters are respectively made of aluminum, tin, and copper. Each filter blocks a portion of the radiation-sensitive aluminum oxide OSL, causing a different degree of attenuation for any radiation striking the badge depending on its energy. The Al filter offers the least absorption, whereas the Cu filter attenuates the most. What this means is that when the exposed aluminum oxide layer

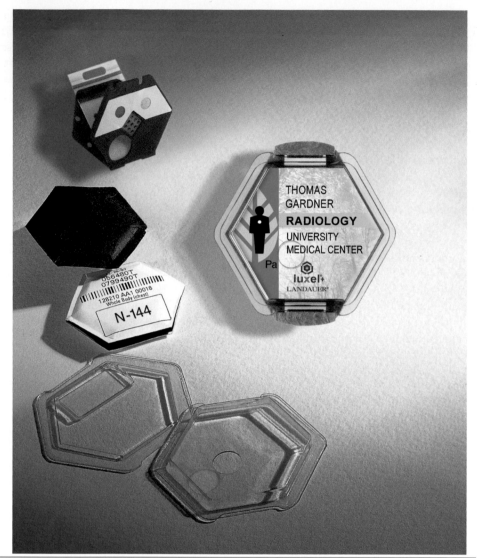

FIG. 10-7. Optically stimulated luminescence (OSL) dosimeter. Disassembled OSL dosimeter demonstrating components of monitor: sensing material holder, preloaded packet incorporating an Al_2O_3 strip sandwiched within a three-element filter pack that is heat sealed within a light-tight black paper wrapper that has been laminated to the white paper label. (All components are sealed inside a tamper-proof plastic blister pack.) (Courtesy Landauer, Inc., Glenwood, Ill.)

is read out by a laser, the degree of luminescence detected in the areas from beneath the filters is a measure of radiation dose occurring within different energy ranges. Thus a situation in which high-energy radiation strikes the badge would show a pretty similar reading through all of the filters. On the other hand, if it was only very low energy radiation that the badge was subjected to, then the laser readout, also known as

a *glow curve*, would be much more pronounced in the region covered by the Al filter than for the other filter-blocked portions. Somewhat more energetic radiation would also enhance the glow curve of the region beneath the tin filter. This therefore is the way that radiation energy discrimination is achieved by the OSL badges. The different energy ranges are typically classified as "deep," "eye," and "shallow" and physically correlate with different penetration depths and therefore different effective radiation energies. In the latest type of OSL badges from one manufacturer,[2] a "bare" or unfiltered portion of the aluminum oxide is used to detect dynamic exposures—i.e., those received when there was rapid motion between the source of radiation and the enhanced dosimeter badge. Examination of the glow curves from this "bare" region will demonstrate a shift or spread in their light frequency that can be correlated with motion (technically classifiable as a Doppler shift).

OSL Dosimeter Sensitivity The OSL dosimeter provides a new degree of sensitivity by giving an accurate reading as low as 1 mrem for x-ray and gamma ray photons with energies ranging from 5 keV to greater than 40 MeV. The maximum equivalent dose measurement for x-ray and gamma ray photons is 1000 rem. For beta particles with energies from 150 keV to in excess of 10 MeV, dose measurement ranges from 10 mrem to 1000 rem. Neutron radiation with energies of 40 keV to greater than 35 MeV has a dose measurement range from 20 mrem to 25 rem. In diagnostic imaging the increased sensitivity of the OSL dosimeter makes it ideal for monitoring employees working in low-radiation environments and for pregnant workers.

Pocket Ionization Chamber

The **pocket ionization chamber (pocket dosimeter)** (Fig. 10-8) is the most sensitive type of personnel dosimeter. However, the use of these monitors in diagnostic imaging is uncommon. Externally the pocket dosimeter resembles an ordinary fountain pen,

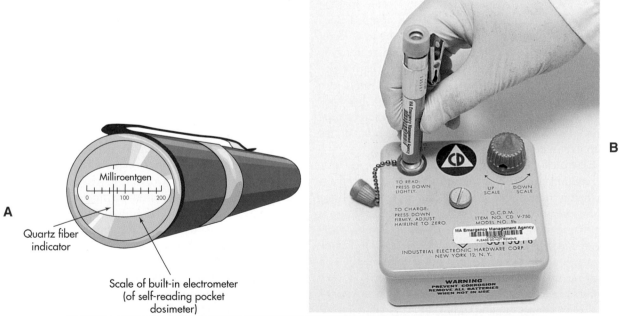

FIG. 10-8. A, The pocket ionization chamber (pocket dosimeter), the most sensitive personnel dosimeter, looks like a fountain pen from the outside but contains an ionization chamber that measures radiation exposure. Viewed through an eyepiece, the quartz fiber indicator of the built-in electrometer of the self-reading pocket dosimeter generally used in radiology indicates exposures of 0 to 5.2×10^{-5} C/kg (0 to 200 mR). Before being used, each pocket dosimeter should be charged to a predetermined voltage by a special charging unit **(B)** so that the charges of the positive and negative electrodes will be balanced and the quartz fiber indicator reads zero (0).

but it contains a thimble ionization chamber that measures radiation exposure. A clip is present on the eyepiece end, allowing the dosimeter to be attached to an individual's apparel (e.g., like a pen in a lab coat pocket).

Types Two types of pocket ionization chambers exist: the self-reading type, which contains a built-in electrometer (a device that measures electrical charge), and the non-self-reading type, which requires a special accessory electrometer to read the device. The self-reading type pocket dosimeter has largely replaced the non–self-reading type for most operations. The operating principle of both types is similar to that of the gold leaf electroscope, which detects the presence and sign of an electric charge.

Components The pocket ionization chamber contains two electrodes, one positively charged (the central electrode) and one negatively charged (the outer electrode). A quartz fiber may form part of the positive electrode and also function as the indicator on the transparent reading scale; in such a system the quartz fiber casts a shadow onto a scale so that the quantity of charge on the positively charged electrode determines the position of the shadow along the scale and is equivalent to the scale reading at that position. When the charged electrodes in the device are exposed to gamma or x-radiation, the air surrounding the central electrode (+) becomes ionized and discharges the mechanism in direct proportion to the amount of radiation to which it has been exposed.

Special charging unit A special charging unit is required for pocket ionization chambers. Each dosimeter must be charged to a predetermined voltage before use so that the quartz fiber indicator shows a zero (0) reading. As the dosimeter is exposed to ionizing radiation, it discharges and the fiber indicator advances along the scale in a linear fashion, thereby showing the net exposure in milliroentgens. Pocket chambers generally used in medical imaging are sensitive to exposures ranging from 0 to 5.2×10^{-5} C/kg (0 to 200 mR).

Advantages The pocket ionization chamber provides an immediate exposure readout for radiation workers who work in high-exposure areas (e.g., a cardiac catheterization laboratory). Such individuals can read the dosimeter on-site to determine the dose received at the completion of a given assignment and, if necessary, alter their working habits. Furthermore, pocket ionization chambers are compact, easy to carry, and convenient to use. Reasonably accurate and sensitive, they are ideal monitoring devices for procedures of relatively short duration.

Disadvantages Pocket ionization chambers are fairly expensive, costing $150.00 or more per unit. If not read each day, the dosimeter may give an inaccurate reading because the electric charge tends to escape (i.e., the fiber indicator drifts with time; thus a false high reading might be obtained from a dosimeter read too late). Also, pocket ionization chambers can discharge if subjected to mechanical shock, which again would result in a false high reading. Because these devices provide no permanent legal record of exposure, health care facilities that use this method to record personnel exposure must delegate someone to keep such a record. This task is generally the responsibility of the RSO.

Thermoluminescent Dosimeter (TLD)

The exterior of a **thermoluminescent dosimeter (TLD)** badge (Fig. 10-9) may look similar to that of a film badge. However, the interior of this monitoring mechanism differs completely. This light-free device usually contains a crystalline form (powder or small chips) of lithium fluoride (LiF), which functions as the sensing material of the TLD.

Ionizing radiation causes the LiF crystals in the TLD to undergo changes in some of their physical properties. When irradiated, some of the electrons in the crystalline lattice structure of the LiF molecule absorb energy and are "excited" to higher energy levels or bands. The presence of impurities in the crystal causes electrons to become trapped within these bands. When the LiF crystals are passed through a special heating process, however, these trapped electrons receive enough energy to rise above their present locations into a region called the *conduction band*. From here the electrons can return to their original or normal state with the emission of energy in the form of visible light. The energy emitted is equal to the difference between the electron-binding energy of the two orbital levels. The intensity of the light is proportional to the amount of radiation that interacted with the crystals.

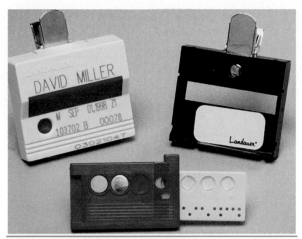

FIG. 10-9. Thermoluminescent dosimeter (TLD) badge containing the sensing material lithium fluoride (LiF).

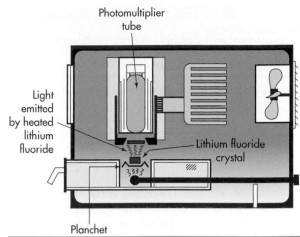

FIG. 10-10. Diagram of a typical analyzer. The analyzer measures the amount of ionizing radiation to which a badge has been exposed by heating the irradiated lithium fluoride (LiF) crystals of the exposed badge with linearly rising temperatures produced by hot gas. This represents a departure from the previously used heating method, which relied on physical contact between the crystals and a heated plate. The new method is a technical improvement because it eliminates any need for contact readjustments.

A device called a **TLD analyzer** (Fig. 10-10) measures the amount of ionizing radiation to which a TLD badge has been exposed by first heating the crystals to free the trapped, highly energized electrons and then recording the amount of light emitted by the crystals (which is proportional to the TLD badge exposure).

Advantages of the TLD Over the Film Badge
The TLD has several advantages over the film badge. The LiF crystals interact with ionizing radiation as human tissue does*; hence this monitor determines dose more accurately. Exposures as low as 1.3×10^{-6} C/kg (5 mR) can be measured precisely. Humidity, pressure, and normal temperature changes do not affect the TLD. Unlike the film in a monthly film badge, which can fog if worn for more than 1 month, the TLD may be worn up to 3 months. After the TLD reading has been obtained, the crystals can be reused. This makes the device somewhat cost effective, even though the initial cost is high (approximately twice the cost of a film badge service).

Disadvantages of the TLD
TLDs have some disadvantages other than their high cost. A TLD can be read only once. The readout process destroys the stored information; the TLD may be reused, but once the crystal is heated, the record of any previous exposure

is gone. The necessity of using calibrated dosimeters with TLDs is also a disadvantage, because the calibrated dosimeters must be prepared and read with each group of TLDs when they are processed.

Summary of Advantages and Disadvantages of Personnel Monitoring Devices
Table 10-2 provides a summary of the advantages and disadvantages of the personnel monitoring devices discussed in this chapter.

RADIATION SURVEY INSTRUMENTS FOR AREA MONITORING

Radiation Detection and Measurement

Radiation survey instruments are area monitoring devices that detect and measure radiation. A detection system indicates the presence or absence of radiation, whereas a dosimeter system measures only cumulative radiation intensity.

---

*The effective atomic number of LiF is equal to 8.2, which is similar to that of soft tissue (Z = 7.4).

TABLE 10-2

Advantages and Disadvantages of Personnel Dosimeters

Monitoring Device	Advantages	Disadvantages
Film badge	Lightweight, durable, easy to carry Cost-efficient monitor for large numbers of people Records radiation exposure accumulated at a low rate over a long period of time Provides permanent, legal record of personnel exposure Detects and records small and large exposure in consistent, reliable manner Performance not affected by heat, humidity, and nonextreme mechanical shock Possible to estimate direction from which radiation came Filters can indicate whether exposure was the result of excessive amounts of scattered radiation or single exposure from the primary beam Control badge indicates whether group badges were exposed in transit to/from health care facility Monitors x-radiation and gamma and all but very low-energy beta radiation Discriminates between type of radiation and energy of x-radiation and gamma and beta radiation	Records only exposure received in the body area where it is worn Not efficient as a monitoring device if not worn High temperatures and excess humidity can cause film in the badge to fog over long periods of time, causing inaccurate exposure readings Film sensitivity decreased at energy levels greater than or less than 50 keV Exposure not determinable on day of occurrence Accuracy limited to ±20%
Optically stimulated luminescence dosimeter (OSL)	Lightweight, durable, easy to carry Integrated, self-contained, preloaded packet Color-coding, graphic formats, and body location icons provide identification Heat, moisture, and pressure will not affect the tamper-proof blister packet Has extended wear frequencies Offers complete reanalysis Gives accurate reading as low as 1 mrem for x-ray and gamma ray photons with energies from 5 keV to 40 MeV Can be used for up to 1 year	Exposure not determinable on the day of occurrence
Pocket ionization chamber	Small, compact, easy to carry and use Reasonably accurate and sensitive Can be used for procedures that last a short time Immediate exposure readout	Not cost-effective for large numbers of personnel Readings may be lost if not carefully recorded Dosimeter must be calibrated to zero or its initial reading must be noted each day it is used Mechanical shock can cause false high reading

TABLE 10-2

Advantages and Disadvantages of Personnel Dosimeters—cont'd

Monitoring Device	Advantages	Disadvantages
Thermoluminescent dosimeter (TLD)	Not affected by humidity, pressure, or normal temperature changes Can be worn up to 3 months After a reading has been obtained, TLD crystals can be reused, making the device somewhat cost-effective	No permanent, legal record of exposure Records only exposure received in body area where worn Initial cost is greater than film badge service Readings may be lost if not carefully recorded Readout process destroys information stored in TLD, which prevents the "read" TLD from serving as a permanent legal record of exposure Calibrated dosimeters must be prepared and read with each group of TLDs as they are processed Records only the exposure received in the body area in which it is worn Not effective as a monitoring device if not worn

Types of Radiation Survey Instruments for Area Monitoring

When in contact with ionizing radiation, survey instruments respond to the charged particles that are produced because radiation interacts with and ionizes the gas (usually air) in the detector. These instruments measure either the total quantity of electrical charge resulting from the ionization of the gas or the rate at which the electrical charge is produced. The ionization chamber-type survey meter ("cutie pie"), the proportional counter, and the Geiger-Müller (GM) detector are three different gas-filled radiation detectors that serve as field instruments. They detect the presence of radiation and, when properly calibrated, give a reasonably accurate measurement of the exposure. Each of these instruments has its own special use, and they are not all equally sensitive in the detection of ionizing radiation.

Requirements

Radiation survey instruments for area monitoring should meet the following requirements:
1. They must be easy to carry so that one person can operate the device in an efficient manner for a period of time.
2. They must be durable enough to withstand normal use, including routine handling that occurs during standard operating procedures.
3. They must be reliable; only in such a case can radiation exposure or exposure rate in a given area be accurately assessed.
4. They should interact with ionizing radiation in a manner similar to the way human tissue reacts. This permits dose to be determined more accurately.
5. They should be able to detect all common types of ionizing radiation. Such a capability increases their usefulness.

6. The energy of the radiation should not significantly affect the response of the detector, and the direction of the incident radiation should not affect the performance of the unit. Such characteristics ensure consistency in unit operation among individual users.

7. They should be cost-effective. The initial cost and subsequent maintenance charges should be as low as possible.

Gas-Filled Radiation Survey Instruments

As mentioned, three types of gas-filled radiation survey instruments exist: the ionization chamber-type survey meter (cutie pie), the proportional counter, and the Geiger-Müller (GM) detector.

Ionization Chamber-Type Survey Meter (Cutie Pie)

The **ionization chamber-type survey meter (cutie pie)** (Fig. 10-11) is both a rate meter device (measures exposure rate) used for area surveys and an accurate integrating or cumulative exposure instrument. This device measures x-radiation and gamma radiation and,

if equipped with a suitable window, can also record beta radiation.

Sensitivity Ranges and Uses In the rate mode, the cutie pie can measure radiation intensities ranging from 1 mR per hour to several thousand roentgens per hour; and in the integrate mode, it can sum exposures from as little as 0.1 mR to as much as 1 R. This device can be used to monitor diagnostic x-ray installations when exposure times of a second or more are chosen and to measure fluoroscopic scatter radiation exposure rates, exposure rates of patients containing therapeutic doses of radioactive materials, exposure rates in radioisotope storage facilities, and the cumulative exposures received outside protective barriers.

Advantage and Disadvantages An advantage of the cutie pie is that it is able to measure a wide range of radiation exposures within a few seconds. The delicate detector and relatively large size of the unit, however, may be considered disadvantages. Another disadvantage is that without adequate warm-up time, its meter will drift and produce an inaccurate reading. This device cannot be used to measure exposures produced by typical diagnostic procedures because the exposure times are too short to permit the meter to respond. Instead, it is most commonly used to measure exposure rates (mR/hr) at various distances from a patient who has received radioactive materials for diagnostic or therapeutic purposes.

Proportional Counter

The **proportional counter** serves no useful purpose in diagnostic imaging. It is generally used in a laboratory setting to detect alpha and beta radiation and small amounts of other types of low-level radioactive contamination. The proportional counter can discriminate between alpha and beta particles. Because alpha radiation travels only a short distance in air, the operator of the proportional counter must hold the unit's probe close to the surface of the object being surveyed to obtain an accurate reading of the alpha radiation emitted by the object.

Geiger-Müller (GM) Detector

Sensitivity and Use The Geiger-Müller (GM) detector (Fig. 10-12) serves as the primary radiation survey instrument for area monitoring in nuclear medicine facilities. With the exception of alpha particle

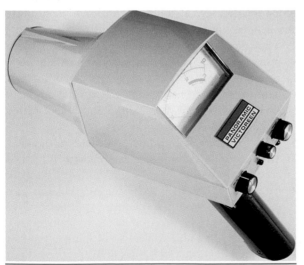

FIG. 10-11. Ionization chamber-type survey meter, or "cutie pie." (Courtesy Victoreen, Inc., Cleveland.)

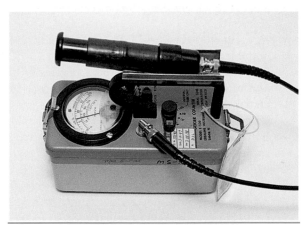

FIG. 10-12. Geiger-Müller (GM) detector.

emission, the unit is sensitive enough to detect individual particles (e.g., electrons emitted from certain radioactive nuclei) or photons. Hence it can easily detect any area contaminated by radioactive material. Because the GM detector allows rapid monitoring, it can be used to locate a lost radioactive source or low-level radioactive contamination.

Components The GM detector has an audible sound system (an audio amplifier and speaker) that alerts the operator to the presence of ionizing radiation. Metal encloses the counter's gas-filled tube or probe, which is the unit's sensitive ionization chamber. When the shield covering the probe's sensitive chamber is open, very-low-energy x-radiation and beta and gamma radiation can be detected. Meter readings are usually obtained in milliroentgens per hour. Because GM tubes tend to lose their calibration over time, the instrument generally has a "check source" of a weak, long-lived radioisotope located on one side of its external surface to verify its constancy daily.

Disadvantages The meter reading of a GM detector is not independent of the energy of the incident photons. This means that photons of widely different energies cause the instrument to respond quite differently, which is a disadvantage in diagnostic imaging. The cutie pie (ionization chamber-type survey meter) exhibits a much flatter, or more constant-response, with varying photon energies. Also, the GM detector

is likely to saturate or jam when placed in a very high-intensity radiation area (such as that associated with a linear accelerator used in radiation therapy), thereby giving a false reading.

CALIBRATION INSTRUMENTS

Ionization chambers can be used to calibrate radiographic and fluoroscopic x-ray equipment. We have seen previously that a cutie pie ionization chamber is used for radiation protection surveys. If this instrument, operating in "rate" mode, were to be placed in the beam emanating from an x-ray tube during a radiographic exposure, the electrical signal produced during the very brief radiographic exposure would be too small to be recorded and measured reliably. An ionization chamber specifically designed for calibration purposes is connected to an electrometer, a device that can measure tiny electrical currents with high precision and accuracy. Such a combination is shown in Fig. 10-11. Both the ionization chamber and the electrometer system must be calibrated periodically to meet state and federal requirements for patient dose evaluation. Several regional calibration laboratories offer this service. A current listing of calibration laboratories is available from the American Association of Physicists in Medicine.*

Ionization chambers connected to electrometers are used by medical physicists to perform the standard measurements required by state, federal, and health care accreditation organizations for radiographic and fluoroscopic devices. These measurements include x-ray output in mR/mAs, reproducibility and linearity of output, timer accuracy, half-value layer, or beam quality, and entrance exposure rates for fluoroscopy units. Furthermore, such a device equipped with a specially calibrated parallel plate chamber is used for similar, but nonfluoroscopic, measurements for mammography x-ray units.

*One Physics Ellipse, College Park, MD 20740-3846 or http://www.aapm.org.

SUMMARY

➤ Personnel monitoring ensures that occupational radiation exposure levels are kept well below the annual effective dose limit.

- Such monitoring is required whenever radiation workers are likely to risk receiving 10% or more of the annual occupational effective dose limit of 50 mSv (5 rem) in any 1 year.
- To keep radiation exposure ALARA, most health care facilities issue dosimeter devices when personnel might receive about 1% of the annual occupational effective dose limit in any month, or approximately 0.5 mSv (50 mrem).
- The working habits and conditions of diagnostic imaging personnel can be assessed over a designated period of time through the use of the personnel dosimeter.
- A radiation worker should wear a personnel monitoring device at collar level during routine radiographic procedures to approximate the maximum radiation dose to the thyroid and the head and neck.
- During high-level radiation procedures, imaging professionals should wear a protective lead apron, with the dosimeter worn outside of the garment at collar level, to provide a reading of the approximate equivalent dose to the thyroid and eyes.
- During special radiographic procedures, two separate personnel dosimeters may be worn, a primary dosimeter worn outside the apron at collar level and a second dosimeter worn beneath the apron at waist level to monitor the approximate equivalent dose to the lower body trunk.
- Pregnant radiation workers should wear a second dosimeter to monitor the abdomen during gestation to provide an estimate of the equivalent dose to the embryo-fetus.
- TLD ring badges are worn under certain conditions to monitor and determine equivalent dose to the hands when they are near the primary beam.
- Health care facilities must maintain a record of exposure recorded by personnel dosimeters as part of each radiation worker's employment record.
- In general, personnel dosimeters must be portable, durable, and cost-efficient.
- Four types of personnel monitoring devices exist: film badges, OSL dosimeters, pocket ionization chambers, and TLDs.
- To meet state and federal regulations, results from personnel monitoring programs must be recorded accurately and maintained by each health care facility.
- The RSO in a health care facility receives and reviews personnel monitoring reports to assess compliance with ALARA guidelines.
- Monitoring reports list the deep, eye, and shallow occupational exposure of each person wearing a monitoring device in the facility as measured by the exposed monitor.

➤ Area monitoring can be accomplished through the use of radiation survey instruments.

- The detection system indicates the presence or absence of radiation, whereas the dosimeter system measures only cumulative radiation intensity.
- Radiation survey instruments for area monitoring must be durable and easy to carry, be able to detect all common types of ionizing radiation, and not be affected by the energy of the radiation or the direction of the incident radiation.
- Types of gas-filled radiation survey instruments include the ionization chamber-type survey meter (cutie pie), the proportional counter, and the GM detector.
- Radiographic and fluoroscopic units can be calibrated with ionization chambers. When used for this purpose, the ionization chamber is connected to an electrometer that can measure tiny electrical currents with high precision and accuracy.

References

1. Gillman M: Shining a light on dosimetry, *RT Image* 13:22, 27, 2000.
2. Landauer, Inc., 2 Science Road, Glenwood, IL 60425-1586. Available at: http://www.landauerinc.com/luxelosl.htm.

GENERAL DISCUSSION QUESTIONS

1. How is exposure monitoring accomplished?
2. Why should a personnel dosimeter be worn outside of a protective apron at collar level on the anterior surface of the body during a fluoroscopic procedure?
3. What must personnel dosimeters be able to detect and record from day to day?
4. Why does a monitoring company supply a control badge with every new batch of badges?
5. What must be done with results from personnel monitoring programs to meet state and federal regulations?
6. When changing employment, what responsibility does a radiation worker have for personal data pertinent to accumulated permanent equivalent dose?
7. How sensitive to x- and gamma radiation is an OSL dosimeter?
8. What are some of the requirements that radiation survey instruments must meet if they are to be used for area monitoring?
9. How does a GM detector alert the operator to the presence of ionizing radiation?
10. What type of diagnostic x-ray equipment would ionization chambers be used to calibrate?

REVIEW QUESTIONS

1. **When laser light is incident on the sensing material in an OSL dosimeter, the material:**
   A. Becomes luminescent in proportion to the amount of radiation exposure received
   B. Fluoresces in proportion to the amount of radiation exposure received and then emits beta particles
   C. Phosphoresces in proportion to the amount of radiation exposure received and then darkens
   D. Turns ice blue and fluoresces in proportion to the amount of radiation exposure received

2. **Which of the following chemicals functions as the sensing material in a thermoluminescent dosimeter?**
   A. Barium sulfate
   B. Calcium tungstate
   C. Lithium fluoride
   D. Sodium iodide

3. **During routine radiographic procedures, when a protective apron is *not* being worn, the primary personnel dosimeter should be attached to the clothing on the front of the body at:**
   A. Collar level to approximate the maximum radiation dose to the thyroid and the head and neck
   B. Chest level to approximate the maximum radiation dose to the heart and lungs
   C. Hip level to approximate the maximum radiation dose to the reproductive organs
   D. Waist level to approximate the maximum radiation dose to the small intestine

4. **Which of the following requirements should radiation survey instruments fulfill?**
   1. **Instruments must be reliable by accurately recording exposure or exposure rate**
   2. **Instruments must be durable enough to withstand normal use**
   3. **Instruments should interact with ionizing radiation in a manner similar to the way in which human tissue interacts**
   A. 1 only
   B. 2 only
   C. 3 only
   D. 1, 2, and 3

5. **During diagnostic imaging procedures, how should the radiation dose to the abdomen of a pregnant radiographer be monitored during gestation?**
   A. It should be estimated from the radiation dose recorded by the primary monitor worn at collar level
   B. It should be obtained from the primary radiation monitor worn at abdominal level
   C. It should be obtained from a second radiation monitor worn at abdominal level
   D. It is not necessary to monitor the radiation dose to the embryo-fetus that results from occupational exposure of a pregnant radiographer during gestation

6. **When a radiologic procedure requires the hands of a radiation worker to be near the primary beam, the equivalent dose to the hands of that individual may be determined through the use of:**
   A. The primary personnel monitor worn at collar level
   B. A pocket ionization chamber attached to the wrist-watch of the radiation worker
   C. A TLD ring badge worn on the hand of the radiation worker
   D. A cutie pie

7. **Which of the following instruments is used to calibrate radiographic and fluoroscopic x-ray equipment?**
   A. Proportional counter
   B. GM detector
   C. Ionization chamber with electrometer
   D. Pocket ionization chamber

8. **For x-ray and gamma ray photons with energies from 5 keV to in excess of 40 MeV, the _____ gives an accurate reading as low as 1 mrem.**
   A. Film badge
   B. OSL dosimeter
   C. Pocket ionization chamber
   D. TLD

9. **Which of the following instruments should be used to locate a lost radioactive source or detect low-level radioactive contamination?**
   A. GM detector
   B. Proportional counter
   C. Ionization chamber-type survey meter (cutie pie)
   D. TLD analyzer

10. **Which of the following instruments should be used in an x-ray installation to assess fluoroscopic scatter radiation exposure rate?**
    A. GM detector
    B. Ionization chamber with electrometer
    C. Proportional counter
    D. TLD

11

Radioisotopes and Radiation Protection

KEY TERMS

annihilation radiation
beta decay
computed axial tomography (CAT)
decontamination
electron capture
Environmental Protection Agency (EPA)
fluorine-18 (^{18}F)
fluorodeoxyglucose (FDG)
Geiger-Müller (GM) detectors
iodine-123 (^{123}I)

iodine-125 (^{125}I)
iodine-131 (^{131}I)
half-value layer
internal contamination
isotopes
neutrino
nuclear medicine
PET/CT scanner
positron
positron emission tomography (PET)
radiation emergency plans

radiation therapy
radioactive contamination
radioactive dispersal device, or "dirty bomb"
radioisotopes
surface contamination
strontium-89 (^{89}Sr)
technetium-99m (^{99m}Tc)

OBJECTIVES

After completing this chapter, the reader will be able to perform the following:

- Explain what causes cancerous growths or tumors to be eliminated or controlled by irradiation
- Describe how therapeutic isotopes may be characterized.
- Describe the process of electron capture.
- Identify the two best radiation safety practices to follow for patients having therapeutic prostate seed implants.
- Explain the process of beta decay.
- Discuss the radiation hazards that may be encountered by personnel caring for a patient who is receiving iodine-131 therapy treatment for thyroid cancer.
- Explain how radioisotopes are used as radioactive tracers in nuclear medicine work.
- Identify the most common radioisotope used in nuclear medicine diagnostic studies.

Continued

Atoms that have the same number of protons within the nucleus but have different numbers of neutrons are called **isotopes.** Most elements in the periodic table (see Appendix D) have associated isotopes, and quite a few of them have many. However, not all of the nuclei of these isotopes represent stable configurations of protons and neutrons. Some have too many neutrons, whereas others have too many protons. Because of this, such isotopes spontaneously undergo changes or transformations to rectify the unstable arrangement. All such atoms or their associated nuclei are referred to as **radioisotopes.**

This chapter provides a brief description of the use of radioisotopes in both diagnostic and therapeutic medical procedures and discusses some relevant radiation safety issues. The use of radiation as a terrorist weapon is also discussed and includes some fundamental principles for dealing with radioactive contamination in a health care setting.

MEDICAL USAGE

Radiation Therapy

As has been discussed in previous chapters, well-oxygenated, rapidly dividing cells are very sensitive to damage by radiation. This causes cancerous growths or tumors to be either eliminated or at least controlled by irradiation of the area containing the growth. Radiation may be delivered internally to such regions by either infusion or implantation of certain radioisotopes. These therapeutic isotopes are characterized by relatively long half-lives that are measured in terms of multiple days or multiple years and, with the exception of a few of them, usually quite high energy radiation. The radiation may be in the form of gamma rays*

---

*Gamma rays are high-energy photons (particles of electromagnetic radiation) that are emitted by the nucleus as a result of an unstable situation. They differ from x-ray photons, which are also particles of electromagnetic radiation, only in the method of how they are produced.

or fast electrons (beta radiation). Several of the most important therapeutic radioisotopes are briefly described here.

Iodine-125 (^{125}I)

Iodine-125 (^{125}**I**) is an unstable, radioactive isotope of the element iodine. It has been used quite extensively in the past decade in the form of titanium-encapsulated cylindrical seeds (4.5 millimeters [mm] long and about the diameter of a paper clip) (Fig. 11-1, A and B) to give a tumoricidal radiation equivalent dose to cancers that are confined within the prostate gland. With the aid of computerized treatment planning and real-time ultrasound imaging, the seeds are permanently inserted into the gland in a calculated prescribed arrangement. The goal is to deliver 145 gray (Gy) to at least 90% of the prostate's volume while limiting radiation dose as much as possible to adjacent structures such as the urethra, bladder, and anterior rectal wall. The process is done in the operating room and typically takes about 2 hours. This is a same-day procedure, and the patient is usually discharged within 4 to 5 hours afterward.

^{125}I has 53 protons and 72 neutrons in its nucleus and has a has a half-life of 59.4 days. It decays by a process called **electron capture,** wherein an inner-shell electron is captured by one of the nuclear protons, followed by the two combining to produce a neutron. There is also the emission of characteristic energy in the form of a 27-keV x-ray generated due to the filling of the inner-electron shell vacancy by a lower-energy electron. The nucleus now has one fewer proton, and thus the decay process leads to the formation of a different element called tellurium-125 (^{125}Te). ^{125}Te, which has 52 protons and 73 neutrons, is produced in an unstable excited energy state; this instability is immediately relieved as its nucleus emits energy in the form of a 35-keV gamma ray. Both the 27-keV characteristic x-rays and the 35-keV gamma rays deliver the radiation equivalent dose to the prostate gland.

Because these radiation emissions have little penetrating power, a very high percentage of the radiation energy is concentrated in the prostate gland. All of the remaining radiation is virtually absorbed by the patient, and yet some detectable radiation emerges from the patient. At a distance of 3 feet, the radiation exposure rate for virtually all prostate seed implants is less than 0.5 milliroentgen per hour (mR/hour), increasing to 25 to 30 mR/hour at the patient's lower abdomen surface.

The concepts of distance and time are the best radiation safety practices to be followed for these types of therapeutic implants. A typical safety recommendation is that ^{125}I patients should significantly limit durations of close contact (<3 feet) with small children and pregnant women for a period of 6 months (3 half-lives) after the implant procedure. They may then resume completely normal behavior.

Strontium-89 (^{89}Sr)

Strontium-89 (^{89}**Sr**) is a radioactive isotope of the element strontium. Because strontium is a member of the same family of elements (called the alkaline *earths*) in the periodic table (see Appendix D) as calcium, it has the same chemical properties. Therefore, just like calcium, strontium—and, in particular, its isotope ^{89}Sr—is a bone-seeker, but with a difference.

For cancer patients who, having failed other methods of treatment, now have metastases (i.e., cancer spread) to bone, ^{89}Sr is used to deliver **radiation therapy** to those areas. It is usually administered by intravenous infusion in the chemical compound strontium chloride (trade name, Metastron). The effect is to give these patients a period of relief (up to 4 months in many cases) from incapacitation and significant pain. Because of its possible side effects (i.e., substantial depression of the patient's white blood cell count and hemoglobin that is cumulatively deleterious over time), Metastron can only be administered to a patient several times over a period of several years and in relatively small doses (typically 4-5 millicuries [mCi] per treatment).

^{89}Sr has 38 protons and 51 neutrons. For stability, this is one neutron too many. To correct this imbalance, the isotope undergoes the process of **beta decay.** In beta decay, a neutron transforms itself into a combination of a proton and an energetic electron (called a beta particle). There is also emission of another particle called a **neutrino,** which has negligible mass and no electric charge but carries away any excess energy. The electron exits the nucleus and interacts with surrounding atoms. The decayed nucleus now has one additional proton that constitutes a different element called yttrium-89 (^{89}Y).

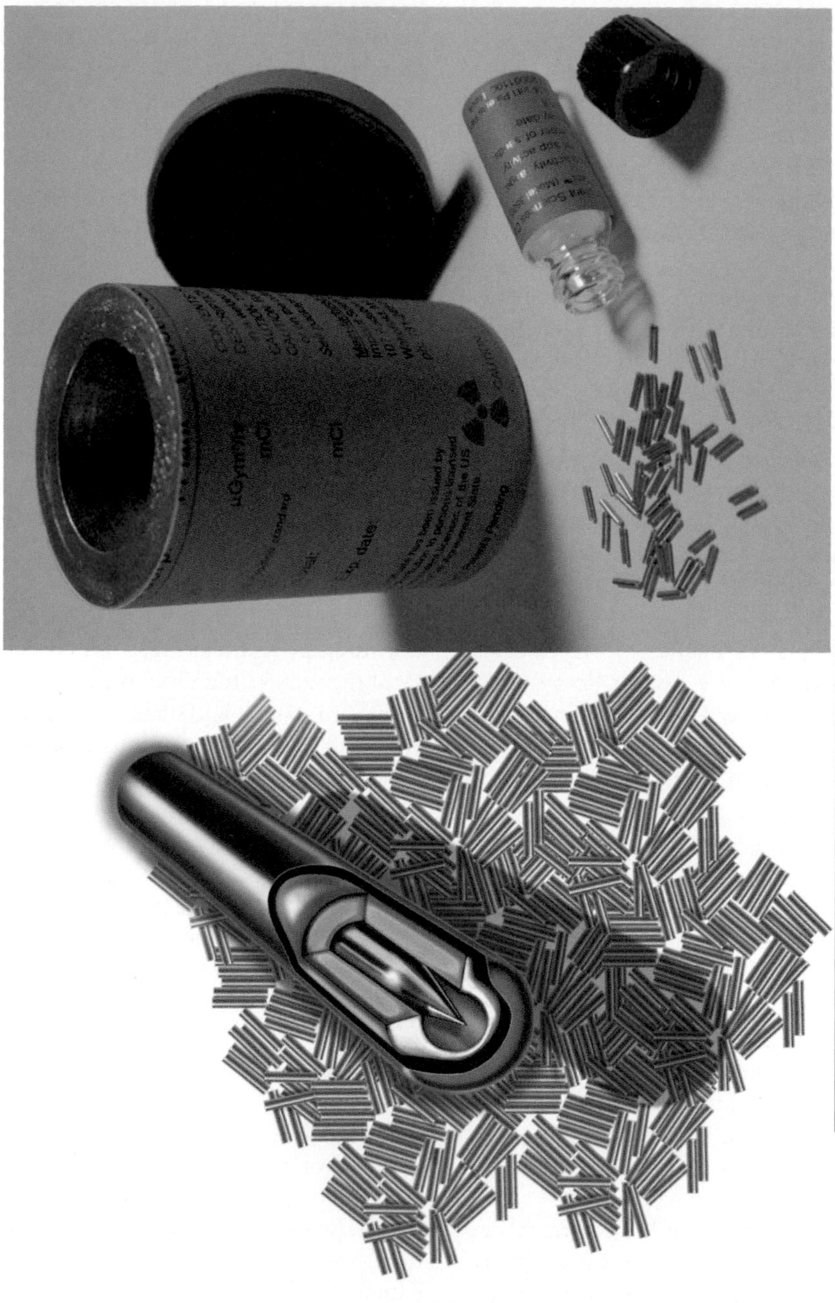

FIG. 11-1. A, ^{125}I-titanium-encapsulated cylindrical seed. **B,** ^{125}I seeds prior to encapsulation. (Courtesy of Implant Sciences Corporation.)

[89]Sr is a pure beta-emitter (i.e., there is no accompanying gamma radiation) with maximum electron energy of 1460 keV. Electrons of this energy can only penetrate through approximately 8 mm of tissue; consequently the radiation exposure levels at 3 feet will typically be less than 1 mR/hour. These patients therefore do not pose a radiation hazard to the general public. Because the isotope is given intravenously, however, there is a potential contamination problem during the first 2 days following the infusion as a result of escape through the pores of the skin and especially from urination. This can be handled easily by having the patient observe some simple precautions, such as urinating carefully, minimizing contact with others, and using separate linen and utensils during that time. After that, the patient, having been encouraged to drink a lot of fluids, essentially will have radioactivity concentrated only in bony regions.

Iodine-131 (^{131}I)

Iodine-131 (^{131}I) is another unstable isotope of the element iodine, with 53 protons and 78 neutrons in its nucleus. It has a half-life of 8 days. During its radioactive decay process (beta decay), it generates both electrons with an approximate mean energy of 192 keV and high-energy gamma rays (mean energy of 365 keV).

[131]I can be joined chemically with sodium to form a radioactive compound called sodium iodide I-131 that can be orally administered in the form of tablets. For a patient who has thyroid cancer, it is desirable to strongly irradiate any residual thyroid tissue not removed by surgery while significantly sparing surrounding tissue and other organs. Because the thyroid gland tends to highly (but not totally) absorb any iodine in the blood, administration of ^{131}I-labeled sodium iodide tablets is an efficient way of delivering a destructive radiation dose to a specific cancer site, in this case the remainder of the thyroid. It is the relatively low-energy electrons that mainly cause the destruction.

The much more penetrating gamma rays, while delivering some radiation dose to more distant body sites, primarily exit the body, presenting a **radiation protection** hazard to both nursing personnel and nuclear medicine technologists. As discussed in earlier chapters, the concepts of time, distance, and shielding should be applied. While the patient is hospitalized (usually no more than two days), a large, up to 1-inch thick, rolling lead shield can be positioned between the patient and any attending personnel for protection. Such patients are also encouraged to drink lots of fluids so that as much ^{131}I, and therefore high-energy gamma radiation, can be removed from the body by urination in as short a time as is possible.

The radioiodide tablets dissolve in the blood stream, permitting passage of radioactive matter through the pores of the skin. This poses yet another radiation safety hazard and a potential lengthy cleanup, or decontamination, task. Therefore, hospital rooms for ^{131}I therapy patients are usually isolated and carefully prepared with absorbent cloths to substantially minimize radiation exposure to both personnel and visitors either from emitted gamma radiation from the patient or from contaminated surfaces. Only trained oncology nurses and nuclear medicine personnel should be allowed in the patient's room.

Nuclear Medicine

Nuclear medicine is the branch of medicine that employs radioisotopes to study organ function in a patient, to detect the spread of cancer into bone, and to treat certain types of disease. Diagnostic techniques in nuclear medicine typically make use of short-lived radioisotopes as radioactive tracers. These radionuclides have been attached to biologically active substances or chemicals, forming radioactive compounds that diffuse predominantly into certain regions or organs where it is medically desired to scrutinize particular physiologic processes.

Iodine-123 (^{123}I)

One of the most common examples of this process makes use of **Iodine-123** (^{123}I), another unstable isotope of the element iodine, which undergoes radioactive decay by the process of electron capture (described in the section on Radiation Therapy) and has an average half-life of 13.3 hours. When chemically coupled with sodium, it forms the radiotracer compound sodium iodide I-123. This compound preferentially concentrates in the thyroid gland, achieving levels of concentration that can be directly correlated with the thyroid gland's performance status. Thus measurement of radioactivity in the region of the thyroid gland, which is due to the relative uptake by the thyroid of ^{123}I-labeled sodium iodide, makes it possible to determine the thyroid's health status.

Technetium-99m (^{99m}Tc)

By far the most common radioisotope used in nuclear medicine diagnostic studies (as much as 80% of all procedures) is **technetium-99m (^{99m}Tc).** This isotope is produced from the radioactive decay of another unstable isotope (molybdenum-99), which relieves its instability by beta decay, during which (as discussed previously) an excess neutron transforms itself into a proton, with the emission of a fast electron from the nucleus. An additional proton within the nucleus means a change in atomic number and consequently a different element. The new element in this case is ^{99m}Tc, with 43 protons and 56 neutrons. Because the beta decay of molybdenum-99 produces technetium in an excited or higher-energy state than normal, it too is unstable. Most isotopes generated in this manner immediately get rid of their excess energy. However, some do not do so for a short period, and these relatively more enduring isotopes are given the designation *m*, which stands for *metastable* (meaning "more lasting"). ^{99m}Tc has a half-life of 6 hours and decays by emission from its nucleus primarily of a gamma ray photon with energy of 140 keV.

^{99m}Tc is an extremely versatile radioisotope because it can be incorporated into a wide variety of different compounds or biologically active substances, each with a specificity for different tissues or organs of the body. For example, in combination with a tin compound it binds to red blood cells and is useful for mapping circulatory system disorders; in combination with a sulfur compound, it is absorbed by the spleen, making it possible to image the structure of the spleen; in another chemical combination, it concentrates in bone, permitting evaluation of potential cancer spread to bony areas; it can also be used to evaluate heart function. All of these studies are possible because either a deficiency of radioisotope uptake (i.e., a cold spot in radioactivity) or an excessive uptake of radioisotope-labeled compound (i.e., hot spots of radioactivity) signals abnormal organ behavior. Because of such capabilities, nuclear medicine offers diagnostic advantages beyond those of ordinary x-ray techniques.

Positron Emission Tomography and Computed Axial Tomography (PET/CT)

Overview

In Chapter 2, when the pair production interaction was discussed, a diagnostic modality called **positron emission tomography (PET)** was also mentioned. Although this modality does not require pair production interaction, it does make use of the **annihilation radiation** events that are a byproduct of this interaction. However, in the case of PET, the annihilation radiation is initiated by the radioactive decay of the nucleus of an unstable isotope. The instability in this case is associated with too many protons residing within the nucleus. Nuclei such as these usually will spontaneously undergo a reaction in which the excess proton is transmuted into a neutron and a positively charged electron **(positron).** This conserves electric charge because the neutron has none. In order to conserve energy as well, the process includes the emission of an additional particle called the neutrino. As mentioned previously, a neutrino has no electric charge and almost negligible mass, but its energy of motion (kinetic energy) balances the energy of the reaction.

As discussed in Chapter 2, a positron, classified as antimatter, when passing close to an electron—normal matter—will interact destructively with the electron. In the process, both particles will disappear, having *annihilated* one another. Their respective masses will be converted into energy that will be carried off by two photons emerging from the annihilation site in opposite directions, each with a kinetic energy of 511 keV. These energies correspond to the mass energies of the former positron and electron.

Imaging

If there is a volume (e.g., a human torso) in which many of these annihilation events are taking place, and if this volume is surrounded by a ring of densely packed detectors that are specifically tuned to 511-keV photon energies, then it is possible, in a manner analogous to that used in **computed axial tomography (CAT)**, to reconstruct diagnostically useful images of the regions within the encompassed volume where the annihilation photons are coming from. This is the concept of PET scanning.

Fluorine-18 (^{18}FI)

By far the most important isotope in PET scanning is the positron-emitter **fluorine-18 (^{18}F)**, which symbolically can be depicted as $_9F^{18}$. The subscript 9 is the atomic number and is equal to the number of protons within the nucleus, whereas the superscript 18 is the mass number and refers to the total number of nuclear particles. Thus there are nine neutrons present in the nucleus of ^{18}F. Nine neutrons are not enough to overcome the electromagnetic repulsion of the tightly packed nuclear protons. More neutrons are needed, and so the unstable nucleus undergoes a change in which, as described previously, there is one less proton present. This can be represented as:

$$p \rightarrow n + e^+ + v$$

where v is the symbol for a neutrino.

If the isotope as a whole is looked at, the process can be represented as:

$$_9F^{18} \rightarrow _8O^{18} + v + 2 \text{ annihilation energy photons}$$

where $_8O^{18}$ is a stable isotope of oxygen having 8 protons and 10 neutrons.

PET is an important imaging modality because it can examine metabolic processes within the body. This is particularly relevant to the proliferation of cancer cells. Such cells seek to reproduce without end and in order to do so require a great deal of sugar, or glucose, to supply the energy for the unlimited growth. Therefore, if it were possible to introduce within the body a radioactive molecule that was very similar to a glucose molecule, then the presence of excessive glucose metabolism sites associated with cancer cell proliferation could be discerned by detecting areas of abnormally high radioactivity.

The great significance of ^{18}F is that it can be attached to a glucose molecule, yielding a compound called **fluorodeoxyglucose (FDG)**. FDG is a radioactive tracer that not only is very similar in chemical behavior to ordinary glucose, and so will be taken up or metabolized by cancerous cells, but also will reveal their locations through its positron emission decay and subsequent generation of oppositely traveling annihilation photons. These annihilation event sites are localizable through the PET scanner's ring of coincidence detectors.

If a PET scanner is physically joined in a tandem configuration with a CAT scanner to produce a single joint imaging device then, in essence, a facility gains the ability not only to detect the presence of abnormally high regions of glucose metabolism, yielding evidence that there is cancer spread, or metastases, into other body areas, but also, at the same time, the means to obtain detailed information about the location and size of these lesions or growths. Such a combined imaging device is called a **PET/CT scanner** (Fig. 11-2).

Radiation Protection

Positron emitters result in the production of high-energy radiation. Each ^{18}F nuclear transformation by positron decay yields two highly penetrating 511-keV photons. These cannot be shielded by an ordinary lead apron. In fact, because the thickness of lead needed to attenuate such high-energy radiation by 50% (known as the **half-value layer [HVL]**) is approximately 0.2 inches, adequate shielding at close distances would require up to an inch of lead. Thus, the design of a PET/CT imaging suite involves significant radiation safety concerns. A discussion of the radiation safety design difficulties with respect to the PET/CT technologist for a minimal, but not zero, radiation exposure facility follows.

Unlike the usual diagnostic imaging suites in which the designer concentrates on protection from the radiation produced by an x-ray machine, the design of a PET/CT imaging suite presents unique additional radiation safety problems. In this situation, the scatter radiation generated by the CT scanner portion is the least of the designer's difficulties. Of far more importance is the high-energy annihilation photons emanating in all directions from the patient having the PET/CT scan. Furthermore, the presence of yet a third source of radiation, also of high energy, must be considered. Every patient who is to have a PET/CT scan requires what is called a "prep" time. During this time ^{18}F, in the form of fluorodeoxyglucose (FDG) with an

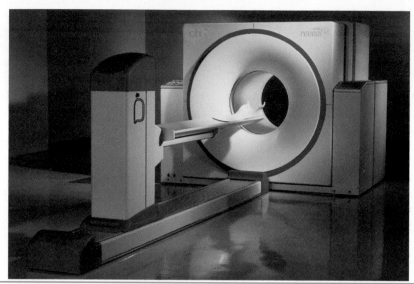

FIG. 11-2. Combined PET/CT System. (From Ballinger PW, Frank ED: *Merrill's atlas of radiographic positions and radiologic procedures,* ed 10, vol 3, St. Louis, 2003, Mosby.)

activity usually of about 15 mCi (555 megabecquerels [mbq]), is injected into the patient. The patient typically remains in the injection or prep room in a semi-reclining position for 45 to 60 minutes so that the FDG can be distributed throughout the body. This implies that in order to have a smooth-flowing, coordinated patient throughput, while one "hot" patient is being scanned, a second "hot" patient is reclining in a nearby room waiting to be scanned. Thus, during this procedure, the technologist and other personnel as well as the general public must be protected from at least two sources of high-energy radiation in addition to the scatter x-radiation from the CAT scanner.

All of this makes the calculations for a practical space-limited shielding design anything but trivial. These problems are greatly simplified when a facility can be designed from scratch instead of being retrofitted into limited existing space. Unfortunately, most often the latter is the case. Earlier it was shown that it takes a considerable amount of lead to attenuate photons with 511-keV energy. Therefore, unless other potentially mitigating factors can be brought to bear, the amount of lead shielding needed to ensure acceptable radiation safety could become unreasonable. However, such mitigating factors do exist. They involve the concepts of weekly workload (W) and

occupancy factor (T),* the decay in activity of the ^{18}F during the prep and scan times, self-attenuation by the patient, and significantly, the distance to each area of occupancy, also known as the inverse square law. Requirements for the protection of a radiographer in a new PET/CT suite shall be briefly considered.

A potential workload for an average facility could be 7 PET/CT patients per daily shift, which amounts to 35 patients per week, with each patient, let us say, receiving at the start of prep time an activity of 15 mCi of ^{18}F. The larger the weekly workload, the more shielding will be necessary in order to maintain permissible maximum equivalent dose levels to personnel and the public. ^{18}F has a physical half-life of 110 minutes; therefore, the patient's degree of radioactivity will decrease naturally throughout the prep time, losing approximately 25% to 30% by the time of scanning. This process will continue during the 45- to 50-minute scan time, with the amount of ^{18}F decreasing through physical decay alone to approximately 50% of its initial activity at the conclusion of the scan. The patient's radioactivity is further decreased by any

*The concepts of *workload* and *occupancy factor* are discussed in Chapter 9.

voiding that may take place just prior to the scanning procedure. The two processes taken together constitute what is known as an effective half-life (T_{eff}), which can be much less than the physical half-life of 110 minutes. Consequently, the patient's remaining radioactivity will typically be about one fourth of its initial value after the scan. This is important for radiation safety of the general public and any family members at the patient's home.

It should be noted that such patients at discharge produce a measured midline surface radiation intensity of 40 to 50 mR/hour, and at a distance of 1 foot a radiation intensity of about 15 mR/hour. After returning home, the patient is encouraged to drink plenty of fluids, so that with frequent urination and little permanent tissue retention, the patient's T_{eff} will be so small that emitted radiation will be almost negligible 1 day later. After this time the patient may resume full contact with all.

A well-designed facility should be arranged so that there are no areas of full occupancy immediately adjacent to a high-energy radiation source; the prep-room and scanning location of the patient are the most important of these sites to have distance from. A secondary but less significant site is the patient's toilet, which could easily acquire some contamination.

In order to determine the equivalent dose rate (millirem [mrem]/hour or microsievert [μSv]/hour) at a particular distance from a person injected with a specific amount of ^{18}F, the shielding planner must make use of a measured quantity called the *dose rate constant*.* This value is 6.96 μSv/hour, or 0.7 mrem/hour, at a distance of 1 meter per mCi of ^{18}F. Thus, if the patient did not self-attenuate any of the ^{18}F radiation, then just after a 15-mCi injection, the equivalent dose rate at 1 meter would be approximately $0.7 \times 15 = 10.5$ mrem/hour (105 μSv/hour). At greater distances, the inverse square law can be applied to obtain a value. For example, at a distance of 4 meters (approximately 13 feet), the equivalent dose rate without any shielding present has diminished to:

---

*The information discussed in this paragraph is based on material presented at the 2004 American College of Medical Physics Annual Meeting in Scottsdale, Arizona by Melissa C. Martin, M.S., FACR, in a workshop entitled "PET/CT—Site Planning and Shielding Design."

$$\frac{10.5}{4^2} = 0.66 \text{ mrem/hour } (6.6 \text{ μSv/hour})$$

Distance is a powerful tool of radiation protection! A well-designed facility will take good advantage of this. Returning to the injected patient, there are other facilitators of radiation protection at hand. Both the patient and nature are the generator of these. It has been found that the body can absorb a substantial amount of ^{18}F annihilation radiation.

The mean maximum equivalent dose rate at 1 meter from the patient per mCi (37 mbq) injected just after the injection is not 0.7 mrem/hour (6.96 μSv/hour), as it would be for an unshielded point source of radiation; rather, it has been determined to be approximately 0.3 mrem/hour (3 μSv/hour) per mCi. At a distance of 4 meters from the patient just after a 15-mCi injection, the equivalent dose rate is now given by:

$$15 \times \frac{0.3}{4^2} = 0.28 \text{ mrem/hour } (2.8 \text{ μSv/hour})$$

The contribution of nature to the radiation protection effort is that ^{18}F has a short half-life. Therefore, the 15-mCi dose injected at 2 PM is about 70% as strong at 3 PM (the approximate time that a scan will start) because of natural radioactive decay. Thus, in actuality the equivalent dose delivered by the hot patient waiting during the prep time at a distance of 4 meters is less than 0.28 mrem. If not this amount, then what effectively would a person at this location receive in 60 minutes? It must be a percentage of the whole, between 100% and 70%. Doing the mathematics of radioactive decay* yields a value of about 83%, or a correction factor of 0.83. Consequently, the equivalent dose at a distance of 4 meters that might be received by a technologist continuously at this location (i.e., occupancy level T = 1) from a 1-hour prep patient in the absence of any added shielding is:

$$0.83 \times 0.28 \text{ mrem} = 0.23 \text{ mrem } (2.3 \text{ μSv})$$

Over the course of a week, then, with all conditions remaining the same, this person will accumulate an equivalent dose of:

---

*Decay correction factor = $1.443 \times (110/60)(1 - e^{-[0.693 \times 60/100]})$

$$35 \times 0.23 \, \text{mrem} = 8.1 \, \text{mrem} \, (81 \, \mu\text{Sv})$$

Over 50 weeks, this would add up to 400 mrem (4000 μSv) from prep patients alone. But it is known that prep patients are not the only sources of high-energy radiation dose to PET/CT personnel. There is also the scan patient and, to a much lesser extent, the patient toilet. The contributions of these sources of radiation dose also need to be factored into the facility's design and shielding plan.

Consider the scan patient in some detail. As always, it is desirable to have a good distance, if at all possible, between personnel and radiation source. That may not be possible if the facility is being fit into a pre-existing area. So let it be assumed that there is only a separation of 3.3 meters from the scan patient midline to the location of the PET/CT technologist. In the absence of additional shielding, what might be the equivalent dose rate from the scan patient? The first thing to be aware of is the lesser activity in the scan patient, namely 70% of the original 15 mCi. However, this is not the whole story. The prep patient is encouraged to void just prior to being scanned. What this means is that the residual ^{18}F in the patient's body at the start of the scan will be less than 70% of the original activity. If it is assumed that about 20% more was removed by voiding, then at the start of the scan, the activity within the patient is just 50% of the original activity, namely $0.5 \times 15 = 7.5$ mCi. If there were no other considerations,* then at the start of the scan, the equivalent dose rate at the location of the technologist with no shielding would be:

$$\frac{7.5 \, \text{mCi} \times 0.3 \, \text{mrem/hour per mCi}}{(3.3)^2} = 0.2 \, \text{mrem/hour} \, (2 \, \mu\text{Sv/hour})$$

However, as seen previously, the activity within the patient will continue to decay all throughout the approximate 1 hour between voiding and his or her departure. Therefore, the equivalent dose to the technologist from the scan patient will actually be 0.83×0.2 mrem/hour, or 0.17 mrem (1.7 μSv). Over the course of a week, this amounts to $35 \times 0.17 = 6$ mrem (60 μSv). At 50 weeks, this equals 300 mrem (3 mSv).

---

*In this discussion any shielding provided by the scanner itself is being neglected.

Assuming that all other sources (e.g., patient toilet and possibly the hot lab) of radiation dose to the technologist might contribute an additional 50 mrem annually, then the unshielded technologist could receive an annual equivalent dose of 750 mrem in this facility.

Shielding can be installed to significantly decrease this amount. Let us seek to reduce this value to a total of 250 mrem (2.5 mSv), or 5 mrem/week (50 μSv/week).

Fig. 11-3 depicts a facility layout schematic that will be referred to for shielding calculations. For simplicity, they shall be restricted to protection of the PET/CT radiographer. In addition, the task will be further confined to reducing the contributions from the patient occupying the prep room and the patient being scanned. Beginning with the scan patient, it is required that both the viewing window and its surrounding wall be shielded so that the 300-mrem (3-mSv) annual equivalent dose contribution decreases to 100 mrem (1 mSv). As mentioned earlier, the amount of lead needed to decrease the intensity of this high-energy radiation by 50% is called its half value layer (HVL). The HVL is equal to 0.2 inches of lead. One HVL will bring the equivalent dose down to 150 mrem, and 2 HVLs will cut it to 75 mrem. Therefore, less than 2 HVLs would be needed. Doing the mathematics* results in:

$$1.56 \, \text{HVLs or } 1.56 \times 0.2 \, \text{inch of lead} = 0.312\text{-inch of lead} \, (5/16\text{-inch})$$

Thus, 5/16-inch of lead must be placed in the wall surrounding the view window, and the view window itself must be composed of 5/16-inch of lead acrylic to achieve the goal. This amount of lead is far more than would be required to shield the operator from the much less penetrating CT scatter radiation. Therefore,

---

*If n is the required number of HVLs, then in order to attenuate the radiation to 1/3 of its value:

$$2^{-n} = 1/3$$

$$\log 2^{-n} = \log(1/3)$$

$$-n \log 2 = \log 1 - \log 3 = -\log 3$$

$$n = \log 3/\log 2$$

$$n = 1.56$$

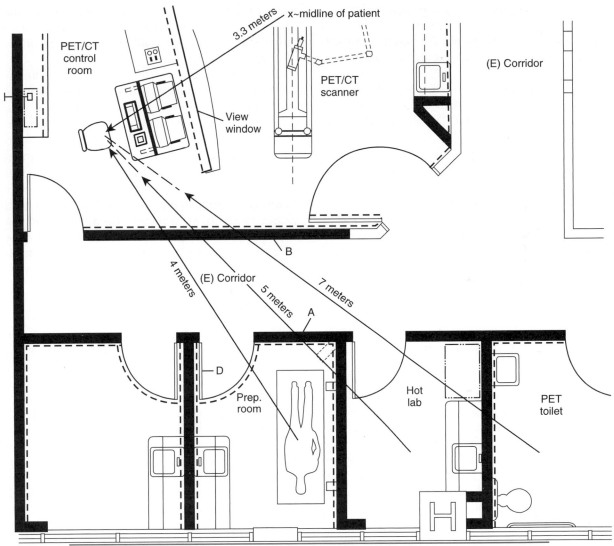

FIG. 11-3. Layout diagram of a PET/CT imaging facility.

the scatter radiation does not have to be additionally accounted for. For the patient in the prep room, the goal is to interpose shielding so that the 400-mrem (4-mSv) annual equivalent dose contribution to the technologist decreases to 100 mrem (1 mSv); this decrease by a factor of 4 clearly requires 2 HVLs, or 0.4-inch (13/32-inch) of lead. Examining the diagram, it is evident that this amount of shielding can be distributed between the prep room corridor wall and door (labeled A and D, respectively) and the scan suite cor-

ridor wall (labeled B). Excluding personnel other than the operator and any other circumstances, a practical solution is to place ¼-inch of lead in A and D and 3/16-inch of lead in B.

In conclusion, it is obvious that there is much to be considered when designing radiation shielding for a PET/CT facility. Other personnel and the general public must also be protected from the high-energy radiation. Their protection involves lower permissible equivalent dose limits than for the occupationally exposed radiographer. If there is the opportunity to design the facility from scratch, then the required shielding can be greatly reduced; if not, then the calculations and the amount of needed shielding can be sizeable.

RADIATION EMERGENCIES: THE USE OF RADIATION AS A TERRORIST WEAPON

Following the attack of the World Trade Center by hijacked airplanes on September 11, 2001, the possibility of the use of other possible terrorist weapons, such as radiation, became a public health concern. Today, most hospitals have **radiation emergency plans** for handling emergency situations involving **radioactive contamination.** Radiologic technologists should make themselves aware of the radiation emergency plans that exist in the facilities in which they work. In this section, some fundamental principles of dealing with radioactive contamination in a health care environment are discussed.

Contamination

A **radioactive dispersal device, or "dirty bomb,"** is a radioactive source mixed with conventional explosives. It is intended to contaminate an area with radioactive material and thereby cause panic. The actual long-term health effects of a dirty bomb are likely to be minimal. If the radioactive material remains in a small area, few people may be affected. However, if enough explosives are used to spread the radioactive material over a broad area, then the radioactivity will be diluted and may not be much higher than background levels.

For example, it would be difficult for terrorists to accumulate as much radioactive material as existed in the Chernobyl nuclear reactor. However, if they were able to do this and exploded the device with the same force as the explosion at Chernobyl, the actual number of radiation injuries would probably be quite small. At Chernobyl, no cases of acute radiation syndrome (ARS) were caused by exposure outside of the immediate vicinity of the reactor. The only cases occurred in emergency workers, primarily firemen, who worked very near the reactor. They had little training and essentially no protective gear to prepare them for a radioactive emergency. In the United States, at the present time emergency responders are equipped to monitor and assess personnel exposure on-site in an emergency situation.

After an explosion of a dirty bomb, some individuals would be contaminated with dust and debris, some of which could contain radioactive materials. The procedure for **decontamination** is surprisingly simple. Removal of contaminated clothing and immersion in a shower is the best method. If a wound contains radioactive material, a simple rinse of the area is usually sufficient to allow medical personnel to provide medical attention. Most hospitals are stocked with **Geiger-Müller (GM) detectors** (described in Chapter 10), and emergency personnel are trained to provide guidance concerning contamination levels. The facility's radiation safety officer (RSO) would also be available to assess contamination levels.

It is unlikely that a dirty bomb would cause contamination with so much radioactive material that a victim could not receive medical attention. The key here is that the same personnel need not be near the patient(s) for any length of time. Most emergency room treatments do not require the staff to be near the patient(s) for as long as an hour. Even if a GM detector shows readings of two to five times natural background radiation, this means an effective dose of only 0.03-0.15 mSv per hour (3–15 mrem per hour) to a physician who is in direct contact with the patient. Therefore, a physician could treat this patient under these circumstances without exceeding normal badge limits. In fact, normal badge limits do not apply in radiation emergency situations.

The **Environmental Protection Agency (EPA)** suggests that, during an emergency situation, individuals engaged in non-lifesaving activities work under a dose limit of 50 mSv (5 rem) per event. For individuals engaged in lifesaving activities, the dose limit rises to 250 mSv (25 rem) per event.[1] Because it may be difficult to monitor all workers involved in a radiation emergency, a dose rate criterion is often used. In this case, if the dose rate in the area is less than 0.1 mSv/hour (10 mrem/hour), emergency personnel may enter an area to perform critical tasks. At a dose rate of 0.1 Sv/hour (10 rem/hour), emergency personnel should await specific instructions from radiation experts on how to proceed.[2]

Cleanup of a Contaminated Urban Area

The EPA sets limits for radioactive contamination that assume that a 1-in-10,000 risk of causing a fatal cancer is unacceptable. This type of regulation requires hospitals, educational facilities, and industries to control accidental exposures so that the health of the population cannot be measurably affected. It also assumes that there are many other carcinogens present and that all are regulated to a similar low level.

However, if radioactive contamination were to result from a dirty bomb, it is hoped that a more realistic evaluation of actual risk would be used. Unnecessary use of resources to clean a large inhabitable area, at the heart of a major city, for example to unreasonably stringent standards would be an unfortunate outcome requiring the expenditure of vast resources that could be used to benefit the public elsewhere. For example, a 1-in-10,000 probability of causing a fatal cancer corresponds approximately to a 2-mSv (200-mrem) effective dose. Recall from Chapter 1 that the effective dose due to average natural background radiation is approximately 3 mSv (300 mrem). Therefore, cleanup of a contaminated site to levels associated with normal radiation protection standards would require heroic measures such as removal of topsoil and digging up of roadways. A practical compromise should be made to allow land use after a reasonable cleanup.

Medical Management of Persons Suffering from Radiation Bioeffects

If **surface contamination** is suspected, personnel should wear gowns, masks, and gloves when working with the patient. The same procedures that control the spread of infection are useful to prevent the spread of radioactive contamination. Clothing of individuals that have been contaminated should be placed in plastic containers and set aside for later evaluation. Removal of surface contamination involves removal of the patient's clothing and the use of a shower to cleanse the skin.

The various stages of ARS were discussed in Chapter 6. (A complete discussion of procedures for dealing with people who suffer from ARS is beyond the scope of this text. The interested reader is referred to several recent publications on this subject.[3,4]) In dealing with patients with ARS, some estimate of the amount of exposure they have received helps predict the clinical course of the syndrome (Table 11-1). For exposures localized to specific regions of the body,

---

TABLE 11-1

Dose-Effect Relation After Acute Whole-Body Radiation from Gamma Rays or X-Rays*

Whole-Body	Absorbed Dose Effect
0.05 Gy	No symptoms
0.15 Gy	No symptoms, but possible chromosomal aberrations in cultured peripheral blood lymphocytes
0.5 Gy	No symptoms (minor decreases in white blood cell and platelet counts in a few persons)
1 Gy	Nausea and vomiting in approximately 10% of patients within 48 hr after exposure
2 Gy	Nausea and vomiting in approximately 50% of persons within 24 hr, with marked decreases in white blood cell and platelet counts
4 Gy	Nausea and vomiting in 90% of persons within 12 hr, and diarrhea in 10% within 8 hr; 50% mortality in the absence of treatment
6 Gy	100% mortality within 30 days due to bone marrow failure in the absence of treatment
10 Gy	Approximate dose that is survivable with the best medical therapy available
>10-30 Gy	Nausea and vomiting in all persons in less than 5 min; severe gastrointestinal damage; death likely in 2 to 3 wk in the absence of treatment
>30 Gy	Cardiovascular collapse and central nervous system damage, with death in 24 to 72 hr

*Data from Gusev et al.[3]

medical management involves prevention of infection and control of pain and may include skin grafts. If beta-emitting radioactive material settles on a patient's skin, the dose is superficial and skin grafts may be successful. Gamma emitting materials can produce a deeper dose that may interfere with healing.

During the first 48 hours of ARS, symptoms such as nausea and vomiting occur. Medical management at this time is simply to treat the symptoms and try to prevent dehydration. The bone marrow becomes depleted (leukopenia and thrombocytopenia) after a few weeks. Bone marrow transplantation has been attempted in individuals such as Chernobyl emergency workers. However, this strategy has not been successful. The current strategy is to administer drugs that stimulate any remaining bone marrow.

In the event of **internal contamination,** various strategies are used, depending upon the clinical and radiologic form of contamination. Some of these strategies include dilution (forcing fluids) and blocking absorption in the gastrointestinal tract (administration of emetics, charcoal, laxatives). If the radionuclide is iodine, administration of potassium iodide to block further uptake in the thyroid is possible if no more than a few hours have elapsed since the contamination.

SUMMARY

➤ Isotopes are atoms that have the same number of protons within the nucleus but have different numbers of neutrons.
  ■ Some nuclei of isotopes have too many neutrons or too many protons.
  ■ Radioactive isotopes spontaneously undergo changes or transformations to rectify their unstable arrangement.
➤ Rapidly dividing cells that are well oxygenated are very radiosensitive.
  ■ When cells are radiosensitive, cancerous growths or tumors can either be eliminated or at least controlled by irradiation of the area containing the growth.
➤ Therapeutic isotopes may be characterized by relatively long half-lives.
➤ Fast electrons are beta radiation.

➤ Gamma rays and x-ray photons differ only in their point of origin.
➤ Iodine-125 decays with a half-life of 59.4 days by a process called electron capture.
➤ The most practical radiation protection to follow for patients having therapeutic prostate seed implants is utilization of the concepts of distance and time.
➤ The radioactive isotope Strontium-89 is a bone-seeker.
➤ A neutrino is a particle that has negligible mass and no electric charge but carries away any excess energy from the nucleus of the atom.
➤ When Iodine-131 is being administered to treat a hospitalized patient for thyroid cancer, a large, up to 1–inch-thick, rolling lead shield can be positioned between the patient and any attending personnel for protection.
➤ Diagnostic techniques in nuclear medicine typically make use of short-lived radioisotopes as radioactive tracers.
  ■ Technetium-99m is the most common radioisotope used in nuclear medicine.
➤ Positron emission tomography (PET) makes use of annihilation radiation events.
  ■ When annihilation occurs, the positron and electron interact destructively and annihilate each other. Their respective masses convert into energy that will be carried off by two photons emerging from the annihilation site in opposite directions, each with a kinetic energy of 511 keV.
  ■ Fluorine-18 is the most important isotope used for PET scanning.
  ■ PET is an important imaging modality because it can examine metabolic processes within the body.
  ■ Fluorodeoxyglucose (FDG) is a radioactive tracer that is taken up or metabolized by cancerous cells and that will reveal their location through positron emission decay and subsequent generation of oppositely traveling annihilation photons.
  ■ A PET/CT scanner can detect the presence of abnormally high regions of glucose metabolism, providing evidence that there is metastasis to

other body areas, and at the same time can obtain detailed information about the location and size of these lesions or growths.

- Positron emitters result in the production of high-energy radiation, and for this reason, design of a PET/CT imaging suite involves significant radiation safety concerns.

➤ Most hospitals have radiation emergency plans for handling emergency situations involving radioactive contamination.

➤ A radioactive dispersal device, or "dirty bomb," is a radioactive source mixed with conventional explosives, the actual long-term health effects of which will most likely be minimal.

- If radioactive material from a dirty bomb remains in a small area, few people may be affected.
- On the other hand, if enough explosives are used to spread the radioactive material over a broad area, radioactivity will be diluted and may not be much higher than background levels.
- If a dirty bomb exploded with the same force as the explosion at Chernobyl, the actual number of radiation injuries could be quite small.

➤ The United States currently has emergency responders that are prepared and equipped to monitor and assess personnel exposure on-site in an emergency situation.

- After an explosion of a dirty bomb, externally contaminated individuals can be decontaminated by removal of contaminated clothing and immersion in a shower.
- Geiger-Müller (GM) detectors may be used by trained emergency personnel to monitor contamination levels.
- During an emergency situation, individuals engaged in non-lifesaving activities are to work under a dose limit of 50 mSv (5 rem) per event, while those persons performing lifesaving activities have a dose limit of 250 mSv (25 rem).
- If surface contamination is suspected, emergency personnel should protect themselves by wearing gowns, masks, and gloves while working with the patient.
- Handling of patients with internal contamination will vary depending on the clinical and radiologic form of contamination. Strategies

may include dilution and blocking absorption in the gastrointestinal tract. Potassium iodide can be administered to block further uptake of radioactive iodine in the thyroid gland.

References

1. Mettler NEJM, Mettler FA, Voelz: Major radiation exposure: what to expect and how to respond, *N Engl J Med*, 346:20, 1554-1561, 2002.
2. National Council on Radiation Protection and Measurements (NCRP): *Report #138, Management of terrorist events involving radioactive material*, Bethesda, MD, 2001, NCRP.
3. Gusev I, Guskova AK, Mettler FA Jr, editors: *Medical management of radiation accidents*, ed 2, Boca Raton, Fla, 2001, CRC Press.
4. Jarrett D, editor: Medical management of radiation casualties: handbook, AFRRI special publication 99-2, Bethesda, Md, 1999. Armed Forces Radiobiology Research Institute. (Also available at http://www.afrri.usuhs.mil.)

GENERAL DISCUSSION QUESTIONS

1. Why do isotopes that have too many neutrons or too many protons spontaneously undergo changes or transformations?
2. What causes cancerous growths or tumors to be eliminated or controlled by irradiation?
3. What difference exists between gamma rays and x-ray photons?
4. What are the best radiation safety practices to follow for patients having therapeutic prostate seed implants?
5. While caring for a hospitalized patient receiving Iodine-131 therapy for cancer, what can hospital personnel do to minimize occupational exposure?
6. What radiation safety concerns are associated with the design of a PET/CT imaging suite and how is radiation protection provided to meet these concerns?
7. What is a radioactive dispersal device, or "dirty bomb," and what are the possible consequences if such a device is detonated?

8. If a wound contains radioactive material, what should be done to decontaminate the wound?

9. At what dose level may an individual engaged in lifesaving activities during a radiation emergency receive?

10. If surface contamination is suspected, what should medical personnel wear when working with a contaminated patient?

REVIEW QUESTIONS

1. **Well-oxygenated rapidly dividing cells are:**
   A. Very insensitive and are not damaged by radiation
   B. Very sensitive to damage by radiation
   C. Moderately sensitive to damage by radiation
   D. Somewhat sensitive to damage by radiation

2. **Iodine-125 decays with a half-life of 59.4 days by a process called:**
   A. Attenuation
   B. Electron capture
   C. Pair production
   D. Photodisintegration

3. **Which of the following steps should be taken for external decontamination from radioactive materials?**
   1. **Removal of contaminated clothing**
   2. **Immersion of contaminated person in a shower**
   3. **Monitoring of the contaminated individual with a Geiger-Müller detector**
   A. 1 and 2 only
   B. 1 and 3 only
   C. 2 and 3 only
   D. 1, 2, and 3

4. **What dose level may an individual who is engaged in non-lifesaving activities during a radiation emergency safely receive?**
   A. 10 mSv (1 rem) per event
   B. 30 mSv (3 rem) per event
   C. 50 mSv (5 rem) per event
   D. 250 mSv (25 rem) per event

5. **Clothing of individuals that has been contaminated should be:**
   A. Aired out on a clothesline to decontaminate
   B. Burned immediately
   C. Placed in plastic containers and set aside for later evaluation
   D. Shaken out and put back on

6. **All of the following statements are true *except*:**
   A. In dealing with patients with acute radiation syndrome (ARS), some estimate of the amount of exposure they have received helps predict the clinical course of the syndrome.
   B. If beta-emitting radioactive material settles on a patient's skin, the dose is very deep and skin grafts will not be very successful
   C. Gamma-emitting radioactive materials may produce a deep dose that may interfere with healing
   D. Current strategy for an ARS patient is to administer drugs that stimulate any remaining bone marrow

7. **Some of the strategies used to treat internal radiation contamination include:**
   1. **Dilution (forcing fluids)**
   2. **Blocking absorption in the gastrointestinal tract (administration of emetics, charcoal, laxatives)**
   3. **Administration of potassium iodide to block further uptake in the thyroid, if the radionuclide is iodine and no more than a few hours have elapsed since the contamination**
   A. 1 only
   B. 2 only
   C. 3 only
   D. 1, 2, and 3

8. **A well-designed PET/CT facility should be arranged so that there are no areas of full occupancy immediately adjacent to a:**
   A. High-energy radiation source
   B. Low-energy radiation source
   C. Patient waiting area
   D. Public corridor

9. **Which of the following is a radioactive tracer that is taken up or metabolized by cancerous cells and that will reveal their location through positron emission decay and subsequent generation of oppositely traveling annihilation photons?**
   A. Technetium-99m
   B. Strontium-89
   C. Iodine-131
   D. Fluorodeoxyglucose

10. **Iodine-125 patients should *significantly* limit durations of close contact (<3 feet) with small children and pregnant women for a period of:**
   A. Six days after their implant procedure
   B. Six weeks after their implant procedure
   C. Six months after their implant procedure
   D. Six years after their implant procedure

BIBLIOGRAPHY

American College of Radiology Bulletin 52:4, 1996.

American Society of Radiologic Technologists: Shields and radiation safety, patient page, Radiol Technol 71:2, 1999.

American Society of Radiologic Technologists: Authors tie CT dose with increased cancer risk, ASRT Scanner 33:6, 2001.

Anderson R: New dose limits boggle the mind, ASRT Scanner 27:1, 1995.

ASRT Scanner 30:27, 1997.

ASRT Scanner 31:10, 1999.

Ballinger PW, Frank ED: Merrill's atlas of radiographic positions and radiologic procedures, ed 10, St. Louis, 2003, Mosby.

Balter M: Children become the first victims of fallout, Science 272:357, 1996.

Barannov A et al: Bone marrow transplantation after the Chernobyl nuclear accident, N Engl J Med 321:205, 1989.

Barcham N, Egan I, Dowd SB: Gonadal protection methods in neonatal chest radiography, Radiol Technol 69:2, 1997.

Barnett MH: The biological effects of ionizing radiation: an overview, HEW Publication FDA 77-8004, Rockville, Md, 1976, USDH.

Baron J et al: Radiation biology: a survey of the measurement of ionizing radiation and the latent effects of low levels of radiation, Chicago, ASRT.

Beebe GW, Kato H, Land CE: Studies of the mortality of A-bomb survivors. 6. mortality and radiation dose, 1950-1974, J Radiat Res 75:138, 1978.

Bethesda Council on Radiation Protection and Measurements: Report 102: medical x-ray, electron beam and gamma-ray protection for energies up to 50 MeV, Bethesda, Md, 1989, NCRP.

Bond VP, Thiessen JW, editors: Reevaluation of dosimetric factors: Hiroshima and Nagasaki, Springfield, Va, 1982, U.S. Department of Energy/U.S. Department of Commerce.

Bonte FJ: Chernobyl retrospective, Semin Nucl Med 18:16, 1988.

Bontrager KL: Textbook of radiographic positioning and related anatomy, ed 5, St. Louis, 2001, Mosby.

Boone JM, Levin DC: Radiation exposure to angiographers under different fluoroscopic conditions, Radiology 180:861, 1991.

Brateman L: Radiation safety considerations for diagnostic radiology personnel, RadioGraphics. Available at: http://radiographics.rsnajnls.org/cgi/com. Accessed March 16, 2000.

Burke PJ: Human oocyte radiosensitivity, Radiol Technol 75:6, 2004.

Bushong S: Radiation protection: Essentials of medical imaging series, New York, 1998, McGraw-Hill.

Bushong S: Radiologic science for technologists: physics, biology, and protection, ed 8, St. Louis, 2004, Elsevier Mosby.

Cameron JR: Radiation hormesis, Phys Today 45:13, 1992 (letter).

Cameron JR: Are x-rays safe? RT Image 13(33):21–22, 31–32, 2000.

Cameron JR: What is TLD? RT Image 14:17, 2001.

Cameron JR: Beyond TLD optically stimulated luminescence, RT Image 14:19, 2001.

Cameron JR: Radiation quantities translating foreign language, RT Image 14:32, 2001.

Cardis E: Long-term health effects. Available at: http://iaea.or.at/worldatom/inforesource/bulletin/ bull383/cardis.html.

Carlton RR, Adler AM: Principles of radiographic imaging: an art and a science, ed 3, Stamford, CT, 2001, Delmar/Thomson Learning.

Chernobyl Accident. Available at http://www.world-nuclear.org/info/chernobyl/inf07print.htm. Accessed December 2, 2004.

Chernobyl: Health impact—Chapter 5. Available at: http://www.nea.fr/html/rp/chernobyl/c05.html. Accessed October 22, 2000.

Chernobyl disaster: health and psychological consequences of Chernobyl. Available at: http://www.chernobyl.co.uk/health.html. Accessed October 22, 2000.

Chernobyl information. Available at http://chernobyl.info/. Accessed June 30 2004 and January 2, 2005.

Children getting too much radiation from CT scans, RT Image 14:6, 2001.

Chu RYL, Parry C, Eaton BG: Entrance skin exposure in PA chest radiography, Radiol Technol 69:3, 1998.

Commission of Life Sciences, Advisory Committee on Biologic Effects of Ionizing Radiation: Biological effects of radiation, Washington, DC, 1980, National Academy Press.

Committee on the Biological Effects of Ionizing Radiations: *The effects on populations of exposure to low levels on ionizing radiation*, Washington, DC, 1990, National Academy Press.

Committee on the Biological Effects of Ionizing Radiations, National Academy of Sciences, National Research Council: *Health effects of exposure to low levels on ionizing radiation (BEIR III Report)*, Washington, DC, 1980, National Academy Press.

Committee on Biological Effects of Ionizing Radiation, National Research Council, Commission of Life Sciences, Board on Radiation Research: *Health effects of exposure to low levels of ionizing radiation (BEIR V Report)*, Washington, DC, 1989, National Academy Press.

Dansak RL: Portable procedures: what RTs should know, *RT Image* 14:41, 2001.

Dowd SB, Ott K: The radiologic technologist's role in patient education, *Radiol Technol* 69:5, 1998.

Duke RC, Ojcius DM, Young J: Cell suicide in health and disease, *Sci Am* 275:80, 1996.

Early PJ, Sodee DB: *Principles and practice of nuclear medicine*, ed 2, St. Louis, 1995, Mosby.

Eastman TR: Portable radiography, *Radiol Technol* 69:5, 1998.

Eddy DM, Hasselblad V, McGivney W, Hendee W: The value of mammography screening in women under age 50 years, JAMA 259:1512, 1988.

ER patients unaware of CT risks and benefits, *ASRT Scanner* 36:10, 2004.

FDA Public Health Advisory: Avoidance of serious x-ray-induced skin injuries to patients during fluoroscopically guided procedures. Available at: http://www.fda.gov/cdrh/fluo.html. Accessed November 4, 1999.

Finch SC: Acute radiation syndrome, JAMA 258:664, 1987.

Fullerton GD et al, editors: *Medical Physics Monograph No. 5*, New York, 1980, American Institute of Physics for the American Association of Physicists in Medicine.

Furlow B: Biological effects of diagnostic imaging, *Radiol Technol* 75:5, 2004.

Gale RP: Immediate medical consequences of nuclear accidents: lessons from Chernobyl, JAMA 258:625, 1987.

Garner J: Screen-film vs. filmless: which yields less radiation?, *RT Image* 18:17, 2005.

Glasstone S, editor, for U.S. Department of Defense: *The effects of nuclear weapons*, rev ed, Washington, DC, 1964, U.S. Atomic Energy Commission.

Gollnick DA: *Basic radiation protection technology*, ed 4, Altadena, Calif, 2000, Pacific Radiation Corporation.

Hagler M: Radiation protection update, *RT Image* 3:10, 1990.

Hall EJ: Risk of cancer causation by diagnostic x-rays, *Cancer Prev Control* 1, 1990.

Hamilton TE, van Belle G, LoGerfo JP: Thyroid neoplasia in Marshall Islanders exposed to nuclear fallout, JAMA 258:629, 1987.

Health Central: Child thyroid cancer rises 10-fold after Chernobyl. Available at: Health Central.com—news. Accessed June 30, 1999.

Hendee WR: Estimation of radiation risks: BEIR V and its significance for medicine, JAMA 268:620, 1992.

Herlitz Publications: Ionizing radiation exposure levels show less than estimated, *Oncology Times* 10:4, 1988.

Hersey J: *Hiroshima*, First Vintage Books Edition, New York, February 1989, Vintage Books.

Hildreth R: *From x-ray martyrs to low level radiation*, Kalamazoo, Mich, 1981, Industrial Graphics Services.

International Atomic Energy Agency: Radiation safety. Available at: http://www.iaea.or.at/worldatom/inforesource/other/radiation/radsafe.html. Accessed November 13, 2000.

International Commission of Radiation Units and Measurements: *Report 33, Radiation quantities and units*, Washington, DC, 1981, ICRU.

International Commission of Radiological Protection: *Protection of the patient in x-ray diagnosis*, ICRP Publication 16, Oxford, England, 1977, Pergamon Press.

International Commission of Radiological Protection: *Recommendations of the ICRP*, ICRP Publication 26, Elmsford, NY, 1977, Pergamon Press.

International Commission of Radiological Protection: *Cost-benefit analysis in the optimization of radiation protection*, ICRP Publication 37, Elmsford, NY, 1983, Pergamon Press.

International Commission of Radiological Protection: *Optimization and decision-making in radiological protection*, ICRP Publication 55, Elmsford, NY, 1989, Pergamon Press.

International Commission of Radiological Protection: *1990 recommendations of the ICRP*, ICRP Publication 60, Elmsford, NY, 1991, Pergamon Press.

International Commission of Radiological Protection: Some more information about ICRP. Available at: http://www.icrp.org/services.asp. Accessed April 26, 2001.

International Conference: One decade after Chernobyl. Available at: http://www.iaea.or.at/worldatom/thisweek/preview/chernobyl/concls17.html. Accessed October 22, 2000.

Jayaraman S et al: Analysis of radiation risk versus benefit in mammography, *Appl Radiol* 68:1, 1996.

Kamm B: Communicating with mammography patients, *Radiol Technol* 71:3, 2000.

Katsuda T, Okazaki M, Kuroda C: Using compensating filters to reduce radiation dose, *Radiol Technol* 68:1, 1996.

Kehoe J: Brilliant science, bitter scandal: the life of Marie Curie, *Biography Magazine*, July 1999, p 88.

Kilthau GF: Cancer risk in relation to radioactivity in tobacco, *Radiol Technol* 67:217, 1996.

Kusza J: Diving into new possibilities: hyperbaric oxygen therapy surfaces as powerful therapy, *RT Image* 17:27, 2004.

Legg JS: Provider efforts to increase mammography screening, *Radiol Technol* 71:435, 2000.

Lessard E et al: *Thyroid absorbed dose for people at Rongelap, Utrik, and Sifo on March 1, 1954*, U.S. Department of Energy publication (BNL) 51882, Upton, NY, 1985, Brookhaven National Laboratory.

Lewis J: The birth of the EPA, U.S. Environmental Protection Agency. Available at: http://www.epa.gov/history/faqs/index.html.

Lindell B, Dunster HJ, Valentin J: *International Commission on Radiological Protection: history, policies, procedures*, Swedish Radiation Protection Institute (SSI), SE-171 16 Stockholm, Sweden. Available at: http://www.icrp.org. Accessed March 3, 2001.

Linnemann RE: Soviet medical response to the Chernobyl nuclear accident, *JAMA* 258:637, 1987.

Loudin A: The radiation debate continues, *RT Image* 3:10, 1990.

March HC: Leukemia in radiologists, *Radiology* 43:275, 1944.

Marples DR: Chernobyl ten years later—the facts. Available at: http://209.82.13.226/history/ chernobyl/marples.

Miller PE: Biological effects of diagnostic irradiation, *Radiol Technol* 48:11, 1976.

Miller RW: Effects of ionizing radiation from the atomic bomb on Japanese children, *Pediatrics* 41:257, 1968.

Miller RW: Delayed radiation effects in atomic bomb survivors, *Science* 166:569, 1969.

Minigh J: Pediatric Radiation Protection, *Radiol Technol* 76:5, 2005.

Mosby's radiographic instructional series: *Radiobiology and radiation protection*, St. Louis, 1999, Mosby.

National Council on Radiation Protection: *Report 39, basic radiation protection criteria*, Washington, DC, 1971, NCRP.

National Council on Radiation Protection: *Report 43, review of the current state of radiation protection philosophy*, Washington, DC, 1975, NCRP.

National Council on Radiation Protection: *Report 68, radiation protection in pediatric radiology*, Washington, DC, 1981, NCRP.

National Council on Radiation Protection: *Report 91, recommendations on limits for exposure to ionizing radiation*, Washington, DC, 1987, NCRP.

National Council on Radiation Protection: *Report 93, ionizing radiation exposure of the population of the United States*, Washington, DC, 1987, NCRP.

National Council on Radiation Protection: *Report 104, the relative biological effectiveness of radiations of different quality*, Washington, DC, 1987, NCRP.

National Council on Radiation Protection: *Report 105, radiation protection for medical and allied health personnel*, Washington, DC, 1990, NCRP.

National Council on Radiation Protection: *Report 107, implementation of the principle of as low as reasonably achievable (ALARA)*, Washington, DC, 1990, NCRP.

National Council on Radiation Protection: *Report 115, risk estimates for radiation protection*, Washington, DC, 1993, NCRP.

National Council on Radiation Protection: *Report 116, limitation of exposure to ionizing radiation*, Washington, DC, 1993, NCRP.

National Council on Radiation Protection: *Commentary 13, an introduction to efficacy in diagnostic radiology and nuclear medicine (justification of medical radiation exposure)*, Bethesda, Md, 1996, NCRP.

National Council on Radiation Protection and Measurements: *Report 49, structural shielding design and evaluation for medical use of x-ray and gamma rays with energies up to 10 meV*, Washington, DC, 1976, NCRP.

National Council on Radiation Protection and Measurements: *Report 54, medical radiation exposure of pregnant and potentially pregnant women*, Washington, DC, 1977, NCRP.

National Council on Radiation Protection and Measurements: *Report 100, exposure of the U.S. population from diagnostic medical radiation*, Washington, DC, 1977, NCRP.

National Council on Radiation Protection and Measurements: *Report 101, exposure of the U.S. population from occupational radiation*, Washington, DC, 1989, NCRP.

National Council on Radiation Protection and Measurements: *Report 147, structural shielding design for medical x-ray imaging facilities*, Bethesda, Md, 2004, NCRP.

National Council on Radiation Protection and Measurements: *The application of ALARA for occupational exposures*, NCRP statement No. 8, issued June 8, 1999.

National Council on Radiation Protection and Measurements: Background information. Available at: http://www.ncrp.com/info.html. Accessed March 8, 2001.

National Safety Council, Environmental Health Center: *How to protect you and your family from radon*, Washington, DC, 2002, NSC.

New Jersey Department of Health, Division of Occupational Environmental Health: *Facts and recommendation on exposure to radon*, Trenton, 1987, New Jersey Department of Health.

Newman J: Radiation protection for radiologic technologists, *Radiol Technol* 71:3, 2000.

Peart O: Radiation protection and ensuring proper positioning, *RT Image* 14:22, 2001.

Perry AR, Iglar HF: The accident at Chernobyl: radiation doses and effects, *Radiol Technol* 61:290, 1990.

Polednak AP, Stehney AF, Rowland RE: Mortality among women first employed before 1930 in the US radium dial-painting industry, *Am J Epidemiol* 107:179, 1978.

Radiation Effects Research Foundation: RERF history—historical perspectives. Available at: http://www.rerf.or.ip/eigol/historic/histpers.htm. Accessed April 26, 2001.

Radiation induced skin injuries can result from fluoroscopy, *ASRT Scanner* 27:22, 1995.

Radiation safety. Available at: http://www.iaea.or.at/worldatom/inforesource/other/radiation/radsafe.html.

Radon. Available at: http://www.nsc.org/issues/radon/. Accessed January 12, 2005.

Reimenschneider J: Rethinking radiation protection standards, *RT Image* 3:1990.

Rowland RE, Stehney AF, Lucas HF Jr: Dose response relationships for female radium dial workers, *Radiat Res* 76:368, 1978.

Saccomanno G, Archer VE, Saunders RP, et al: Lung cancer of uranium miners on the Colorado plateau, *Health Phys* 10:1195, 1964.

Schleipman AR: Occupational radiation exposure: population studies, *Radiol Technol* 76(3):185-191, 2005.

Seeram E: Digital image processing, *Radiol Technol* 75(6): 435-452, 2004.

Seeram E: Radiation dose in computed tomography, *Radiol Technol* 70(6):534, 1999.

Seltser R, Sartwell PE: The influence of occupational exposure to radiation on the mortality of American radiologists and other medical specialists, *Am J Epidemiol* 81:2, 1965.

Shcherbak YM: Ten years of the Chernobyl era. Available at: http://www.sciam.com/0496issue/0496shcherbak.html. Accessed October 22, 2000.

Shymko M: Minimizing occupational exposure, *Radiol Technol* 70:89, 1998.

Sinclair WK: Radiation protection recommendations on dose limits: the role of the NCRP and ICRP and future developments, *Int J Radiat Oncol Biol Phys* 31:387, 1995.

Statkiewicz MA: Communication skills for the radiologic technologist, *Radiol Technol* 54:449, 1983.

Stone R: The explosions that shook the world, *Science* 272:352, 1996.

Straume T, Dobson RL: Implication of new Hiroshima and Nagasaki dose estimates: cancer risk and neutron RBE, *Health Phys* 41:666, 1981.

Sullivan CA: Chromosome aberrations as a means to determine occupational exposure: an alternative, *Radiol Technol* 52:185, 1980.

The Three Mile Island (TMI-2) recovery and decontamination collection. Available at: http://www. libraries/psu.edu/crsweb/tmi/questions.htm.

Tilke B: Navajo miners battle long-term effects of radiation, *ADVANCE for Radiologic technologists* 3:3, 1990.

Tsuya A, Wakano Y, Otake M, Dock DS: Capillary microscopic observation of the superficial minute vessels of atomic bomb survivors, Hiroshima, 1972-73, *Radiat Res* 72:353, 1977.

U.S. Department of Health and Human Services, Public Health Service, Food and Drug Administration, Bureau of Radiological Health: *The correlated lecture laboratory series in diagnostic radiological physics*, FDA Publication 81-8150, Rockville, Md, 1981, HHS.

U.S. Department of Health, Education, and Welfare, Public Health Service, Food and Drug Administration, Bureau of Radiological Health: *The biological effects of ionizing radiation: an overview*, Publication FDA 77-8004, Rockville, Md, 1976, HEW.

U.S. Department of Health, Education, and Welfare, Public Health Service, Food and Drug Administration, Bureau of Radiological Health, Division of Compliance (HFX-400): *A practitioner's guide to the diagnostic x-ray equipment standard*, FDA Publication 78-8050, Rockville, Md, 1975, HEW.

U.S. Department of Health, Education, and Welfare, Public Health Service, Food and Drug Administration, Bureau of Radiological Health, Division of Compliance X-ray Products Branch: *Assembler's guide to diagnostic x-ray equipment*, Publication FDA 75-8002, Rockville, Md, 1975, HEW.

U.S. Department of Health, Education, and Welfare, Public Health Service, Food and Drug Administration, Bureau of Radiological Health, Division of Compliance X-ray Products Branch: *Gonadal shielding in diagnostic radiology*, FDA Publication 75-8024, Rockville, Md, 1975, HEW.

U.S. Department of Health, Education, and Welfare, Public Health Service, Food and Drug Administration, Bureau of Radiological Health, Division of Compliance X-ray Products Branch: *Analysis of retakes: understanding, managing, and using an analysis of retakes program for quality assurance*, FDA Publication 79-8097, Rockville, Md, 1980, HEW.

U.S. Department of Health, Education, and Welfare, Public Health Service, Food and Drug Administration, Bureau of Radiological Health, Division of Compliance X-ray Products Branch: *Quality assurance programs for diagnostic radiology facilities*, FDA Publication 80-1110, Rockville, Md, 1980, HEW.

U.S. Department of Health, Education, and Welfare, Public Health Service, Food and Drug Administration, Bureau of Radiological Health, Division of Compliance X-ray Products Branch: *The selection of patients for x-ray examinations*, FDA Publication 80-8104, Rockville, Md, 1980, HEW.

U.S. Environmental Protection Agency: Indoor air—radon (Rn), Available at: http://www.epa.gov/iaq/radon/index. html. Accessed January 12, 2005.

U.S. Environmental Protection Agency—History Office: Agency mission statement, Available at: http://www. epa.gov/history/org/origins/documents.htm. Accessed April 26, 2001.

U.S. Environmental Protection Agency—History Office: Duties transferred to EPA, Available at: http://epa.gov/ history/org/origins/duties.htm. Accessed April 26, 2001.

U.S. Food and Drug Administration—Center for Devices and Radiological Health: Radiological health item. Available at: http://www.fda/gov/cdrh/radhealth.html. Accessed April 26, 2001.

U.S. Government Printing Office: *Pre-surgical chest x-ray screening examination*, FDA Publication 86-8265, Superintendent of Documents, Washington, DC, 1986, U.S. Government Printing Office.

Vann JM: *Radiation effects of Three Mile Island*, New Jersey Society of Radiologic Technologists, November 28, 1979, State of NJ Nuclear Engineers, Bureau of Radiation Protection (lecture).

Walker JS: *Permissible dose: a history of radiation protection in the twentieth century*, Berkeley and Los Angeles, Calif, 2000, University of California Press.

Watson E: Radiation dose limits lowered, *ASRT Scanner* 27:15, 1994.

Webster EW et al: *A primer on low-level ionizing radiation and its biological effects*, American Association of Physicists in Medicine (AAPM) Report No 18, New York, 1986, American Institute of Physics (published for the AAPM).

Williams N, Balter M: Chernobyl research becomes international growth industry, *Science* 272:355, 1996.

Wilson BG: The evolution of PET-CT, *Radiol Technol*, 76:4, 2005.

Women's breast health, *RT Image*, 17:35, 2004.

X-ray guided interventional procedures rarely result in radiation injury, *RT Image* 14:28, 2001.

APPENDIX A

Chance of a 50-KeV photon interacting with atoms of tissue as it travels through 5 cm of soft tissue

[1]

Let N_0 be the number of x-ray photons incident on a uniform slab of tissue of thickness "y." The probability that there will be an interaction of any sort between a photon and an atom within the slab is, in the simplest case, proportional to the slab thickness and the number of incident photons and the mean target size presented by a slab atom to an x-ray photon.

MATHEMATICALLY, ONE MAY PROCEED AS FOLLOWS:

1) Let dN be the change in the number of photons in the x-ray beam after the beam has passed through an infinitesimal distance dy. Because the number of photons decreases with every interaction, dN is a negative quantity.

2) At any depth within the phantom the number of interactions that will occur in the next incremental thickness dy is proportional to the remaining number of photons N at that depth and the distance of penetration dy. In mathematical terms:

$$dN = -\mu N dy$$

where the symbol μ is the constant of proportionality and is known as the linear attenuation coefficient. It is defined by the previous equation and has the following unit: 1/cm.

3) Rearranging the previous equation, one performs the following integration:

$$\int_{N_0}^{N} dN/N = -\mu \int_{0}^{y} dy$$

which leads to the following relation:

$$\ln(N/N_0) = -\mu y$$

4) If one uses the properties of logarithms and raises both sides of the last equation to the power "e," the x-ray attenuation equation is as follows:

$$N = N_0 e^{-\mu y}$$

5) For 50-KeV photons passing through 5 cm of soft tissue:

$$\mu_{\text{soft tissue}} = 0.214 \text{ and } y = 5$$

Substituting these values into the last equation and rearranging the equation a bit, the following is obtained:

$$N/N_0 = e^{-(0.214 \times 5)} = 0.34$$

which shows that only 0.34, or 34%, of the initial number of photons in the 50-KeV beam remain (i.e., have not undergone an interaction) after traversing a 5-cm slab of tissue. In other words, *66% of the incident x-ray beam has interacted with a tissue atom*.

APPENDIX B

Relationship among photons, electromagnetic waves, wavelength, and energy

Before 1900, all attempts to use current theories and concepts in physics to explain the measured energy distribution of radiation from a heated body had failed grievously. In that year a German physicist, Max Planck, introduced the concept of a "quantum," or discrete unit of energy, to resolve these discrepancies. According to Planck's theory, whenever radiation is emitted or absorbed by a hot object, the energy of that radiation is emitted or absorbed in discrete amounts, which he called *quanta*.

Mathematically a single such amount or energy quantum is given by the following equation:

$$(1) \quad E = hf$$

where f is the frequency of the radiation and h is a proportionality constant called, appropriately, *Planck's constant*. This quantum of energy has since received the name *photon*. Thus the energy of a photon varies directly as the frequency of the radiation. Because the frequency f and the wavelength w of any type of radiation are related by the simple expression

$$(2) \quad c = fw$$

where c is the speed of light (300,000,000 meters per second in a vacuum), then

$$(3) \quad E = hf = hc/w$$

This last result shows that the energy of a photon decreases as the wavelength of the radiation increases (e.g., photons of infrared light are less energetic than those of ultraviolet light because infrared wavelengths are longer than ultraviolet wavelengths). Einstein used these ideas to explain the emission of electrons from a metallic surface when visible light radiation was directed at it. This is called the *photoelectric effect*. The light-produced electrons, or photoelectrons, were found to have energies that depended on the wavelength of the focused light but were completely independent of the intensity or brightness of that light. This phenomenon could not be explained by traditional physics. However, it was fully explicable in terms of the new concept of radiation energy (quanta or photons) and the energy relation given in equation (3). That relation contains no reference to the brightness of the light. For his work in this area, Einstein received the Nobel Prize in Physics in 1921.

To summarize, photons are the particles associated with the electromagnetic (EM) radiation spectrum (within which visible light and x-rays are included). When energy is transferred from an EM wave through interaction with matter, the energy is transferred by photons in discrete, or integral, amounts. Each such discrete amount is directly proportional to the frequency of the EM radiation.

APPENDIX C
Compton interaction

The principle of conservation of mass-energy is that for an isolated system (i.e., a system on which no external energy source or energy drain is active), the total mass plus energy of all the particles composing the system remains constant. This restraint, however, does not prevent mass-energy transfers between individual particles.

The *linear momentum* of a particle is defined as the product of its mass and its velocity. A photon, which is the particle associated with electromagnetic radiation, moves at the speed of light; consequently, according to Einstein's theory of relativity, a photon must be a massless entity. Because of the equivalence between mass m and energy E given by the famous relation

$$E = mc^2$$

where c is the speed of light in a vacuum, one can associate a mass equivalent with the photon given by

$$E/c^2$$

Then the photon can be considered to have a linear momentum given by the product of the mass equivalent and the velocity of the photon.* The principle of conservation of linear momentum states that for an isolated system the sum of the linear momenta of all its particles is constant. Exchanges of linear momentum between particles within the system can, of course, occur.

---

*From Appendix B, here is the following energy relation:

$$E = hc/w$$

Then the linear momentum expression for the photon becomes

$$P = (E/c - squared)c = (h/cw)c = h/w.$$

The Compton interaction is, most simply, a collision between an incident x-ray photon and the weakly bound outer electron of a target atom. Application of the principles of the conservation of mass-energy and the conservation of linear momentum to the x-ray photon and outer electron system leads to equations that can be used to predict the energies and angles of scattering of both particles following their collision. If the energy of the incident photon is E, the following energy balance relation can be written:

$$E = E' + K$$

where E' is the photon's energy after the collision and K is the recoil energy of the "struck" electron.

Several important types of Compton interactions will now be described. These effects depend on the size of E and the angle at which the photon interacts with the electron.

Case 1: The photon makes a head-on collision with the electron.
    Result: The electron travels or scatters directly forward, and the photon backward (180-degree scatter angle).
    Energy Situations:
    a) $E \ll 511$ keV (low energy range):
       E' is approximately equal to E
       K is almost zero
    b) $E = 511$ keV:
       $E' = E/3$
       $K = (2/3)$ E
    c) $E \gg 511$ keV (high energy range):
       E' is approximately zero
       K = E to good approximation

295

Case 2: The photon grazes the electron.

Result: The photon emerges from the collision nearly undeflected from its initial direction, and the electron scatters at right angles.

Energy Situation:

E′ is approximately equal to E

K is approximately zero

Collisions of this nature, in which the incident photon loses little or no energy, are especially important in the planning of radiation shielding for therapeutic x-ray suites.

Periodic table of the elements

Outer Electrons located in	Period	Group I	Group II	Group III	Group IV	Group V	Group VI	Group VII	Group VIII		
K shell	1	1 **H** Hydrogen 1.09							2 **He** Helium 4.00		
L shell	2	3 **Li** Lithium 6.94	4 **Be** Beryllium 9.02	5 **B** Boron 10.82	6 **C** Carbon 12.01	7 **N** Nitrogen 14.09	8 **O** Oxygen 16.00	9 **F** Fluorine 19.00	10 **Ne** Neon 20.18		
M shell	3	11 **Na** Sodium 23.0	12 **Mg** Magnesium 24.32	13 **Al** Aluminum 26.97	14 **Si** Silicon 28.06	15 **P** Phosphorus 30.98	16 **S** Sulfur 32.06	17 **Cl** Chlorine 35.46	18 **A** Argon 39.99		
N shell	4	19 **K** Potassium 39.096	20 **Ca** Calcium 40.08	21 **Sc** Scandium 45.10	22 **Ti** Titanium 47.90	23 **V** Vanadium 50.95	24 **Cr** Chromium 52.01	25 **Mn** Manganese 54.93	26 **Fe** Iron 55.85	27 **Co** Cobalt 58.94	28 **Ni** Nickel 58.69
		29 **Cu** Copper 63.57	30 **Zn** Zinc 65.38	31 **Ga** Gallium 69.72	32 **Ge** Germanium 72.60	33 **As** Arsenic 74.91	34 **Se** Selenium 79.00	35 **Br** Bromine 79.92	36 **Kr** Krypton 83.7		
O shell	5	37 **Rb** Rubidium 85.48	38 **Sr** Strontium 87.63	39 **Y** Yttrium 88.92	40 **Zr** Zirconium 91.22	41 **Cb** Columbium 92.91	42 **Mo** Molybdenum 96.0	43 **Tc** Technetium 99	44 **Ru** Ruthenium 101.7	45 **Rh** Rhodium 102.9	46 **Pd** Palladium 106.7
		47 **Ag** Silver 107.88	48 **Cd** Cadmium 112.41	49 **In** Indium 118.70	50 **Sn** Tin 121.77	51 **Sb** Antimony 127.6	52 **Te** Tellurium 126.93	53 **I** Iodine 126.92	54 **Xe** Xenon 131.3		
P shell	6	55 **Cs** Cesium 132.9	56 **Ba** Barium 137.4	Rare Earths 57-71	72 **Hf** Halfnium 178.6	73 **Ta** Tantalum 180.9	74 **W** Tungsten 183.9	75 **Re** Rhenium 186.3	76 **Os** Osmium 190.2	77 **Ir** Iridium 193.1	78 **Pt** Platinum 195.2
		79 **Au** Gold 197.2	80 **Hg** Mercury 200.6	81 **Tl** Thallium 204.4	82 **Pb** Lead 207.2	83 **Bi** Bismuth 209.0	84 **Po** Polonium 210	85 **At** Astatine 211	86 **Rn** Radon 222		
Q shell	7	87 **Vi** Virginium 224	88 **Ra** Radium 226.05	Actinide Series 89-103							

	Rare Earths Series	57 **La** Lanthanum 138.91	58 **Ce** Cerium 140.12	59 **Pr** Proseodymium 140.91	60 **Nd** Neodymium 144.24	61 **Pm** Promethium 147	62 **Sm** Samarium 150.35	63 **Eu** Europium 151.96	64 **Gd** Gadolinium 157.25	65 **Tb** Terbium 158.92	66 **Dy** Dysprosium 162.50	67 **Ho** Holmium 164.93	68 **Er** Erbium 167.26	69 **Tm** Thulium 168.93	70 **Yb** Ytterbium 173.04	71 **Lu** Lutetium 174.97
	Actinide Series	89 **Ac** Actinium 227	90 **Th** Thorium 232.04	91 **Pa** Protactinium 231	92 **U** Uranium 238.03	93 **Np** Neptunium 237	94 **Pu** Plutonium 242	95 **Am** Americium 243	96 **Cm** Curium 245	97 **Bk** Berkelium 249	98 **Cf** Californium 251	99 **Es** Einsteinium 254	100 **Fm** Fermium 255	101 **Md** Mendelevium 256	102 **No** Nobelium 254	103 **Lr** Lawrencium 257

APPENDIX E
Metric system equivalents for length

Length	Symbol	Power of Ten Fractional Form	Power of Ten Decimal Form	Scientific Notation
yottameter	Ym		1,000,000,000,000,000,000,000,000	10^{24} (m)
zettameter	Zm		1,000,000,000,000,000,000,000	10^{21} (m)
exameter	Em		1,000,000,000,000,000,000	10^{18} (m)
petameter	Pm		1,000,000,000,000,000	10^{15} (m)
terameter	Tm		1,000,000,000,000	10^{12} (m)
gigameter	Gm		1,000,000,000	10^{9} (m)
megameter	Mm		1,000,000	10^{6} (m)
kilometer	km		1,000	10^{3} (m)
hectometer	hm		100	10^{2} (m)
dekameter	dam		10	10^{1} (m)
meter	m		1	10^{0} (m)
decimeter	dm	1/10	0.1	10^{-1} (m)
centimeter	cm	1/100	0.01	10^{-2} (m)
millimeter	mm	1/1,000	0.001	10^{-3} (m)
micrometer	μm	1/1,000,000	0.00001	10^{-6} (m)
nanometer	nm	1/1,000,000,000	0.000000001	10^{-9} (m)
picometer	pm	1/1,000,000,000,000	0.000000000001	10^{-12} (m)
femtometer	fm	1/1,000,000,000,000,000	0.000000000000001	10^{-15} (m)
attometer	am	1/1,000,000,000,000,000,000	0.000000000000000001	10^{-18} (m)
zeptometer	zm	1/1,000,000,000,000,000,000,000	0.000000000000000000001	10^{-21} (m)
yoctometer	ym	1/1,000,000,000,000,000,000,000,000	0.000000000000000000000001	10^{-24} (m)

APPENDIX F
Revision of 10 CFR Part 35*

§ 35.50 TRAINING FOR RADIATION SAFETY OFFICER

Except as provided in § 35.57, the licensee shall require an individual fulfilling the responsibilities of the Radiation Safety Officer (RSO) as provided in § 35.24 to be an individual who:

(a) Is certified by a specialty board whose certification process includes all of the requirements in paragraph (b) of this section and whose certification has been approved by the Commission or;

(b) (1) Has completed a structured educational program consisting of both:
    (i) 200 hours of didactic training in the following areas:
        (A) Radiation physics and instrumentation;
        (B) Radiation protection;
        (C) Mathematics pertaining to the use and measurement of radioactivity;
        (D) Radiation biology; and
        (E) Radiation dosimetry; and
    (ii) One year of full-time radiation safety experience under the supervision of the individual identified as the RSO on a Commission or Agreement State license that authorized similar types(s) of use(s) of byproduct material involving the following;
        (A) Shipping, receiving, and performing related radiation surveys;
        (B) Using and performing checks for proper operation of dose calibrators, survey meters, and instruments used to measure radionuclides;
        (C) Securing and controlling byproduct material;
        (D) Using administrative controls to avoid mistakes in the administration of byproduct material;
        (E) Using procedures to prevent or minimize radioactive contamination and using proper decontamination procedures; and
        (F) Disposing of byproduct material; and

    (2) Has obtained written certification, signed by a preceptor RSO, that the requirements in paragraph (b) (1) of this section have been satisfactorily completed and that the individual has achieved a level of competency sufficient to independently function as an RSO for medical uses of byproduct material; and

    (3) Following completion of the requirements in paragraph (b) of this section, has demonstrated sufficient knowledge in radiation safety commensurate with the use requested by passing an examination given by an organization or entity approved by the Commission in accordance with Appendix A of this part; or

(c) Is an authorized user, authorized medical physicist, or authorized nuclear pharmacist identified on the licensee's license and has experience with the radiation safety aspects of similar types of use of byproduct material for which the individual has RSO responsibilities.

*Training is the same as described in current 10 CFR Part 35.

APPENDIX G

Consumer-patient radiation health and safety act of 1981*

SUBTITLE-I—CONSUMER-PATIENT RADIATION HEALTH AND SAFETY ACT OF 1981

Short title
[42 USC 10001.] note

SEC. 975. This subtitle may be cited as the "consumer-patient radiation health and safety act of 1981."

Statement of findings
[42 USC 10001.]

SEC. 976. The congress finds that . . .

(1) it is in the interest of public health and safety to minimize unnecessary exposure to potentially hazardous radiation due to medical and dental radiologic procedures;

(2) it is in the interest of public health and safety to have a continuing supply of adequately educated persons and appropriate accreditation and certification programs administered by state governments;

(3) the protection of the public health and safety from unnecessary exposure to potentially hazardous radiation due to medical and dental radiologic procedures and the assurance of efficacious procedures are the responsibility of state and federal governments;

(4) persons who administer radiologic procedures, including procedures at federal facilities, should be required to demonstrate competence by reason of education, training, and experience; and

(5) the administration of radiologic procedures and the effect on individuals of such procedures have a substantial and direct effect upon United States interstate commerce.

Statement of purpose
[42 USC 10002.]

SEC. 977. It is the purpose of this subtitle to–

(1) provide for the establishment of minimum standards by the federal government for the accreditation of education programs for persons who administer radiologic procedures and for the certification of such persons; and

(2) ensure that medical and dental radiologic procedures are consistent with rigorous safety precautions and standards.

Definitions
[42 USC 10003.]

SEC. 978. Unless otherwise expressly provided, for purposes of this subtitle, the term–

(1) "radiation" means ionizing and nonionizing radiation in amounts beyond normal background levels from sources such as medical and dental radiologic procedures;

(2) "radiologic procedure" means any procedure or article intended for use in-

    (A) the diagnosis of disease or other medical or dental conditions in humans (including diagnostic x-rays or nuclear medicine procedures); or

---

*Modified from Consumer-Patient Radiation Health and Safety Act of 1981, Chapter 107, Secs. 10001-8 (Aug. 13, 1981).

(B) the cure, mitigation, treatment, or prevention of disease in humans that achieves its intended purpose through the emission of radiation;

(3) "radiologic equipment" means any radiation electronic product that emits or detects radiation and is used or intended for use to-

(A) diagnose disease or other medical or dental conditions (including diagnostic x-ray equipment); or

(B) cure, mitigate, treat, or prevent disease in humans that achieves its intended purpose through the emission or detection of radiation;

(4) "practitioner" means any licensed doctor of medicine, osteopathy, dentistry, podiatry, or chiropractic who prescribes radiologic procedures for other persons;

(5) "persons who administer radiologic procedures" means any person, other than a practitioner, who intentionally administers radiation to other persons for medical purposes and includes medical radiologic technologists (including dental hygienists and assistants), radiation therapy technologists, and nuclear medicine technologists;

(6) "Secretary" means the Secretary of Health and Human Services; and

(7) "State" means the several states, the District of Columbia, the Commonwealth of Puerto Rico, the Commonwealth of the Northern Mariana Islands, the Virgin Islands, Guam, American Samoa, and the Trust Territory of the Pacific Islands.

Promulgation of standards
[Regulation. 42 USC 10004.]

SEC. 979. (a) Within 12 months after the date of enactment of this act, the Secretary, in consultation with the Radiation Policy Council, the Administrator of Veterans' Affairs, the Administrator of the Environmental Protection Agency, appropriate agencies of the States, and appropriate professional organizations, shall by regulation promulgate minimum standards for the accreditation of educational programs to train individuals to perform radiologic procedures. Such standards shall distinguish between programs for the education of (1) medical radiologic technologists (including radiographers), (2) dental auxiliaries

(including dental hygienists and assistants), (3) radiation therapy technologists, (4) nuclear medicine technologists, and (5) such other kinds of health auxiliaries who administer radiologic procedures as the Secretary determines appropriate. Such standards shall not be applicable to educational programs for practitioners.

[Regulation.]

(b) Within 12 months after the date of enactment of this act, the Secretary, in consultation with the Radiation Policy Council, the Administrator of Veterans' Affairs, the Administrator of the Environmental Protection Agency, interested agencies of the States, and appropriate professional organizations, shall by regulation promulgate minimum standards for the certification of persons who administer radiologic procedures. Such standards shall distinguish between certification of (1) medical radiologic technologists (including radiographers), (2) dental auxiliaries (including dental hygienists and assistants), (3) radiation therapy technologists, (4) nuclear medicine technologists, and (5) such other kinds of health auxiliaries who administer radiologic procedures as the Secretary determines appropriate. Such standards shall include minimum certification criteria for individuals with regard to accredited education, practical experience, successful passage of required examinations, and such other criteria as the Secretary shall deem necessary for the adequate qualification of individuals to administer radiologic procedures. Such standards shall not apply to practitioners.

Model statute
[42 USC 10005.]

SEC. 980. In order to encourage the administration of accreditation and certification programs by the states, the Secretary shall prepare and transmit to the states a model statute for radiologic procedure safety. Such model statute shall provide that—

(1) it shall be unlawful in a state for individuals to perform radiologic procedures unless such individuals are certified by the state to perform such procedures; and

(2) any educational requirements for certification of individuals to perform radiologic procedures shall be limited to educational programs accredited by the state.

Compliance
[42 USC 10006.]

SEC. 981. (a) The Secretary shall take all actions consistent with law to effectuate the purposes of this subtitle.

(b) A state may utilize an accreditation or certification program administered by a private entity if–

(1) such state delegates the administration of the state accreditation or certification program to such private entity;

(2) such program is approved by the state; and

(3) such program is consistent with the minimum federal standards promulgated under this subtitle for such program.

(c) Absent compliance by the states with the provisions of this subtitle within 3 years after the date of enactment of this act, the Secretary shall report to the Congress recommendations for legislative changes considered necessary to ensure the states' compliance with this subtitle.

[Report to Congress.]

(d) The Secretary shall be responsible for continued monitoring of compliance by the states with the applicable provisions of this subtitle and shall report to the Senate and the House of Representatives by January 1, 1982, and January 1 of each succeeding year the status of the states' compliance with the purposes of this subtitle.

(e) Notwithstanding any other provision of this section, in the case of a state that has, prior to the effective date of standards and guidelines promulgated pursuant to this subtitle, established standards for the accreditation of educational programs and certification of radiologic technologists, such state shall be deemed to be in compliance with the conditions of this section unless the Secretary determines, after notice and hearing, that such state standards do not meet the minimum standards prescribed by the Secretary or are inconsistent with the purposes of this subtitle.

Federal radiation guidelines
[42 USC 10007.)

SEC. 982. The Secretary shall, in conjunction with the Radiation Policy Council, the Administrator of Veterans' Affairs, the Administrator of the Environmental Protection Agency, appropriate agencies of the states, and appropriate professional organizations, promulgate Federal radiation guidelines with respect to radiologic procedures. Such guidelines shall–

(1) determine the level of radiation exposure due to radiologic procedures that is unnecessary and specify the techniques, procedures, and methods to minimize such unnecessary exposure;

(2) provide for the elimination of the need for retakes of diagnostic radiologic procedures;

(3) provide for the elimination of unproductive screening programs;

(4) provide for the optimum diagnostic information with minimum radiologic exposure; and

(5) include the therapeutic application of radiation to individuals in the treatment of disease, including nuclear medicine applications.

Applicability to federal agencies
[42 USC 10008.]

SEC. 983. (a) Except as provided in subsection (b), each department, agency, and instrumentality of the executive branch of the federal government shall comply with standards promulgated pursuant to this subtitle.

[Regulations.]
[38 USC 101 *et seq.*]

(b) (1) The Administrator of Veterans' Affairs, through the Chief Medical Director of the Veterans' Administration, shall, to the maximum extent feasible consistent with the responsibilities of such Administrator and Chief Medical Director under subtitle 38, United States Code, prescribe regulations making the standards promulgated pursuant to this subtitle applicable to the provision of radiologic procedures in facilities over which the Administrator has jurisdiction. In prescribing and implementing regulations pursuant to this subsection, the Administrator shall consult with the Secretary in order to achieve the maximum possible coordination of the regulations, standards, and guidelines, and the implementation thereof, which the

Secretary and the Administrator prescribe under this subtitle.

[Report to congressional committees.]
(2) Not later than 180 days after standards are promulgated by the Secretary pursuant to this subtitle, the Administrator of Veterans' Affairs shall submit to the appropriate committees of Congress a full report with respect to the regulations (including guidelines, policies, and procedures thereunder) prescribed pursuant to paragraph (1) of this subsection. Such report shall include–

(A) an explanation of any inconsistency between standards made applicable by such regulations and the standards promulgated by the Secretary pursuant to this subtitle;

(B) an account of the extent, substance, and results of consultations with the Secretary respecting the prescription and implementation of regulations by the Administrator; and

(C) such recommendations for legislation and administrative action as the Administrator determines are necessary and desirable.

[Publication in Federal Register.]
(3) The Administrator of Veterans' Affairs shall publish the report required by paragraph (2) in the Federal Register.

ANSWERS TO REVIEW QUESTIONS

Chapter 1

1. D
2. C
3. B
4. A
5. B
6. B
7. D
8. D
9. A
10. D

Chapter 2

1. B
2. C
3. A
4. B
5. A
6. B
7. A
8. D
9. A
10. C

Chapter 3

1. B
2. B
3. C
4. A
5. B
6. C
7. D
8. A

9. B
10. C

Chapter 4

1. C
2. C
3. B
4. B
5. B
6. D
7. D
8. D
9. C
10. B

Chapter 5

1. C
2. B
3. A
4. C
5. B
6. D
7. B
8. D
9. C
10. D

Chapter 6

1. A
2. B
3. A
4. A
5. C

6. C
7. C
8. C
9. C
10. D

Chapter 7

1. B
2. B
3. C
4. A
5. B
6. B
7. A
8. A
9. A
10. B

Chapter 8

1. B
2. B
3. C
4. C
5. D
6. A
7. B
8. B
9. A
10. D

Chapter 9

1. D
2. D

3. C
4. A
5. C
6. A
7. D
8. B
9. B
10. D

Chapter 10

1. A
2. C
3. A
4. D
5. C
6. C
7. C
8. B
9. A
10. B

Chapter 11

1. B
2. B
3. D
4. C
5. C
6. B
7. D
8. A
9. D
10. C

GLOSSARY

Aberration Deviation from normal development or growth.

Absolute risk Model predicting that a specific number of excess cancers will occur as a result of exposure to ionizing radiation.

Absorbed dose (D) The deposition of energy per unit mass by ionizing radiation in the patient's body tissue. This absorbed energy is responsible for whatever biologic damage occurs as a result of tissues being exposed to x-radiation. The gray (Gy) is the SI unit of this radiation quantity.

Absorption Transference of electromagnetic energy from an x-ray beam to the atoms or molecules of the matter through which it passes.

Acid-base balance State of equilibrium or stability between acids and bases.

Acids Hydrogen-containing compounds that can attack and dissolve metal (e.g., HNO_3, nitric acid).

Action limits Limits to occupational exposure that are set by the medical facility well below the regulatory values as they appear in state or federal regulations. These limits are set so that a facility can take preemptive action to find the cause of unusual exposures before they reach the regulated limits.

Acute Something that begins suddenly and runs a short but severe course (e.g., an acute disease).

Acute radiation syndrome (ARS) Radiation sickness that occurs in humans after whole-body reception of large doses of ionizing radiation (1 Gy [100 rads] or more) delivered over a short period of time.

Acute somatic effects (See *Early somatic effects*.)

Added filtration Sheets of aluminum (or its equivalent) of appropriate thickness interposed outside the glass window of the x-ray tube housing above the collimator shutters.

Adenine (A) One of two purine bases found in both DNA and RNA.

Adenosine triphosphate (ATP) High-energy-releasing phosphate compound essential for life. This compound plays a role in active transport within the cell.

Agreement states Individual states of the United States that have entered into an agreement with the Nuclear Regulatory Commission (NRC) to assume responsibility for enforcing radiation protection regulations through their respective health departments.

Air gap technique An alternative procedure to the use of a radiographic grid for reducing scattered radiation during certain examinations.

ALARA concept/principle Precept holding that occupational exposure of the radiographer and other occupationally exposed persons should be kept "as low as reasonably achievable." An ALARA program should also be established and maintained for patients. Radiation exposure should always be kept ALARA for all medical imaging procedures.

Alkali A member of a group of elements that includes lithium, sodium, and potassium.

Alkaline earth A member of a group of elements including calcium, magnesium, and strontium.

Alpha particle A positively charged particle of radiation that is ejected by certain radioactive elements. It consists of two protons and two neutrons.

Aluminum (Al) The metal most frequently selected as a filter material because it effectively removes low-energy (soft) x-rays from a polyenergetic x-ray beam.

Aluminum oxide (Al_2O_3) Sensing material found in optically stimulated luminescence dosimeters.

American Association of Physicists in Medicine (AAPM) Professional organization that is the primary scientific and educational body for medical physicists and is also responsible for accrediting calibration laboratories that measure radiation exposure in medical radiology.

American College of Radiology (ACR) Major professional organization of American radiologists.

Amino acids The structural units of protein.

Ampere The SI unit of electric charge. One ampere represents the quantity of electrons amounting to a charge of 1 coulomb crossing unit area per second.

Analog image A visible image produced by x-radiation on radiographic film. An analog image is not limited by any pixel size. The microscopic film grain size is much smaller than the size of pixels used in digital images. Therefore, a recording and storage medium such as film is considered to be continuously variable in optical density.

Anaphase The phase of mitosis during which two chromatids repel each other and migrate along the mitotic spindle to opposite sides of the cell.

Anemia A condition characterized by a lack of vitality and caused by a decrease in the number of red blood cells in the circulating blood.

Anion A negatively charged ion.

Annihilation radiation Radiation in the form of two oppositely moving 511 keV photons generated as the result of the mutual annihilation of matter and antimatter (i.e., an electron and a positron).

Annual occupational effective dose (EfD) limit An upper boundary limit for radiation workers for yearly whole body exposure (excluding personal medical and natural background exposure) of 50 millisievert (mSv) (5 rem).

Anode The positively charged target in the x-ray tube.

Antibodies Materials developed by the body in response to the presence of foreign antigens such as bacteria or a flu virus. Once the skin is penetrated, they provide a primary defense mechanism against such antigens.

Antimatter Matter composed of the counterparts of ordinary matter that does not exist freely in the universe and is unstable in the presence of ordinary matter.

Aperture diaphragm A simple beam limitation device that consists of a flat piece of lead with a hole of a designated size and shape cut in its center.

Aplastic anemia Anemia resulting from bone marrow failure.

Apoptosis A nonmitotic or nondivision form of cell death that occurs when cells die without attempting division during the interphase portion of the cell life cycle.

Artificial radiation (See *Man-made radiation*.)

Atom The smallest portion of an element that has all of its chemical properties.

Atomic Energy Commission (AEC) (See *U.S. Nuclear Regulatory Commission*.)

Atomic number The number of protons contained within the nucleus of an atom.

Atrophy A wasting caused by lack of nutrition in any part.

Attenuation Any process decreasing the intensity of the primary photon beam that was directed toward a destination.

Audible sound system An audio amplifier and speaker, such as in a Geiger-Müller detector.

Auger electron When a vacancy exists in an inner electron shell of an atom (as the result of photoelectric effect, Compton scattering, or bombardment by other electrons) an outer-shell electron drops into the vacancy, and energy equal to the difference in binding energy between the two shells must be released by the atom. This energy may be released as a characteristic photon, or it may be released as an electron, an outer-shell electron that is ejected from its shell. Any energy beyond the energy required to release the Auger electron appears as kinetic energy of the Auger electron.

Axon Nerve cell process that extends out from the cell body and conducts impulses away from the cell body.

Background equivalent radiation time (BERT) Method to compare the amount of radiation received from a radiologic procedure with natural background radiation received over a given period of time.

Backscatter Photons that have interacted with the atoms of an object and as a result are deflected backward (toward the x-ray tube).

Bases Alkali or alkaline earth OH compounds that can neutralize acids.

Beam direction factor (See *Use factor*.)

Beam limiting device A device that limits the parameters of the useful beam to a designated size and shape before it enters the area of clinical interest.

Becquerel The SI unit of radioactivity. It is equal to 1 disintegration per second.

Beta decay The process wherein a nucleus relieves an instability by a neutron converting to a proton and an electron and a neutrino with the emission of both the electron and the neutrino.

Beta particles   High-speed electrons ejected from a nucleus that undergoes beta decay.

Binding energy   Force that holds the components of an atom or a nucleus together.

Biologic damage   Damage in living tissue.

Biologic dosimetry   A method of dose assessment in which biologic markers or effects of radiation exposure are measured and the dose to the organism is inferred from previously established dose-effect relationships. Examples include white blood cell counts and chromosomal aberrations.

Biologic effects   Damage to living tissue of animals and humans exposed to radiation.

Biologic radiation   Radiation from radionuclides deposited in the human body via natural processes.

Biology   A science that explores living things and life processes.

Birth defects   (See *Embryologic effects.*)

Blebs   Tiny membrane-enclosed structures that are produced when cells shrink in apoptosis.

Bone marrow dose   (See *Mean marrow dose.*)

Bone marrow syndrome   (See *Hematopoietic syndrome.*)

Bragg-Gray theory   Relates the ionization produced in a small cavity in an irradiated medium or object to the energy absorbed in that medium as a result of its radiation exposure.

Bremsstrahlung   Ionizing electromagnetic radiation that is nonuniform in energy and wavelength and that is produced when a bombarding beam of electrons in an x-ray tube undergoes deceleration by interaction with the nuclei of the x-ray tube target atoms.

Bucky slot shielding device   A protective device that automatically covers the Bucky slot opening in the side of the x-ray table during a fluoroscopic examination when the Bucky tray is positioned at the foot end of the table, thus protecting the radiographer and the radiologist from radiation exposure to the gonads.

Bureau of Radiological Health (BRH)   (See *Center for Devices and Radiological Health.*)

Calibration instrument   Device used to measure the output of a piece of equipment so that a comparison may be made with expected values. In radiography an ionization chamber connected to an electrometer is used to measure the x-ray output of radiographic equipment.

Candela per square meter   Unit used to describe luminance. One candela corresponds to 3.8 million billion photons per second being emitted from a light source through a cone-like field of view.

Carbohydrates   Compounds composed entirely of carbon, hydrogen, and oxygen. Carbohydrates such as sugars and starches are involved in energy-releasing processes in animals and plants.

Carbon   Nonmetallic element that is the basic constituent of all organic matter.

Carcinogenesis   The production or origin of cancer.

C-Arm fluoroscope   A portable device for producing real-time (motion) images of a patient. The opposite ends of the C-shaped support arm hold the x-ray tube and the image intensifier.

Catalyst   Agent that affects the speed of a chemical reaction without being altered itself.

Catalytic failure   The inability to influence the speed of a required chemical reaction (e.g., during protein synthesis).

Cataract   Opacity of the eye lens.

Cataractogenesis   The production or origin of cataracts.

Cathode   The negatively charged source of the high-speed electrons in an x-ray tube.

Cation   A positively charged ion.

Cell division   The multiplication process in which one cell divides to form two or more cells.

Cell membrane   The structure that surrounds the cell and functions as a barricade to protect cellular contents from their outside environment and controls the passage of water and other materials into and out of the cell.

Cell metabolism   The series of chemical reactions that modifies foods for cellular use.

Cells   The basic units of all living matter.

Cell survival curve   Method of displaying the radiation sensitivity of a particular type of cell.

Cellular damage   Injury on the cellular level resulting from sufficient exposure to ionizing radiation at the molecular level.

Center for Devices and Radiological Health (CDRH)   Known before 1982 as the Bureau of Radiological

Health (BRH), this agency is responsible for conducting an ongoing electronic product radiation control program.

Centigray (cGy) One one-hundredth of a gray (1/100 Gy).

Centrioles A pair of small, hollow, cylindrical structures located adjacent to the nucleus that are believed to play a part in the formation of the mitotic spindle during cell division.

Centromere A clear region on a chromosome where its two (or four) arms join.

Centrosomes Structures located in the center of the cell near the nucleus that contain the centrioles.

Cerebrovascular syndrome Form of acute radiation syndrome, usually fatal, that results when the central nervous system and cardiovascular system receive doses of 50 Gy (5000 rad) or more of ionizing radiation.

Characteristic curve A graph that represents the response of an image receptor to some probe. A film-screen characteristic curve plots the optical density of the developed film on the vertical axis as a function of the exposure on the horizontal axis.

Characteristic photon A quantum or quantity of radiant energy given off by the parent atom when an electron from an outer shell drops down to fill an inner-shell vacancy after the atom has interacted with an x-ray photon and lost an inner-shell electron as a result. The energy of a characteristic photon is equivalent to the difference in energy level between the two electron shells.

Characteristic radiation Radiation released as a result of a photoelectric interaction between an x-ray photon and an atom. The radiation consists of photons whose energies represent the electron energy level structure of electrons within the atom. Characteristic radiation comprises about 10% of primary radiation, between 80 and 100 kVp.

Charge-coupled device (CCD) A device that, when struck by visible light, produces electrical signals in proportion to the brightness of the light. CCDs are used in indirect types of digital x-ray detectors. Indirect digital detectors use a phosphor to convert the x-ray energy to visible light, after which the CCD converts the visible light into electrical signals.

Chromatid A highly coiled strand; one of the two duplicate portions of DNA that appear during cell division.

Chromatid aberrations Lesions that result when irradiation of individual chromatids occurs later in interphase, after DNA synthesis has taken place.

Chromosome aberrations Lesions that result when irradiation occurs early in interphase, before DNA synthesis takes place.

Chromosome breakage The breaking of one or both of the sugar-phosphate chains of a DNA molecule, which can be caused by exposure of the molecule to ionizing radiation.

Chromosomes Tiny, rod-shaped bodies that contain genes.

Chronic Something that continues for a long time (i.e., a chronic disease).

Cinefluorography An imaging technique in which serial radiographic images are recorded over a short period of time (typically less than 30 seconds) on a strip of 16- or 35-mm film. The images allow study of motion within the patient, such as the spread of contrast material through vessels or the motion of structures within the heart.

Classical scattering (See *Coherent scattering*.)

Clear lead Transparent lead-plastic material that has been impregnated with approximately 30% lead by weight.

Cleaved chromosome A broken chromosome.

Code of Standards for Diagnostic X-Ray Equipment Effective as of August 1, 1974, this code established equipment performance standards for complete systems and major components manufactured after that date.

Coherent scattering The process wherein a low-energy photon (typically less than 30 keV) interacts with an atom as a whole, and the atom responds by releasing the excess energy it has received in the form of a scattered photon that has the same wavelength and energy as the original incident photon but emerges from the atom moving in a slightly different direction. Also known as *Rayleigh scattering*, *classical scattering*, *elastic scattering*, and *unmodified scattering*.

Collective effective dose (ColEfD) Term used to describe radiation exposure of a population or group from low doses of different sources of ionizing radiation.

Compensating filter A material such as aluminum or lead-acrylic inserted between the x-ray source and the patient to modify the quality (penetrating power, spectrum) of the beam across the field of view.

Compton scattered electron An energetic electron dislodged from the outer shell of an atom of the irradiated object as a result of interacting with an incoming x-ray photon.

Compton scattering An interaction between an incoming x-ray photon and a loosely bound outer-shell electron of an atom in the irradiated object. The photon surrenders a portion of its kinetic energy to dislodge the electron from its outer-shell orbit and then continues in a new direction. This process accounts for most of the scattered radiation produced during diagnostic procedures.

Computed radiography Process in which the invisible or latent image generated in conventional radiography is produced in a digital format using computer technology. The digital image can be displayed on a monitor for viewing and it can be printed on a laser film when hard copy is needed

Computed axial tomography (CAT) (See *Computed tomography [CT].)*

Computed tomography (CT) Process by which a computer-reconstructed transverse (or axial) image of a patient is created by an x-ray tube and detector assembly rotating 360 degrees about a specific part of the body. CT may also be referred to as *computerized axial tomography (CAT)*.

Cone A circular metal tube that attaches to the x-ray tube housing or variable rectangular collimator to limit the beam to a predetermined size and shape.

Congenital abnormalities Defects existing at birth that are not inherited, but rather acquired during development in utero.

Consumer-Patient Radiation Health and Safety Act of 1981 Provides federal legislation requiring the establishment of minimum standards for accreditation of educational programs for persons who administer radiologic procedures and the certification of such persons.

Contrast media (negative) The use of air or gas to enhance visualization of body structures during a radiologic procedure.

Contrast media (positive) A liquid solution containing an element with a higher atomic number than surrounding tissue (e.g., barium or iodine) that is either ingested or injected into biologic tissues or structures to be visualized.

Control badge Badge provided by the monitoring company with each batch of badges to serve as a basis for comparison with the remainder of the badges after they have been returned to the monitoring company for processing. The control badge determines whether the batch of badges has been exposed to radiation in transit to or from the health care facility.

Control-booth barrier A permanently secured protective barrier for the radiographer that is located in an x-ray room housing stationary (fixed) radiographic equipment.

Controlled area A hospital area occupied by workers who have been trained in radiation safety procedures and who wear radiation monitoring devices.

Cosmic radiation (cosmic rays) Very-high-speed particles, mainly protons, that are generated as a result of high-energy particle reactions within stars.

Coulomb (C) SI unit of electric charge equal to 1 ampere-second (the quantity of electric charge transferred across unit area by a current of 1 ampere in 1 second).

Coulomb per kilogram (C/kg) SI unit of radiation exposure: 1 coulomb per kilogram (C/kg) of air equals 1 SI unit of exposure, or $1/(2.58 \times 10^{-4})$ R = 3.88×10^3 R.

Covalent bond A chemical union between atoms that arises as a result of the sharing of one or more pairs of electrons.

Covalent cross-link (See *Covalent bond*.)

Cross-over Process occurring during meiosis in which the chromatids exchange some chromosomal material (genes).

Cumulative effect (1) An effect that increases with additional exposure to ionizing radiation; (2) an effect that results from several different causes or from repeated or long-term application of one or more agents.

Cumulative timing device A required device on a fluoroscopic x-ray unit that times the x-ray exposure and sounds an alarm or temporarily interrupts the exposure after the fluoroscope has been activated for 5 minutes.

Cumulative whole-body effective dose (CumEfD) limit A radiation worker's lifetime EfD must be limited to his or her age in years times 10 mSv (years × 1 rem).

Curie The standard unit of radioactivity in use before the SI system of units was established. One curie is equal to 3.7×10^{10} disintegrations per second.

Cutie pie Nickname for an ionization chamber-type survey meter.

Cyclotrons Units that produce high-energy charged particles such as protons.

Cytoplasm The protoplasm that exists outside of the cell's nucleus.

Cytoplasmic organelles Small structures present in the cytoplasm of the cell.

Cytosine (C) One of two pyrimidine bases found in both DNA and RNA.

Daughter cell A cell resulting from division of an individual parent cell.

Dead-man–type fluoroscopic exposure switch A fluoroscopic exposure switch (operated by foot pressure) that requires continuous pressure from the operator. The exposure automatically terminates if the operator becomes incapacitated.

Decontamination Removal of radioactive material from an area, clothing, or person.

Deep equivalent dose External whole-body exposure at a tissue depth of 1 cm (1000 mg/cm²).

Deletion A part of the chromosome or chromatid that is lost at the next cell division, creating an aberration known as an *acentric fragment*.

Dendrites Nerve cell processes that extend outward from the cell body and conduct impulses toward the cell body.

Densitometer An instrument that can be used to determine the amount of radiation to which a film badge dosimeter has been exposed.

Deoxyribonucleic acid (DNA) A type of nucleic acid that carries the genetic information necessary for cell replication and directs the building of proteins.

Deoxyribose A five-carbon sugar molecule.

Desquamation Shedding of the outer layer of skin.

Deterministic effects (See *Nonstochastic effects*.)

Diagnostic efficacy The degree to which a diagnostic study accurately reveals the presence or absence of disease in the patient.

Diagnostic-type protective tube housing The lead-lined metal housing enclosing the x-ray tube that protects both the radiographer and the patient from leakage radiation by restricting the emission of the x-rays to the area of the useful beam or primary beam.

Dicentric chromosomes Chromosomes that have two centromeres.

Diffusion The motion of liquid, gas, or solid particles from an area of relatively high concentration to an area of lower concentration.

Digital fluoroscopy A technique in which the fluoroscopic image exists in digital form at some point in the image acquisition process. In nondigital fluoroscopy, an image intensifier and an analog television camera are used. Typical approaches to digital fluoroscopy include replacement of the image intensifier with a digital detector, replacement of the analog television camera with a digital video camera, and digitization of the analog signal from an analog television camera.

Digital image Image produced by computer representation of anatomical information.

Digital radiography The use of a flat panel detector to record a radiographic image and render it in digital form without developing or scanning the image receptor.

Direct action Biologic damage occurring as a result of radiation interacting without an intermediary on master, or key, molecules (DNA). This interaction causes molecules to become either inactive or functionally altered.

Direct radiation (See *Primary radiation*.)

Direct transmission Primary x-ray photons that traverse an object without interacting.

Dirty bomb (See *Radioactive dispersal device*.)

Distance One of the most important methods of radiation protection (e.g., if one doubles a person's distance from a point-like or localized source of radiation, then that person is only exposed to one fourth of the radiation intensity level present at the previous location).

DNA synthesis The building-up of DNA macromolecules.

Dominant mutation A genetic mutation that will probably be expressed in offspring.

Dose The amount of radiant energy absorbed by an irradiated object per unit mass.

Dose commitment The dose that could ultimately be delivered from a given intake of radionuclide.

Dose limitation Restriction of the amount of ionizing radiation received during a period of time to a specified limit.

Double-emulsion x-ray film X-ray film with emulsion coated on both sides.

Double-strand break The ionization of a DNA macromolecule that results in the rupture of one or more of its chemical bonds, thereby creating one or more breaks in each of the two sugar-phosphate chains of the DNA ladderlike molecular structure.

Doubling dose The radiation dose that causes the number of spontaneous mutations occurring in a given generation to increase to two times their original number.

Early somatic effects Effects of ionizing radiation that appear within minutes, hours, days, or weeks of the time of exposure; also called *acute effects*.

Effective atomic number (Zeff) A composite atomic number for a material that consists of different chemical elements.

Effective communication An interaction that produces a satisfactory result through an exchange of information.

Effective dose (EfD) A quantity that is used for radiation protection purposes to provide a measure of the overall risk of exposure to ionizing radiation. Effective dose takes into account the dose for all types of ionizing radiation to organs or tissues in the human body being irradiated and the overall harm, or weighting factor, of those biologic components for developing a radiation-induced cancer (or for the reproductive organs, the risk of genetic damage).

Effective dose (EfD) limit A level of radiation effective dose that has been recommended as an upper boundary dose of ionizing radiation that results in a negligible risk of bodily injury or genetic damage. These limits may be expressed for whole-body exposure, partial-body exposure, and exposure of individual organs. Separate limits are set for occupationally exposed individuals and for the general public. The sum of both the external and internal whole-body exposures is considered when these limits are established. These upper limits are designed to minimize the risk to humans in terms of nonstochastic and stochastic effects, and they do not include natural background and medical exposure. For occupationally exposed persons these upper limits are associated with risks that are similar to those encountered by employees in other industries such as manufacturing, trade, or government that are generally considered to be reasonably safe.

Effective dose (EfD) limiting system The current method for assessing radiation exposure and associated risk of biologic damage to radiation workers and the general public. It is a set of numeric dose limits that are based on calculations of the various risks of cancer and genetic effects on tissues or organs exposed to radiation.

Effective half-life (T_{eff}) The actual half-life of a radioactive material in a patient's body resulting from a combination of natural decay and physical removal due to bodily functions. T_{eff} is usually substantially less than T (natural decay).

Elastic scattering (See *Coherent scattering*.)

Electrical potential difference (voltage difference) The change in electrical potential energy per unit electrical charge experienced by a charged particle as it moves from one position to another. The unit of electrical potential difference is called a *volt*.

Electrical potential energy The electrical energy acquired by a charged particle as a result of its position relative to other charged particles. The unit of electrical potential energy is the *joule*.

Electrolytes (See *Salts*.)

Electromagnetic radiation Radiation composed of interacting, varying electric and magnetic fields that propagate through space at the speed of light. Examples include radio waves, microwaves, visible light, ultraviolet rays, x-rays, and gamma rays.

Electromagnetic spectrum The complete range of frequencies and energies of electromagnetic radiation.

Electromagnetic wave Electric and magnetic fields that fluctuate rapidly as they travel through space, including radio waves, microwaves, visible light, and x-rays.

Electrometer   A device used to measure electrical charge.

Electron capture   A process wherein an inner-shell electron is captured by one of the nuclear protons, which is followed by the two combining to produce a neutron, thereby creating a different element.

Electron volt (eV)   A unit of energy equivalent to the quantity of kinetic energy an electron acquires as it moves through a potential difference of 1 volt.

Electrons   Negatively charged atomic particles.

Element   A substance made up of atoms that all have the same atomic number and hence the same chemical properties.

Emaciation   The state of being extremely thin.

Embryologic effects   Damage to an organism that occurs as a result of exposure to ionizing radiation during the embryonic stage of development. Also known as *birth defects.*

Endoplasmic reticulum   A vast, irregular network of tubules and vesicles spreading and interconnecting in all directions throughout the cytoplasm, enabling the cell to communicate with the extracellular environment and transfer food from one part of the cell to another.

Energy   The ability to do work.

Enhanced natural sources   Natural sources of ionizing radiation that become increased because of accidental or deliberate human actions.

Entrance exposure   Quantity of radiation, given in SI units of coulombs per kilogram or in traditional units of roentgens, incident upon an object. Backscatter radiation is excluded.

Environmental Protection Agency (EPA)   U.S. government agency that facilitates the development and enforcement of regulations pertaining to the control of radiation in the environment. This agency sets limits for radioactive contamination that assume that a risk of one in ten thousand of causing a fatal cancer is unacceptable. The EPA provides direction to federal agencies, oversees the general area of environmental monitoring, and has authority in specific areas such as determination of the action level for radon.

Enzymatic proteins   Proteins that control the cell's various physiologic activities by functioning as catalysts.

Epidemiologic studies   Observations and statistical analysis of data, such as incidence of disease within groups of people.

Epilation   Loss of hair.

Epithelial tissue   A substance that lines and covers body tissue; the cells that compose this tissue are highly radiosensitive.

Equivalent dose (EqD)   A quantity used for radiation protection purposes that attempts to take into account the variation in biologic harm that is produced by different types of radiation. The EqD is the product of the average absorbed dose in a tissue or organ in the human body and its associated radiation weighting factor chosen for the type of radiation in question. Equivalent dose enables the calculation of the effective (EfD) dose.

Erg   A unit of energy and work.

Erythema   Diffused redness over an area of skin after irradiation.

Erythroblasts   Red blood stem cells.

Erythrocytes   Red blood cells.

ETHOS Project   A 3-year pilot research project that began in 1996 in the Republic of Belarus in the aftermath of the Chernobyl nuclear power plant accident. The local citizens of the contaminated territories were empowered to make their own decisions to facilitate reconstruction of their overall quality of life. They were given the authority to manage their radiologic risk. Through this program, local citizens are engaging in cooperative problem solving as they reconstruct their environment.

Excess cancers   Cancers that would not have occurred in a population without exposure to ionizing radiation.

Excitation   The addition of energy to a system, transforming it from a calm, or low-energy, state to an excited, or higher-energy, state.

Exit, or image formation, radiation   All of the x-ray photons that reach their destination (the image receptor) after passing through the object being radiographed; previously known as *remnant radiation.*

Exposure   The total electrical charge per unit mass that x-ray and gamma ray photons with energies up to 3 MeV generate in air only; the amount of ionizing radiation that may strike an object, such as the human body, when in the vicinity of a radiation source. Measured in coulombs per kilogram (C/kg) or roentgens (R).

Exposure linearity Consistency in radiation intensity stated in milliroentgens per milliampere-seconds (mR/mAs) when changing from one milliampere station to another, with a variance of not more than 10%.

Exposure reproducibility Consistency in output of radiation intensity from an individual exposure to other subsequent exposures having the same technique factors.

Extension cylinder A cylindrical metal tube that possesses a 10- to 20-inch metal extension at the far end of the barrel to limit the size of the useful beam.

Extremity dosimeter A device that monitors the equivalent dose of radiation to the hands.

Eye equivalent dose External exposure of the lens of the eye at a tissue depth of 0.3 cm (300 mg/cm^2).

Fallout Radiation produced as a consequence of nuclear weapons testing and chemical explosions in nuclear power plants.

Fats Compounds composed of carbon, hydrogen, and oxygen, with the ratio of hydrogen atoms to oxygen atoms much greater than 2 to 1; a rich energy source.

Fatty acids Compounds formed when fat combines with an acidic group of atoms (e.g., the carboxyl group); a constituent of amino acids from which proteins are built.

Fetus A developing human in utero.

Fiber A protracted, threadlike structure.

Fibril A minute fiber or strand that is frequently part of a compound fiber.

Fibrosis Abnormal formation of fibrous tissue.

Film badge dosimeter An economical type of personnel monitoring device, it records radiation exposure accumulated by radiosensitive film at a low rate over a long period of time.

Filmless cassette Reusable rectangular imaging plate containing a photostimulable phosphor such as europium-activated barium fluorohalide. This cassette is used in computed radiography.

Filtration Elements that are part of or added to the x-ray tube to reduce exposure to the patient's skin and superficial tissue. Filtration elements function by absorbing most of the lower-energy photons from the heterogeneous beam, thereby increasing its mean energy.

Fission The splitting of the nuclei of atoms whereby some mass is converted into energy.

Fixed radiographic equipment Radiologic equipment that is installed in and cannot be moved from a specific place in an imaging facility. It may also be referred to as *stationary equipment.*

Flat contact shield Uncontoured lead strip or lead-impregnated material placed directly over the patient's reproductive organs to provide protection from exposure to ionizing radiation.

Fluorescent radiation (See *Characteristic radiation.*)

Fluorescent yield The number of characteristic x-rays emitted by an atom per created inner-shell vacancy.

Fluorine 18 Radioactive isotope used for PET scanning. It decays by positron emission and has a half-life of 110 minutes.

Fluorodeoxyglucose (FDG) Radioactive tracer compound similar in chemical behavior to ordinary glucose; therefore, it will be taken up or metabolized by cancerous cells and reveal their location through its radioactive decay process.

Fluoroscopic exposure switch (foot pedal) A dead-man type of switch that causes the fluoroscopic tube to emit x-radiation as long as the operator continues to apply pressure to the pedal.

Fluoroscopy Process in which an x-ray examination is performed that demonstrates dynamic, or active, motion of selected anatomic structures by producing a temporary image of these structures on a television monitor working in conjunction with an image intensifier system under low-light conditions.

Focal spot The area on the anode of the x-ray tube from which the x-rays emanate.

Forward scatter Photons that have interacted with the atoms of an object and consequently are deflected forward (toward the radiographic film). See also *Small-angle scatter.*

Free air ionization chamber An instrument used in a calibration laboratory to obtain a precise measurement of exposure to x-radiation.

Free radical A solitary atom or most often a combination of atoms that behaves as an extremely reactive single entity as a result of the presence of an unpaired electron.

Frequency The number of vibrations or waves per second (crests or cycles per second).

Gadolinium A rare-earth phosphor used in rare-earth intensifying screens.

Gamma rays Short-wavelength, high-energy electromagnetic waves emitted by the nuclei of radioactive substances. Although generally shorter in wavelength than x-rays and with a different point of origin, their other characteristics are identical to those of diagnostic x-rays.

Gastrointestinal (GI) syndrome A form of acute radiation syndrome that appears in humans at a whole-body threshold dose of approximately 6 Gy (600 rads) and that peaks after a dose of 10 Gy (1000 rads).

Geiger-Müller (GM) detector A device that detects individual radioactive particles or photons and that serves as the primary radiation survey instrument for area monitoring in nuclear medicine facilities.

Genes Segments of DNA that serve as the basic units of heredity.

Genetic cells (germ cells) Cells of the human body associated with reproduction.

Genetic damage Radiation damage to generations yet unborn.

Genetic effects Biologic effects of ionizing radiation or other agents on generations yet unborn.

Genetic mutations (See *Mutations*.)

Genetically significant dose (GSD) The equivalent dose to the reproductive organs that, if received by every human, would be expected to cause an identical gross genetic injury to the total population as does the sum of the actual doses received by exposed individual population members. For the U.S. population, this dose is estimated to be about 0.20 mSv (20 mrem).

Germ cells Male and female reproductive cells.

Glucose A form of sugar that is the primary energy source for the cell.

Glycerine A sweet, colorless, odorless, syrupy liquid obtained from fats that are soluble in water; often used as a moistening agent.

Golgi apparatus Tiny sacs located near the cell nucleus, the Golgi apparatus synthesizes glycoproteins and transports enzymes and hormones through the cell membrane.

Gonadal dose Radiation exposure received by the male and female reproductive organs.

Gonadal shielding devices Devices used during radiologic procedures to protect the reproductive organs from exposure to the useful beam when they are in or within approximately 5 cm of a properly collimated beam, unless this would compromise the diagnostic value of the examination.

Gonads Male and female reproductive organs.

Gram (g) A unit of mass of the metric system. An object near the earth's surface that has a mass of 454 grams will weigh 1 pound.

Granule A small particle such as the insoluble, nonmembranous particles found in cytoplasm.

Granulocyte A scavenger type of white blood cell that fights bacteria.

Gray (Gy) SI unit of absorbed dose. An energy absorption of 1 joule (J) per kilogram (kg) of matter in the irradiated object.

Guanine (G) One of two purine bases found in both DNA and RNA.

Half-life Statistical quantity equal to the amount of time associated with a 50% decrease in the radioactivity of a sample containing a very large number of radioactive atoms.

Half-value layer (HVL) The thickness of a designated absorber (customarily a metal such as aluminum) required to decrease the intensity of the primary beam by 50% of its initial value.

Helical CT (See *spiral CT*.)

Hematopoietic syndrome A form of acute radiation syndrome that occurs when humans receive whole-body doses of ionizing radiation ranging from 1 to 10 Gy (100 to 1000 rads) and in which the reduction of the number of blood cells in the circulating blood results in a loss of the body's ability to clot blood and fight infection; also called *bone marrow syndrome*.

Hemoglobin A protein; the oxygen-carrying pigment of the red blood cells (erythrocytes).

Hemorrhage Abnormal escape of blood; heavy bleeding.

Heritable effects (See *Genetic effects*.)

High contrast resolution The ability of a system to make two dissimilar adjacent objects visually distinguishable.

High-LET radiation Includes particles that possess substantial mass and charge such as alpha particles, ions of heavier nuclei, and charged particles released from interactions between neutrons and atoms. Low-energy neutrons, which carry no electrical charge, are also a high-LET radiation.

High-level control fluoroscopy (HLCF)   An operating mode of fluoroscopic equipment in which exposure rates are significantly higher than normally allowed for routine fluoroscopic procedures, allowing for visualization of smaller and lower-contrast objects than are normally visible during fluoroscopy.

Highly differentiated cells   Mature or more specialized cells.

High-speed image receptor system   A relative term that describes an image receptor that requires less exposure to obtain a response, such as generation of a digital image or production of a chemical change displayed as an increase in optical density (darkening) of film.

Holistic approach to patient care   Treating the whole person rather than just the area of concern.

Homeostasis   A state of equilibrium between the different elements of an organism or a tendency toward such a state; the ability of the body to return to and maintain normal functioning despite the changes it has undergone.

Hormones   Chemical secretions manufactured by various endocrine glands and carried by the bloodstream to influence activities of other parts of the body, such as regulating growth and development.

Human genome   The total amount of genetic material (DNA) contained in the chromosomes of a human being.

Hydrocephaly   Abnormal fluid in the brain.

Hydrogen peroxide   A cellular poison that can result from the radiolysis of water.

Hydroperoxyl radical   A substance toxic to the cell that can result from the radiolysis of water.

Hyperbaric oxygen   High-pressure oxygen sometimes used in radiotherapy treatment of certain types of cancerous tumors to increase their radiosensitivity.

Hypoxic cells   Cells that lack an adequate amount of oxygen.

Image intensification fluoroscopy   Use of an image intensifier to increase the brightness of the real-time image produced on a fluorescent screen during fluoroscopy.

Image intensifier   A device that increases the brightness of an image.

Image matrix   The array of pixels that comprise a digital image. Examples of matrix sizes are 256×256 or 512×512.

Image receptor   Radiographic film or phosphorescent screen.

Incident photon   Incoming photon.

Incoherent scattering   (See *Compton scattering.*)

Indirect action   The effect of reactive free radicals created by the interaction of radiation with water molecules; cell death can result.

Indirect transmission   Primary photons that undergo Compton and/or coherent interactions and are scattered or deflected after they traverse an object and then reach the image receptor.

Inelastic scatter   The interaction of an incident photon with a loosely bound outer-shell electron of the target atom in which the photon surrenders some of its kinetic energy to free the electron from its orbit and then continues on its way in a new direction.

Inherent filtration   The glass envelope (0.5-mm aluminum equivalent) encasing the x-ray tube, the insulating oil surrounding the tube, and the glass window in the tube housing.

Inorganic compounds   Compounds that do not contain carbon. The inorganic compounds found in the human body occur in nature independent of living things.

Instant cell death   Immediate death of large numbers of cells occurring when a volume is irradiated with an x-ray or gamma ray dose of about 1000 Gy (100,000 rads) in a period of seconds or a few minutes.

Intensifying screens   By amplifying the effect of the exit, or image formation, radiation reaching the radiographic film, intensifying screens enhance the action of x-rays on the film. They convert x-ray energy into visible light.

Intensity (of radiation)   Quantity, or amount, of radiation crossing unit area per unit time.

Interference of function   Permanent or temporary interference of cellular function independent of the cell's ability to divide can be brought about by exposure to ionizing radiation.

Intermittent fluoroscopy (pulsed fluoroscopy)   Manual or automatic periodic activation of the fluoroscopic tube by the fluoroscopist rather than lengthy or continuous activation.

Internal contamination Ingestion or inhalation of radioactive material within the body.

International Commission on Radiological Protection (ICRP) Radiation protection standards organization considered to be the international authority regarding the safe use of sources of ionizing radiation. The ICRP is responsible for providing clear and consistent radiation protection guidance through its recommendations on occupational and public dose limits.

International system of units (SI) System of units that allows an interchange of units among all branches of science throughout the world.

Interphase The period of cell growth that occurs before actual cell division.

Interphase death (See *Apoptosis*.)

Interslice scatter Radiation that scatters from the CT slice being scanned into adjacent slices.

Interstrand cross-link A cross-link formed between complementary DNA strands or between entirely different DNA molecules.

Interventional procedures Medical procedures, such as inserting catheters into vessels or tissues for the purpose of drainage, biopsy, or alteration of vascular occlusions, performed by a physician during an imaging procedure such as fluoroscopy.

Intrastrand cross-link A cross-link formed between two places on the same DNA strand.

Inverse square law (ISL) The relationship between distance and intensity (quantity) of radiation (e.g., the intensity of the radiation at any location decreases with the square of its change of distance from the source of radiation). The resulting tripling a person's separation from a radiation source causes the exposure received by that person to decrease by a factor of 3^2, or 9.

Investigational levels Defined as Level I and Level II in the ALARA concept. In the U.S., these levels are traditionally one tenth to three tenths the applicable regulatory limits.

Involuntary motion Motion that cannot be willfully controlled. It is caused by muscle groups such as those of the digestive organs and the heart.

Iodine-123 (^{123}I) Unstable isotope of the element iodine used for monitoring thyroid gland function.

Iodine-125 (^{125}I) A radioactive isotope of the element iodine with a half-life of approximately 60 days. It

decays by the method of electron capture, emitting a low-energy gamma ray and a low energy characteristic photon in the process.

Iodine-131 (^{131}I) An unstable isotope of the element iodine. It has 53 protons and 78 neutrons in its nucleus. It undergoes beta decay with a half-life of 8.1 days.

Ionization The conversion of atoms to ions.

Ionization chamber A device that measures the amount of electrical charge resulting from the presence of all the ions of one sign produced during the irradiation of a specific volume of air.

Ionization chamber-type survey meter ("cutie pie") An exposure rate meter normally used for area surveys as well as an accurate integrating or cumulative exposure device for x-radiation and gamma radiation.

Ionize To remove electrons.

Ionizing radiation Radiation that produces positively and negatively charged particles (ions) when passing through matter.

Ion pair Two oppositely charged particles.

Ions Positively and negatively charged particles.

Isotope An atom that contains a different number of neutrons but the same number of protons in its nucleus as does the reference atom (e.g., helium-3 and helium-4, whose nuclei contain one and two neutrons, respectively). Radioactive isotopes of atoms that make up biologic materials may be used in medical imaging nuclear medicine studies.

Joule (J) The work done or energy expended when a force of 1 newton acts on an object along a distance of 1 meter.

Key molecule (See *Master molecule*.)

Kiloelectron volt (keV) A unit used to measure the kinetic energy of an individual electron in the high-speed electron beam within the x-ray tube; equivalent to 1000 electron volts (1 keV = 1000 eV). Also used to measure the energies of x-rays.

Kilogram (kg) 1000 grams (g).

Kilovolt (kV) Electrical potential equal to 1000 volts.

Kinetic energy Energy of motion.

Lanthanum A rare-earth phosphor used in rare-earth intensifying screens.

Last-frame-hold feature An optional equipment feature in which the most recent fluoroscopic image remains in view as a guide to the radiologist when the x-ray beam is not activated.

Late nonstochastic (deterministic) somatic effects Late effects directly related to the dose received that occur months or years after a high-level radiation exposure.

Late somatic effects Nongenetic effects that appear months or years following exposure to ionizing radiation.

Late stochastic (probabilistic) somatic effects Late effects that do not have a threshold, that occur in an arbitrary or probabilistic manner, whose severity does not depend on dose, and that occur months or years after high-level and possibly after low-level radiation exposure.

Latent period The period after the prodromal stage of acute radiation syndrome, during which no visible effects or symptoms of radiation exposure occur.

Law of Bergoiné and Tribondeau The radiosensitivity of cells is directly proportional to their reproductive activity and inversely proportional to their degree of differentiation.

LD 50/30 A quantitative measurement signifying the whole-body dose of radiation that can be lethal to 50% of the exposed population within 30 days.

LD 50/60 A quantitative measurement signifying the whole-body dose of radiation that can be lethal to 50% of the exposed population within 60 days.

Lead-equivalent Thickness of radiation-absorbing material that produces an attenuation equivalent to that which would be accomplished by a specified amount of lead.

Leakage radiation Photons that instead of coming out of the collimator opening with the useful beam emerge in multiple directions, through the protective housing of the x-ray tube.

LET (See *Linear energy transfer*.)

Leukemia Neoplastic overproduction of white blood cells.

Leukemogenesis The production or origin of leukemia.

Leukocytes White blood cells.

Leukopenia An abnormal decrease of white blood corpuscles, usually below 5000/mm^3.

Lifetime effective dose limit Dose that does not exceed 10 times the occupationally exposed person's age in years.

Linear dose-response curve A model used to calculate the occurrence of cancer by extrapolating from information associated with high levels of radiation to determine the risk associated with low doses: the linear dose-response curve describes current high-dose information satisfactorily but exaggerates the actual risk or danger at low doses and dose rates.

Linear energy transfer (LET) The amount of energy transferred on average by incident radiation to an object per unit length of track through the object. It is expressed in units of keV/μm.

Linear, nonthreshold dose-response relationship The chance of sustaining biologic damage and the amount of that biologic damage are directly proportional to the magnitude of the ionizing radiation exposure; even the most minuscule radiation dose has the potential to cause some damage.

Linear-quadratic dose-response curve A model used to calculate the occurrence of cancer by extrapolating from information associated with high levels of radiation to determine the risk associated with low doses. This model fits the current high-dose information satisfactorily but may underestimate risk at low doses.

Linear, threshold dose-response relationship The relationship between dose and response is such that a biologic response does not occur below a specified level of radiation dose.

Lipids Water-insoluble macromolecules that consist only of carbon, hydrogen, and oxygen; lipids store energy in the body for long periods of time.

Lithium fluoride (LiF) The sensing material of the thermoluminescent dosimeter (TLD).

Log, or logarithmic, scale A method used to graph data that cover several orders of magnitude (the powers of ten; e.g., 1, 10, 100, 1000).

Long scale of radiographic contrast Radiographic contrast in which there are many shades of gray. A wide range of exposures will produce a wide range of shades of gray when a long scale image receptor or display is used.

Long-term or late somatic effect Effects of ionizing radiation that appeared months or years following exposure to ionizing radiation.

Low-LET radiations External electromagnetic radiations such as x-rays and gamma rays that have neither mass nor charge.

Low-level radiation An absorbed dose of (0.1 Sv) 10 rem or less delivered over a short period of time or a larger dose delivered over a long period of time, for instance (0.5 Sv) 50 rem in 10 years.

Luminance A scientific term that refers to the brightness of a surface. Luminance quantifies the intensity of a light source (i.e., the amount of light per unit area coming from its surface).

Lymphocyte A type of white blood cell that plays an active role in producing immunity for the body by producing antibodies to combat disease; the most radiosensitive blood cells in the human body.

Lysosomes Small, pealike sacs within the cytoplasm whose primary function appears to be the breaking down of large molecules.

M On a personnel monitoring report, this letter signifies that an equivalent dose below the minimum measurable quantity of radiation has been received during the interval of time covered by the report.

Macromolecule Large molecule built up from smaller chemical structures.

Mammography Radiographic study of the breast.

Manifest illness The stage of acute radiation syndrome when symptoms become visible.

Man-made radiation Ionizing radiation created by humans for various uses, including nuclear fuel for generation of power, consumer products containing radioactive material, and medical radiation; also called *artificial radiation*.

Man-rem Traditional radiation unit for the quantity collective effective dose (ColEfD).

mAs (See *Milliampere-seconds*.)

Mass density Quantity of matter per unit volume. It is generally specified in units of kilograms per cubic meter (kg/m^3) or grams per cubic centimeter (g/cc).

Master molecule A molecule vital to the survival of the cell that maintains normal cell function. It is also referred to as a *key molecule*.

Maximum permissible dose (MPD) A term used in the past to indicate the maximum dose equivalent of ionizing radiation that an occupationally exposed person could absorb in a specified time period without sustaining appreciable bodily injury.

Mean energy The average energy of an x-ray beam.

Mean marrow dose The average radiation dose to the entire active bone marrow.

Medical exposure Exposure to ionizing radiation incurred for the purpose of obtaining medical diagnosis or undergoing treatment.

Megakaryocytes Platelet stem cells.

Meiosis The process of germ (genetic) cell division, which reduces the chromosomes in each daughter cell to half the number of chromosomes in the parent cell.

Mesons Penetrating, unstable, subatomic particles that are components of cosmic radiation.

Messenger RNA (mRNA) The substance responsible for making proteins out of amino acids.

Metabolism Chemical reactions that modify foods for cellular use.

Metaphase The phase of cell division during which the mitotic spindle is completed.

Microcephaly Abnormally small head circumference.

Milliampere (mA) Unit of measurement. X-ray tube current.

Milliampere-seconds (mAs) The product of electron tube current and the amount of time in seconds that the x-ray tube is on.

Milligray (mGy) One one-thousandth of a gray (1/1000 Gy).

Millirad (mrad) One one-thousandth of a rad (1/1000 rad).

Millirem (mrem) One one-thousandth of a rem (1/1000 rem).

Millisievert (mSv) One one-thousandth of a sievert (1/1000 Sv).

Mitochondria Large bean-shape structures containing highly organized enzymes in their inner membrane, which function as "powerhouses" for the cell.

Mitosis The process of somatic cell division wherein a parent cell divides to form two daughter cells identical to the parent cell.

Mitotic death (genetic death) Cell death occurring after one or more divisions following irradiation.

Mitotic delay The failure of a cell to start dividing on time; this can occur when a cell is exposed to as little as 0.01 Gy (1 rad) of ionizing radiation just before it normally would begin to divide.

Mitotic spindle The delicate fibers attached to the centrioles and extending from one side of the cell to the other.

Mobile radiographic equipment Manually portable radiographic equipment.

Modified scattering (See *Compton scattering.*)

Molecular change An alteration in the basic structure of a molecule caused by some type of destructive process, such as exposure to ionizing radiation.

Molecular damage Injury on the molecular level resulting from exposure to ionizing radiation.

Molecular lesions (See *Point lesions.*)

Molecule The smallest unit of a specific substance composed of one or more atoms.

Molten Melted or liquefied by heat.

Monitoring A means of overseeing occupational radiation exposure to ensure that such exposure is kept well below the annual effective dose limit.

Muscle tissue Tissue that contains fibers that affect movement of an organ or part of the body; muscle tissue does not divide and is relatively insensitive to radiation.

Mutagenesis Birth defects that can be caused by irradiation of reproductive cells (sperm and ova) before conception.

Mutagens Agents that increase the frequency of occurrence of mutations, such as elevated temperatures, ionizing radiations, viruses, and chemicals.

Mutation frequency The number of spontaneous or mutagen-caused mutations that occur in a given generation.

Mutations Changes in genes caused by the loss or change of a base in the DNA chain.

Myeloblasts Precursors of granulocytes, a type of white blood cell.

National Academy of Science/National Research Council Committee on the Biological Effects of Ionizing Radiation (NAS/NRC-BEIR) Reviews studies of the biologic effects of ionizing radiation and risk assessment and provides the information to other organizations for evaluation.

National Council on Radiation Protection and Measurements (NCRP) Reviews regulations formulated by the ICRP and decides how to include them in U.S. radiation protection criteria; recommendations are published in the form of various NCRP Reports.

National Institute of Standards and Technology (NIST) Professional organization responsible for accrediting calibration laboratories that measure radiation exposure in medical radiography.

Natural background radiation Ionizing radiation from environmental sources, including radioactive materials in the earth, cosmic radiation from space, and radionuclides deposited in the human body.

Necrosis Death of areas of tissue or bone surrounded by healthy parts.

Negatron A normal electron carrying a negative charge.

Negligible individual dose (NID) An annual effective dose that provides a low-exposure cut-off level so that regulatory agencies may dismiss a level of individual risk as negligible.

Neonatal death Death at birth.

Nervous tissue Conductive tissue found in the brain and spinal cord.

Neuron A nerve cell consisting of a cell body and two kinds of very fine stringlike tissue segments that extend outward called processes and dendrites, and the axon.

Neuron organogenesis In the embryo-fetus, a period of development and change of the nerve cells, which extends into the beginning of the fetal period.

Neutrino An electrically neutral particle that according to current theory has almost negligible mass. The neutrino shows an exceedingly small tendency to interact with any type of matter.

Neutron An electrically neutral particle located within the nucleus of the atom; one of the fundamental constituents of the atom. It has approximately the same mass as a proton.

Neutrophils Leukocytes that fight infection.

Newton Unit of force in the meter-kilogram-second system of physical units. One newton corresponds to approximately one fourth of a pound.

Nit (See *Candela per square meter.*)

Nitrogen A tasteless, odorless, colorless gaseous chemical element found free in the air; an integral part of protein and nucleic acids and thus found in every living cell.

Nitrogenous bases Organic bases that contain the element nitrogen.

Nonagreement states Individual U.S. states in which both the state Department of Environmental Protection and the Nuclear Regulatory Commission (NRC) enforce radiation protection regulations.

Nonoccupational exposure Radiation exposure received by members of the general population who are not employed as radiation workers.

Nonoccupational person Any person not employed as a radiation worker.

Non–self-reading pocket dosimeter A pocket ionization chamber that requires a special accessory electrometer to read the device and is used for personnel monitoring in areas of low radiation exposure when immediate readout is not necessary.

Nonspecific life span shortening A reduction in the life cycle of small laboratory animals resulting from nonlethal exposure to ionizing radiation. Early demise actually resulted from radiation-induced cancer.

Nonstochastic effects Biologic somatic effects of ionizing radiation that can be directly related to the dose received. These cell-killing effects exhibit a threshold dose below which the effect does not normally occur and above which the severity of the biologic damage increases as the dose increases. These effects are also known as *deterministic effects*.

Nonverbal messages Unconscious actions, or body language.

Nuclear medicine Branch of medicine that employs radioisotopes to study organ function within a patient, to detect the spread of cancer into bone, and to treat certain types of diseases.

Nuclear medicine procedure The administration, either orally or intravenously, of a radioactive isotope for the purpose of conducting a diagnostic study of a body area.

Nuclear reactor A mechanism for creating and continuing a controlled nuclear chain reaction in a fissionable fuel for the production of energy or supplementary fissionable material.

Nuclear Regulatory Commission (NRC) A federal agency (formerly known as Atomic Energy Commission) that has the authority to control the possession, use, and production of atomic energy in the interest of national security. This agency also has the power to enforce radiation protection standards.

Nucleic acids Large, complex macromolecules made up of nucleotides.

Nucleotides Units formed from a nitrogenous base such as adenine, guanine, cytosine, or thymine; a five-carbon sugar molecule, deoxyribose; and a phosphate molecule. Several nucleotides make up a nucleic acid.

Nucleus The center of the cell; a spherical mass of protoplasm containing the genetic material (DNA), which is stored in its molecular structure.

Occupancy factor (T) A factor used to modify the shielding requirement for a particular barrier by taking into account the fraction of the x-ray unit's workload for which there is occupancy beyond that barrier.

Occupational and nonoccupational dose limits Upper boundary doses of ionizing radiation that will result in a negligible risk of bodily injury or genetic damage.

Occupational exposure Radiation exposure received by radiation workers in the course of exercising their professional responsibilities.

Occupational risk (1) The probability of injury, ailment, or death resulting from an activity that takes place in the workplace. (2) The possibility of developing a radiogenic cancer or the induction of a genetic defect as a consequence of the radiation exposure received.

Occupational Safety and Health Administration (OSHA) Organization that functions as a monitoring agency in places of employment, predominantly in industry. OSHA regulates occupational exposure to radiation and is responsible for regulations concerning the "right to know" of employees with regard to hazards that may be present in the workplace.

Occupationally exposed person Individual employed as a radiation worker.

Off-focus radiation X-rays emitted from parts of the tube other than the focal spot; also called *stem radiation*.

Oncology Branch of medicine dealing with cancer.

Oocytes Immature female germ cells.

Oogonium Female germ cell.

Optical density The intensity of light transmitted through a given area of the medical imaging film.

Optically stimulated luminescence (OSL) dosimeter A device for monitoring occupational exposure that contains an aluminum oxide detector. When the dosimeter is "read out," optically stimulated luminosity occurs when the dosimeter is struck by laser light at selected frequencies. When such laser light is incident on the sensing material, it becomes luminescent in proportion to the amount of radiation exposure received.

Optimization for radiation protection (ORP) (See *ALARA concept/principle*.)

Organic acids Organic compounds containing the carboxyl (COOH) group.

Organic compounds All carbon compounds, both natural and artificial.

Organic damage Genetic or somatic changes in a living organism, such as mutations, cataracts, and leukemia, caused by excessive cellular damage from exposure to ionizing radiation.

Organogenesis (1) Period of gestation from the 10th day to the 6th week after conception during which the nerve cells in the brain and spinal cord of the fetus develop and the fetus is most susceptible to radiation-induced congenital abnormalities. (2) The stage in which undifferentiated cells are implanted in the uterine wall.

Osmotic pressure The force created when a semipermeable membrane separates two solutions of different concentrations.

Osteogenic sarcoma Bone cancer.

Osteoporosis Decalcification of the bone.

Oxidation Most simply, the combining of a substance with oxygen. The definition of oxidation, however, has been broadened to include reactions in which electrons are lost by an atom.

Oxygen enhancement ratio (OER) A ratio of the radiation dose required to cause a particular biologic response of cells or organisms in any oxygen-deprived environment to the radiation dose required to cause an identical response under normally oxygenated conditions.

Pair production Interaction between an incoming photon of at least 1.022 MeV and an atom of the irradiated object in which the photon approaches, strongly interacts with the nucleus of the atom of the irradiated material, and disappears. In the process, the energy of the incoming photon is transformed into two new particles—a negatron and a positron—after which these particles exit from the atom, carrying away some of the momentum of the absorbed photon when the photon's energy is greater than 1.022 MeV.

Particulate radiation As opposed to x-rays and gamma rays, examples of particulate radiation are electrons, protons, neutrons, and alpha particles (nuclei of helium).

Patient restraint Immobilization of the patient by a mechanical device or human restraint during an imaging procedure.

Peak voltage Maximum voltage directed across an x-ray tube.

Peptic bond Chemical bond connecting two amino acids.

Peptide bond A chemical link that connects each amino acid in long, chainlike molecular complexes.

Permeable Penetrable.

Personnel dosimeter A device that provides an indication of the exposure received by radiation workers as a result of their working habits and working conditions.

Personnel dosimetry Monitoring of radiation exposure of any person occupationally exposed on a regular basis.

Personnel monitoring report A written report of occupational radiation exposure of personnel prepared by a monitoring company.

Person-sievert SI radiation unit for the quantity, collective effective dose (ColEfD).

PET/CT scanner A unit in which a PET scanner is physically joined in a tandem configuration with a CT scanner to produce one joint imaging device. This unit can, using FDG fluorine-18, detect the presence of abnormally high regions of glucose metabolism, which are evidence of cancer spread or metastatic disease in other body areas, while at the same time giving detailed information about the location and size of these lesions or growths.

Photodisintegration An interaction that occurs above 10 MeV in high-energy radiation therapy machines in which a high-energy photon collides with the nucleus of an atom, absorbing all of the photon's energy. This energy excess in the nucleus creates an instability that can be alleviated by the emission of a neutron by the nucleus. If sufficient energy is absorbed by the nucleus, another type of emission is possible: a proton or proton-neutron combination (deuteron).

Photoelectric absorption An interaction between an x-ray photon and an inner-shell electron in which the photon surrenders all its kinetic energy to the orbital electron and ceases to exist. As a result, the electron escapes its inner shell and leaves the atom. Photoelectric absorption is the process most responsible for the contrast between bone and soft tissue in diagnostic radiographs.

Photoelectron   The electron ejected from its inner-shell orbit during the process of photoelectric absorption.

Photon   A particle associated with electromagnetic radiation that has neither mass nor electric charge.

Photopic vision   Cone vision (daytime vision).

Photostimulable phosphor   The image receptor of a computed radiography (CR) system. When struck by x-rays, electrons within the phosphor become trapped at energy levels that are quasi-stable. When a laser strikes the surface of the phosphor, visible light is emitted in proportion to the x-ray exposure that had been received by the phosphor. A photomultiplier tube then records the visible light intensity, which corresponds to the brightness of a picture element, or pixel, in the CR image.

Picocurie   A very small quantity of radioactivity equivalent to one trillionth (10^{-12}) of a curie.

Pixels   Individual picture elements that when taken together represent the total information contained in a slice or a volume of tissue. Each pixel makes up a small part of the image matrix of the digital image.

Platelets   Circular or oval disks found in the blood of all vertebrates. Platelets initiate blood clotting and prevent hemorrhage.

Pocket ionization chamber (pocket dosimeter)   A personnel monitoring device that contains a positively and a negatively charged electrode; when these electrodes are exposed to ionizing radiation, the air around the positively charged electrode is ionized and discharges the mechanism in direct proportion to the amount of radiation to which it has been exposed.

Point lesions   Altered areas in molecules caused by the breaking of a single chemical bond.

Point mutations   Genetic mutations in which the chromosome is not broken but the DNA within it is damaged. (See *Single-strand break*.)

Portable radiographic equipment   (See *Mobile radiographic equipment*.)

Positive beam limitation (PBL)   A feature of current radiographic collimators that automatically adjusts the collimators so that the radiation field size matches the film size.

Positron   A positively charged electron, which is a form of antimatter.

Positron emission tomography (PET)   A modality that produces axial images by making use of annihilation radiation that is initiated by the positron radioactive decay of the nucleus of an unstable atom. This modality examines metabolic processes within the human body.

Potential difference   The difference in electrical potential or voltage between two points in a circuit.

Potential risk   The possibility of inducing a radiogenic cancer or genetic defect after irradiation.

Precursor cells   (See *Stem cells*.)

Preimplantation stage   About 0 to 9 days after conception.

Primary beam   (See *Primary radiation*.)

Primary protective barrier   (1) A barrier designed to prevent primary, or direct, radiation from reaching personnel or members of the general public on the other side of the barrier. (2) A barrier located perpendicular to the undeflected line of travel of the primary x-ray beam.

Primary radiation   Radiation that emerges directly from the x-ray tube collimator and moves without deflection toward a wall, door, viewing window, and so on. Also called *direct radiation*.

Probabilistic effects   (See *Stochastic effects*.)

Prodromal syndrome   The first stage of acute radiation syndrome, which occurs within hours after a whole-body absorbed dose of 1 Gy (100 rads) or more; characterized by nausea, vomiting, diarrhea, fatigue, and leukopenia.

Programmed cell death   (See *Apoptosis*.)

Prophase   The phase of cell division during which the nucleus and the chromosomes enlarge and the DNA begins to take structural form.

Proportional counter   A radiation survey instrument generally used in a laboratory setting to detect alpha and beta radiation and small amounts of other types of low-level radioactive contamination.

Protective apparel   Special garments such as aprons, gloves, and thyroid shields that are conventionally made of lead-impregnated vinyl and worn during fluoroscopic and certain selective radiographic procedures.

Protective barrier   Any medium of adequate composition and thickness that absorbs primary and/or secondary radiation, thereby reducing exposure of persons located on the other side of the barrier.

Protective eyeglasses   Eyeglasses with optically clear lenses that contain a minimum lead-equivalent protection of 0.35 mm.

Protective shielding   A structure or device made of certain materials such as concrete, lead, or lead-impregnated material that will adequately attenuate ionizing radiation.

Protein   Amino acids linked in various patterns and combinations. Proteins contain carbon, hydrogen, nitrogen, oxygen, and occasionally other elements, such as sulfur.

Protein synthesis   The making of new proteins.

Proton   One of the three main constituents of an atom, the proton carries a positive electrical charge equal in magnitude to that of an electron.

Protoplasm   The building material of all living things, protoplasm consists of inorganic substances, such as water and mineral salts, and organic substances, including proteins, carbohydrates, lipids, and nucleic acids.

Pulsed fluoroscopy   (See *Intermittent fluoroscopy*.)

Purines   A class of nitrogenous bases found in DNA and RNA. These bases include adenine (A) and guanine (G).

Pyrimidines   A class of nitrogenous bases found in DNA and RNA. These bases include cytosine (C), thymine (T), and in the case of RNA, uracil (U), which replaces thymine.

Quantum mottle   Faint blotches in the recorded radiographic image produced by an intrinsic fluctuation in the incident photon intensity. This effect is more noticeable when very-high-speed rare-earth systems are used.

Rad (radiation-absorbed-dose)   The unit that indicates the amount of radiant energy transferred to an irradiated object by any type of ionizing radiation. One rad is equivalent to an energy transfer of 100 erg per gram of irradiated object and 1/100 gray.

Radiant energy   Energy that moves in the form of a wave and is transmitted by radiations such as x-rays and gamma rays.

Radiation   Energy in transit from one location to another; a transfer of energy that results from either a change occurring naturally within an atom (see *Radiation decay*) or a process caused by the interaction of a particle with an atom.

Radiation biology   The science concerned with the effects of ionizing radiations on living systems.

Radiation Control for Health and Safety Act of 1968   Law passed by the U.S. Congress to protect the public from the hazards of unnecessary radiation exposure resulting from electronic products such as microwave ovens, color televisions, and diagnostic x-ray equipment.

Radiation decay   A naturally occurring process in which atoms with unstable nuclei relieve that instability by various types of nuclear spontaneous emissions, including charged particles, uncharged particles, and photons.

Radiation dose   The amount of radiation received by an individual. The amount of energy transferred to electrons in biologic tissue by ionizing radiation is the basis of this concept.

Radiation dose-response curve   A graph that maps out the effects of radiation observed in relation to the dose of radiation received.

Radiation dosimetry film   Radiographic film in a film badge that is sensitive to doses ranging from as low as 0.1 mSv (10 mrem) to as high as 5000 mSv (500 rem).

Radiation Emergency Plan   Plan that hospitals can implement for handling emergency situations involving radioactive contamination.

Radiation hormesis effect   A beneficial consequence of radiation for populations continuously exposed to moderately higher levels of radiation.

Radiation-induced malignancy   Cancerous neoplasm caused by exposure to ionizing radiation.

Radiation monitoring device   A device worn by diagnostic imaging personnel to indicate occupational exposure by measuring the quantity of radiation to which it has been exposed over time.

Radiation permeability   The ability of a structure to be penetrated by radiation.

Radiation protection   Effective measures employed by radiation workers to safeguard patients, personnel, and the general public from unnecessary exposure to ionizing radiation.

Radiation safety committee (RSC)   Group that assists in the development of the radiation safety program in a health care facility; provides guidance for the program, and facilitates its ongoing operation.

Radiation safety officer (RSO) An individual such as a medical physicist or radiologist, qualified through adequate training and experience, who is designated by a health care facility and approved by the NRC and state to ensure that internationally accepted guidelines for radiation protection are followed in the facility. The RSO is responsible for developing and implementing an appropriate radiation safety program for the facility and maintaining radiation monitoring records for all personnel.

Radiation survey instruments Area monitoring devices that detect and/or measure radiation.

Radiation therapy Use of x-rays or gamma rays, usually with energies much greater than those employed for diagnostic purposes, to destroy the cells composing a tumor while sparing the surrounding nontumor tissues.

Radiation weighting factor (W_R) A dimensionless factor (a multiplier) used for radiation protection purposes to account for differences in biologic impact between various types of ionizing radiations. This factor places risks associated with biologic effects on a common scale.

Radicals Groups of atoms that remain together during a chemical change and behave almost like a single atom. Atoms in a radical are held together by covalent bonding.

Radiodermatitis Reddening of the skin caused by exposure to ionizing radiation.

Radioactive contamination Radioactive material that is attached to or associated with dust particles or is a in liquid form on various surfaces. Removal of the liquid or dust accomplishes removal of the radioactive material. Radioactive contamination may consist of surface, internal (inhaled, ingested), internal wound, or external wound contamination.

Radioactive dispersal device A radioactive source mixed with conventional explosives. When detonated, this device explodes, spreading radioactive material through a specific area, causing contamination and panic; also called a "dirty bomb."

Radiogenic malignancies Cancerous neoplasms induced by exposure to ionizing radiation.

Radiographer A person qualified through formal education and certification to practice medical imaging procedures and provide related patient care.

Radiographic beam-light beam coincidence Both physical size (length and width) and alignment between the radiographic beam and the localizing light beam must correspond to within 2% of the source-image distance (SID).

Radiographic contrast Differences in density level between the radiographic images of objects in a radiograph.

Radiographic density The degree of overall blackening on the finished radiograph.

Radiographic fog Undesirable, additional density on a processed radiographic film caused by scattered radiation reaching the film.

Radiographic grid A device (made of parallel radiopaque lead strips alternated with low-attenuation strips of aluminum, plastic, or wood) placed between the patient and the film to remove scattered x-ray photons that emerge from the object being radiographed before they reach the film. Use of a grid improves image contrast.

Radiographic image receptor Radiographic film or phosphorescent screen.

Radioisotopes Isotopes of a particular element that are unstable because of their neutron-proton configuration.

Radiologist A qualified physician who specializes in diagnosis and treatment through the use of radiant energy.

Radiolucent Transparent to radiation; a material that allows radiation to pass through.

Radiolysis of water Interaction of radiation with water.

Radionuclide An unstable nucleus that emits one or more forms of ionizing radiation to achieve greater stability.

Radon The first decay product of radium; a colorless, odorless, heavy radioactive gas that along with its decay products, polonium-218 and polonium-214 (solid form), is always present to some degree in the air.

Rare-earth screens Radiographic intensifying screens made with rare-earth phosphors—namely, gadolinium, lanthanum, and yttrium.

Rayleigh scattering (See *Coherent scattering.*)

Recessive mutation   A genetic mutation that probably will not be expressed for a number of generations because both parents must possess the same mutation.

Relative biologic effectiveness (RBE)   Describes the relative capabilities of radiation with differing LETs to produce a particular biologic reaction. Simply defined, it is the ratio of the dose of a reference radiation (conventionally, 250-kVp x-rays) to the dose that is necessary to produce the same biologic reaction in a given experiment. The reaction is produced by a dose of the test radiation delivered under the same conditions.

Relative risk   Model predicting that the number of excess cancers will increase as the natural incidence of cancer increases in a population with advancing age.

Rem (*radiation-equivalent-man*)   Traditional unit for the radiation quantity currently in use (equivalent dose [EqD]); defined as the dose that is equivalent to any type of ionizing radiation that produces the same biologic effect as 1 rad of x-radiation.

Remnant radiation   (See *Exit, or image formation, radiation*.)

Repair enzymes   Enzymes that can mend damaged molecules.

Repeat analysis program   An attempt to record the various causes of inadequate quality on occasions when an image has to be retaken.

Repeat radiograph   Any radiograph that must be taken more than once because of a human or mechanical error in the process of producing the initial radiograph.

Reproductive cells   Male and female germ cells (relatively radiosensitive).

Reproductive death   The permanent loss of a cell's ability to reproduce because of exposure to doses of ionizing radiation (1 to 10 Gy, or 100 to 1000 rads).

Restitution   A process in which chromosome breaks rejoin in their original configuration with no visible damage.

Retina   The rod- and cone-containing area of the eye; the retina receives the image formed by the lens.

Ribonucleic acid (RNA)   Type of nucleic acid that carries genetic information from the DNA in the cell nucleus to the ribosomes located in the cytoplasm.

Ribosomes   Small, spherical, cytoplasmic organelles that attach to the endoplasmic reticulum. They are the cell's "protein factories."

Right-to-Know Act (Employee)   A series of statutes passed by individual states requiring that employees be made aware of the hazards in the workplace, including hazardous substances, infectious agents, and ionizing and nonionizing radiation.

Risk   In general terms, the probability of injury, ailment, or death resulting from an activity. In the medical industry with reference to the radiation sciences, risk is the possibility of inducing a radiogenic cancer or genetic defect after irradiation.

Roentgen (R)   Internationally accepted unit of measurement of exposure to x-radiation and gamma radiation. One roentgen is the photon exposure that produces under standard conditions of pressure and temperature a total positive or negative ion charge of 2.58×10^{-4} coulombs per kilogram of dry air.

Rung   A step in the DNA ladderlike structure composed of a pair of nitrogenous bases.

Salts (electrolytes)   Chemical compounds that result from the action of an acid and a base on each other.

Scattered radiation   All the radiation that arises from the interactions of an x-ray beam with the atoms of an object in the path of the beam.

Scattering   The process wherein x-ray photons undergo a change in direction after interacting with the atoms of an object.

Scotopic vision   Rod vision (night vision).

Secondary protective barrier   A barrier that affords protection from secondary radiation (leakage and scattered radiation) only; as such, it is not designed to intercept the direct x-ray beam or to provide adequate attenuation of the beam.

Secondary radiation   The radiation that results from the interaction between primary radiation and the atoms of the irradiated object and the off-focus or leakage radiation that penetrates the x-ray tube protective housing. Secondary radiation consists of scattered radiation and leakage radiation.

Self-reading pocket dosimeter   A pocket ionization chamber that contains a built-in electrometer and provides an immediate exposure readout for radiation workers who work in high-exposure areas.

Semipermeable membrane   A film that permits the passage of a pure solvent such as water but does not allow material dissolved by the solvent to pass through it.

Shadow shield   A shield of radiopaque material suspended from above the radiographic beam-defining system; this shield hangs over the area of clinical interest to cast a shadow in the primary beam over the patient's reproductive organs.

Shallow equivalent dose   The external exposure of the skin or extremity at a tissue depth of 0.007 cm ($7 \ mg/cm^2$) averaged over an area of $1 \ cm^2$.

Shaped contact shield   A cup-shaped radiopaque shield that encloses the scrotum and penis to protect the male reproductive organs from exposure to ionizing radiation.

Short-term somatic effects (early or acute effects)   Somatic effects that appear within minutes, hours, days, or weeks of the time of radiation exposure.

Side scatter   Photons that interact with the atoms of an object and consequently are deflected to the side.

Sievert (Sv)   The SI unit of measure for the radiation quantity of equivalent dose (EqD). One sievert equals 1 joule of energy absorbed per kilogram of tissue (for x-radiation, Q = 1). This unit is used *only* for radiation protection purposes. It provides a common scale whereby varying degrees of biologic damage caused by equal absorbed doses of different types of ionizing radiation can be compared with the degree of biologic damage caused by the same amount of x-radiation or gamma radiation.

Signal-to-noise ratio (SNR)   The comparison of the average CT number in a region with the statistical variation of CT numbers throughout that region.

Single-strand break   The ionization of a DNA macromolecule resulting in a break of one of its chemical bonds, thereby severing one of the sugar-phosphate chain side rails or strands of the ladderlike DNA molecular structure.

Skin dose   The absorbed radiation dose, stated in Gy or rad, delivered to the most superficial layers of the skin as a result of a radiation exposure. Backscatter radiation contribution is included in this measurement.

Skin erythema dose   The received quantity of radiation (corresponding roughly to a moderate dose of several Gy [several hundred rad]) that causes diffused redness over an area of skin after irradiation.

Small-angle scatter   Photons that pass through the object being radiographed interact with the atoms of the object and are deflected at such a small angle that they can reach the film, thereby degrading the radiographic image by producing small amounts of radiographic fog.

Somatic cells   All the cells in the human body other than female and male germ cells.

Somatic damage   Biologic damage to the body of the exposed individual.

Somatic effects   Biologic damage sustained by living organisms (such as human beings) as a consequence of exposure to ionizing radiation.

Source-image receptor-distance   The distance from the anode focal spot to the radiographic image receptor.

Source-skin-distance (SSD)   The distance from the anode focal spot to the skin of the patient.

Source-to-tabletop distance   The distance from the anode focal spot to the top of the radiographic table.

Specific area shielding   The use of lead or lead-impregnated material to protect selective body areas from exposure to ionizing radiation.

Spermatogonium   The male germ cell.

Spiral CT   Also known as *helical CT*, this is a technique in computed tomography in which the patient couch moves in or out of the bore of the scanner while the x-ray tube rotates around the patient.

Spontaneous mutations   A natural phenomenon involving alterations in genes and DNA. These mutations occur at random and without a known cause.

Spot-film device protective curtain   A sliding panel with a minimum of 0.25-mm lead equivalent attached to the front of the spot-film device of a fluoroscopic x-ray unit for the purpose of intercepting scattered radiation before it reaches the fluoroscopist.

Stationary control-booth barrier   A nonmoveable enclosure where x-ray equipment controls are located. This booth is designed to intercept leakage and scatter radiation only; it may be regarded as a secondary protective barrier.

Stem cells Immature or precursor cells.

Stem radiation (See *Off-focus radiation*.)

Stochastic effects Mutational, nonthreshold, randomly occurring biologic somatic changes in which the chance of occurrence of the effect rather than the severity of the effect is proportional to the dose of ionizing radiation. Examples include cancer and genetic effects. Also called *probabilistic effects*.

Strontium-89 (^{89}Sr) A radioactive isotope of the element strontium. It has a half-life of 50.5 days and undergoes beta decay, emitting a high-speed electron (1.46 MeV) in the process.

Structural proteins Those proteins from which the body acquires its shape and form.

Sunspots Dark spots that occasionally appear on the surface of the sun. Sunspots indicate regions of increased electromagnetic field activity and are sometimes responsible for ejecting particulate radiation into space.

Surface contamination External contamination of the skin or clothing of an individual with radioactive material.

Syndrome A collection of symptoms.

Technetium-99m (^{99m}Tc) A gamma-emitting radioisotope with a 6-hour half-life produced from the radioactive decay of another unstable isotope, molybdenum-99, which relieves its instability by beta decay.

Target theory The theory that the cell will die if inactivation of the master molecule occurs as a result of exposure to ionizing radiation.

Telangiectasis Dilation of capillaries and sometimes of terminal arteries of an organ.

Telophase The phase of mitosis during which cell division is completed with the formation of two new daughter cells, each of which contains exactly the same genetic material as the parent cell.

Teratogenesis Birth effects induced by irradiation in utero.

Terrestrial radiation Long-lived radioactive elements such as uranium-238, radium-226, and thorium-232 that emit densely ionizing radiations. These sources are present in variable quantities in the crust of the earth.

Thermal neutron Nominally classified as a neutron whose kinetic energy is approximately less than or equal to 1 eV. Typically, these are neutrons whose kinetic energy has been significantly degraded as a result of multiple energy loss collisions.

Thermoluminescent dosimeter (TLD) badge A personnel monitoring device that most often contains a crystalline form of lithium fluoride as its sensing material. When this device is placed in a TLD analyzer and heated, the crystals emit visible light in proportion to the amount of radiation to which the TLD badge was exposed. It is most frequently used to directly measure skin dose.

Thompson scattering The elastic scattering of an x-ray photon by a free electron.

Threshold (1) The point at which a response or reaction to an increasing stimulation first occurs. (2) A dose level below which an individual has a negligible chance of sustaining specific biologic damage.

Thrombocytes (See *Platelets*.)

Thymine (T) A pyrimidine base found only in DNA.

Thymus gland An organ of the lymphatic system, located in the mediastinal cavity anterior to and above the heart. It plays a critical role in the body's defense against infection.

Thyroid gland A gland located in the neck just below the larynx. The hormone produced by this gland helps regulate the body's metabolic rate and the process of growth.

Thyroid shield (See *Protective apparel*.)

Title 10 of the Code of Federal Regulations, Part 20 A document prepared and distributed by the U.S. Office of the Federal Register. The rules and regulations of the Nuclear Regulatory Commission (NRC) and fundamental radiation protection standards governing occupational radiation exposure are included in this document.

Tissue weighting factor (W_T) A value denoting the percentage of the summed stochastic (cancer plus genetic) risk stemming from irradiation of tissue (T) to the all-inclusive risk, in which the entire body is irradiated in a uniform fashion. This factor assigns risk for potential biologic responses from various types of ionizing radiation on a common scale and takes into account the relative detriment to each organ and tissue.

TLD analyzer A device that measures the amount of ionizing radiation to which a TLD badge has been exposed.

TLD ring badge (See *Extremity dosimeter*.)

Tolerance dose A radiation dose to which occupationally exposed persons could be continuously subjected without any apparent harmful acute effects such as erythema of the skin.

Total filtration Inherent filtration plus added filtration.

Traditional units Special units associated with radiation protection and dosimetry, namely, the roentgen and the rem.

Trimester A 3-month period of gestation—i.e., 1st, 2nd, and 3rd trimester.

Tubule A small tube.

Tungsten A metal with a high melting point (greater than 3400° C) and a high atomic number (Z = 74). The anode in the x-ray tube is usually made primarily of this metal.

Ulceration The process of pus formation on a free surface, such as the skin or a mucous membrane, to form an ulcer.

Umbra (See *Primary radiation*.)

Uncontrolled area Area in which members of the general public (i.e., individuals who are not trained to work with radiation) may be found.

Undifferentiated cells Immature or nonspecialized cells.

Unit A fixed amount of some property or characteristic (e.g., distance-meter, time-second, energy-joule) used as a measure for which other amounts of that property or characteristic can be described.

United Nations Scientific Committee on the Effects of Atomic Radiation (UNSCEAR) Organization that evaluates human and environmental ionizing radiation exposure and derives radiation risk assessments from epidemiologic data and research conclusions; provides information to other organizations, such as the ICRP, for evaluation.

U.S. Code of Federal Regulations Document prepared and distributed by the U.S. Office of the Federal Register, which contains the rules and regulations of the Nuclear Regulatory Commission (NRC) and the radiation protection standards governing occupational radiation exposure.

U.S. Environmental Protection Agency (EPA) (See *Environmental Protection Agency [EPA]*.)

U.S. Food and Drug Administration (FDA) U.S. regulatory agency. The FDA is conducting an ongoing electronic products radiation control program regulating the design and manufacture of products such as x-ray equipment.

U.S. Nuclear Regulatory Commission (NRC) Federal agency (formerly known as the Atomic Energy Commission [AEC]) that, in the interest of national security, has the authority to control the possession, use, and production of atomic energy.

U.S. Occupational Safety and Health Administration (OSHA) A monitoring agency functioning in places of employment, predominantly in industry, that regulates occupational exposure to radiation.

Unmodified scattering (See *Coherent scattering*.)

Unnecessary exposure Any radiation exposure that does not benefit a person in terms of diagnostic information obtained or any radiation exposure that does not enhance the quality of the study.

Unnecessary radiologic procedure Radiologic examination for which there is no sufficient justification to subject a patient to the minimal risk of the absorbed radiation dose resulting from the procedure.

Uracil (U) A pyrimidine base found only in RNA. It replaces thymine (T) as the nitrogenous base in ribonucleic acid.

Use factor (U) The proportional amount of time during which an x-ray beam is energized or directed toward a particular barrier.

Useful beam (See *Primary radiation*.)

Variable rectangular collimator A box-shaped device containing the radiographic beam-defining system; the device is most often used to define the size and shape of the radiographic beam.

Verbal messages Spoken words.

Vesicle A small cavity or sac-containing liquid.

Volt (V) SI unit of electric potential and potential difference.

Voltage Electrical potential at a point or position relative to ground potential.

Voluntary motion Motion controlled by will (i.e., skeletal muscle).

Wavelength Distance between two consecutive crests or troughs in a wave.

Wave-particle duality In some experiments, light behaves as if it is composed of waves (electromagnetic waves) and, in other experiments, light behaves as if it is composed of tiny particles, called photons. The current interpretation of these observations is that light and matter both have some properties in common with waves and with particles.

Workload (W) Essentially the radiation output weighted time during the week that the unit is actually delivering radiation. It is specified either in units of mA seconds per week or mA minutes per week.

X-ray photons Particles associated with electromagnetic radiation that have neither mass nor electric charge, and travel at the speed of light.

X-rays Electromagnetic radiation that emerges from the anode of an x-ray tube after bombardment by high-speed electrons in a highly evacuated glass tube or from an atom that has experienced a photoelectric interaction.

Yttrium A rare-earth phosphor used in rare-earth intensifying screens.

INDEX